Oxford Medical Publications
Health for All Children

Health for All Children

FOURTH EDITION (REVISED)

Edited by

David M. B. Hall

Emeritus Professor of Community Paediatrics,
University of Sheffield,
Honorary Consultant, Sheffield Children's NHS Trust

and

David Elliman

Consultant in Community Child Health,
Islington PCT and
Great Ormond Street
Hospital for Children

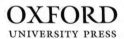

OXFORD
UNIVERSITY PRESS

OXFORD

UNIVERSITY PRESS

Great Clarendon Street, Oxford ox2 6DP

Oxford University Press is a department of the University of Oxford.
It furthers the University's objective of excellence in research, scholarship,
and education by publishing worldwide in

Oxford New York

Auckland Cape Town Dar es Salaam Hong Kong Karachi
Kuala Lumpur Madrid Melbourne Mexico City Nairobi
New Delhi Shanghai Taipei Toronto

With offices in

Argentina Austria Brazil Chile Czech Republic France Greece
Guatemala Hungary Italy Japan Poland Portugal Singapore
South Korea Switzerland Thailand Turkey Ukraine Vietnam

Oxford is a registered trade mark of Oxford University Press
in the UK and in certain other countries

Published in the United States
by Oxford University Press Inc., New York

The moral rights of the authors have been asserted
Database right Oxford University Press (maker)

First edition Published 1989
Second edition 1991
Third edition 1996
Reprinted 1996 (three times) (once with corrections), 1998, 1999
Fourth edition 2003

British Library Cataloguing in Publication Data

Data available

Library of Congress Cataloging in Publication Data

Data available

Typeset by Newgen Imaging Systems (P) Ltd., Chennai, India
Printed in Great Britain
on acid-free paper by
Ashford Colour Press Ltd., Gosport, Hampshire

ISBN 978–0–19–857084–4 (Pbk: alk paper) 0–19–857084–8

10 9 8 7 6 5 4 3 2 1

Preface to the revised 4th edition

The fourth edition of *Health For All Children* was published three years ago, in 2003. In order to avoid the book growing to an unmanageable size, we decided that some additional material should be published on our website, http://www.health-for-all-children.co.uk/—for example, background reading and references.

Three factors prompted our decision to update this fourth edition—first, we had received a number of requests for clarification of various issues in the light of experience with implementing the proposals of the fourth edition; second, some of the material on the website clearly now belonged in the book; and third, we needed to draw the attention of all health professionals to the emergence of new evidence and evolving Government policies. Among the important changes summarised in this updated edition are the new guidance on *Working Together to Safeguard Children*, the publication of the *National Service Framework for Children, Young People and Maternity Services*, and the results from the National Evaluation of Sure Start, which present professionals with some important challenges that must be addressed in the new Children's Centres.

We have consulted various colleagues on points arising from this update but have not involved the complete working groups or their professional bodies as listed in the original fourth edition, so any errors that remain and any points on which our readers may disagree are entirely our responsibility.

We have indicated the new material in the revised 4th edition by placing "4r" in the margin. Within the next few years we anticipate that a full revision will be needed to create a fifth edition but we hope that in the meantime this updated fourth edition will be helpful to our readers.

David Hall and David Elliman (Editors)

Preface to the fourth edition

Fifteen years ago, the British Paediatric Association[1] set up a multidisciplinary working party to review routine health checks for young children. Their report was published in 1989 under the title *Health for all children*. We now present the fourth edition of this work, which targets two distinct audiences. First, we have provided guidance for those responsible for planning, commissioning, and funding community-based services for children. Second, the report offers a framework of practice and prioritization for health professionals working with children in the community.

The fourth edition takes further the gradual shift from a highly medical model of screening for disorders to a greater emphasis on health promotion, primary prevention and active intervention for children at risk, whether for medical or social reasons. This change results from the increasing interest in the social and educational dimensions of child development. In the past decade we have experienced unparalleled prosperity, yet this has been accompanied by increasing levels of violence, family breakdown, disaffection, and alienation. The gap between rich and poor has widened in many countries, including the UK.

There has been an explosion of interest in the causes of these social changes and their impact on children. At the same time, advances in neuroscience, social and political science, and education are beginning to suggest that we do not have to accept this deterioration of our social fabric as inevitable. The phrase 'neurons to neighborhoods'[2] captures the excitement of researchers, governments, professionals, and parents who believe that new insights into the relationships between early brain development, infant experiences, and social circumstances can be applied to the benefit of our children.

While this fourth edition was in preparation, the Secretary of State for Health, the Rt Hon Alan Milburn, announced that a National Service Framework (NSF) for Children would be developed. It is anticipated that this will take 1 to 2 years to complete. This presented our working party with a

---

[1] The British Paediatric Association became the Royal College of Paediatrics and Child Health (RCPCH) in August 1996.

[2] J.P. Shonkoff and D.A. Phillips (2000). *Neurons to neighborhoods—the science of early development*. Institute of Medicine. Website: www.nap.edu

dilemma. We knew that the fourth edition was eagerly awaited by many colleagues who were keen to modernize their child health services in the light of changes already occurring in line with various Government initiatives. On the other hand, we did not wish to constrain the creative thinking of the group that would be asked to develop the NSF by setting out a policy direction that would be difficult to alter.

Previous editions have been endorsed by all the parent organizations represented on the joint working party and have had the backing of the Department of Health. On this occasion, with the agreement of all the organizations concerned, we have decided to publish this fourth edition without any such formal endorsement in order to expedite publication. We believe that the proposals set out in this book command the support of most professional colleagues working with children and are not aware of any areas of conflict with Government policy, but at the same time we recognize that there will inevitably be many points on which there could be disagreement.

Like the three previous editions, we expect and hope that the fourth will have a short life—indeed, we assume that it will be overtaken within a couple of years by the National Service Framework. We do not claim that it is a final or definitive statement on preventive child health programmes. Its immediate aims are to bring together current evidence and suggest how we should use resources in the best interest of children. If it focuses attention on neglected and marginalized children, raises clinical standards, challenges cherished beliefs, and stimulates new research, it will have served its purpose. And if it is judged to be useful by those working on the National Service Framework, we will be delighted.

October 2002   David Hall
                                                                                      David Elliman

Acknowledgements

As the volume of evidence and literature grows, the preparation of each successive edition of *Health for all children* becomes ever more difficult. Development of this fourth edition has been coordinated and the text edited primarily by David Hall and David Elliman, who are responsible for the final version.

Reviews of the literature and current practice were carried out by separate groups as follows (many people also contributed to general discussion as well as that around specific topics).

1 **Pre-school health surveillance, screening and health promotion**—chair David Hall

   Members of the working group, contributors, and correspondents included Obi Amadi, Ian Bashford, John Boyle, Margaret Boyle, Jean Chapple, Neil Corrigan, Hilton Davis, Naomi Eisenstadt, Penny Gibson, Muir Gray, Mary Hickman, Mustafa Kapasi, Zarrina Kurtz, Caroline Lindsay, Jane Ludlow, Roddy Macfaul, Sam Richmond, David Sowden, Carol Youngs

2 **Secondary care services for children and young people of school age**—chair Leon Polnay

   Group members: Zoe Dunhill, David Elliman, Penny Gibson, Honey Heussler, Tom Hutchison, Geoff Lindsay, Margaret Lynch, Jane Naish, Mary Slevin, Carol Youngs

3 **Universal services for school-age children**—chair Jane Naish

   Group members: Helen Bedford, Sarah Stewart-Brown, Chris Donovan, David Elliman, Alison Hadley, Pat Jackson, Judy McRae, Katrina MacNamara

4 **Personal Child Health Record**—chair Helen Bedford

   Group members: David Elliman, Derinda Fitton, Helen Hammond, Del Howard, Sue Latchem, Kate Saffin, Mary Slevin, Jacqui Williams

5 **Information and core public health data set**—Brent Taylor with members of the Child Health Informatics Consortium (CHIC).

Cathy Hill and John Hayward made a substantial contribution to Chapter 15.

David Elliman, who was chair of the Child Health Sub-Group of the National Screening Committee from 1999 onwards, coordinated the screening recommendations.

In parallel with the preparation of this edition of *Health for all children*, a separate working group on adolescent health was chaired by John Tripp and a group on 'Helpful Parenting' was chaired by Malcolm Chiswick. Although their reports will be published separately, we acknowledge the importance of their contributions, which will be accessible via the Health for All Children website (*www.health-for-all-children.co.uk*).

Many others also offered useful advice and in some cases contributed significantly to the final text. We wish to thank the following.

Individuals

Lilias Alison
Gillian Baird
Mitch Blair
Colette Bridgman
Tim Cole
Adrian Davies
Carol Dezateux
Diane DeBell
Alistair Fielder
Peter Fleming
Linda Fox
Frances P. Glascoe
Mark Haggard
Peter Hannon
John Hayward
Cathy Hill
Peter Hill
Sally Inch
Jenny Keen
Danny Lang
James Law
Jane Lightfoot
Stuart Logan
Lynne Murray

Cliona Ni Bhrolchain
Margaret Oates
Frank Oberklaid
Heather Payne
Caroline Pickstone
Jugnoo Rahi
Mary Rudolf
Steven Scott
Jo Sibert
Nick Spencer
Alison Streetly
Pat Tookey
Stuart Tanner
Liz Towner
Evelyn Tseng
Kate Verrier-Jones
Jenny Walker
Tony Waterston
Elspeth Webb
Hilary Williams
Tony Williams
Mike Woolridge
Christopher Wren
Charlotte Wright

Organizations

Association of Directors of Social Services—access to the report *Outcomes are everything*

Child Growth Foundation
Department of Health
Department for Education and Skills
Infectious Diseases Group affiliated to the Royal College of Paediatrics and
   Child Health
Members of the British Association of Community Doctors in Audiology
   (BACDA)
Members of the Child Health Informatics Consortium (CHIC)
National Children's Bureau
Sure Start Parenting Education and Support Forum Unit
The Child Health Sub-Group of the National Screening Committee

If we have inadvertently omitted any individual or organization from this list, we offer our apologies. The list will be displayed on our website and updated from time to time.

Website

The website (see page 2) was created for us by Harlow Printing Ltd, South Shields, NE33 4PU.

A note on Devolution

Health care policies and statutory duties are similar but not identical across the four countries of the UK. Wherever possible we refer to equivalent policies and legislation in England, Scotland, Wales, and N. Ireland, but in some cases more detailed information and links will be found on the website.

The Editors thank all those who contributed, but accept full responsibility for the contents of this report and for any errors that remain.

Contents

Preface to the revised fourth edition *v*

Preface to the fourth edition *vii*

Acknowledgements *ix*

Executive summary of the fourth edition of
  Health for all children xviii

1 Health for *all* children? *1*

A decade of change *3*

Definitions and concepts *6*

Terms and concepts used in public health *10*

Statutory duties *16*

Interprofessional working *17*

User and carer involvement *17*

Children's service plans *18*

Partnership in action *19*

Children in need *19*

What works? The need for evidence and the 'best-buy' concept *23*

Recommendations *25*

2 Child health promotion—focus on parents *27*

Child health promotion—an overview *28*

A holistic approach *29*

Social support—concepts, benefits, and implications for targeting *31*

Quality health visiting *34*

Adult health issues and their impact on children *41*

A summary of the evidence—what works in child
  health promotion? *51*

Recommendations *52*

3 Promoting child development *53*

Helpful parenting *55*

Education for parenthood *56*

Primary prevention of behavioural and
  psychological problems *58*

The relationship between social isolation, parental
  depression, and child development 60
Promoting child development and language acquisition 64
Motor development and coordination 65
Child protection—primary prevention of child abuse and neglect 66
The effectiveness of primary prevention programmes 70
Summary and recommendations 75

4 Child health promotion—opportunities for
primary prevention 77
Reducing the incidence of infectious diseases 77
Prevention of sudden infant death syndrome (SIDS)
  and sudden unexpected death in infancy (SUDI) 82
Reducing smoking by parents 85
Unintentional injury prevention 86
Nutrition 95
Dental and oral disease 100
Special situations 104
Recommendations 105

5 Health promotion and health care for school-age
children and young people 106
Children's views 107
Starting school 108
Pre-school services 108
Health in school 110
Public health focus 118
Vulnerable children and young people 118
Young mothers and teenage pregnancy 120
Recommendations 125

6 Secondary prevention: early detection and the
role of screening 127
Does early detection matter? 127
How early detection is achieved 129
All parents need help sometimes—the role of professional advice 131
The role of formal screening programmes 132
The need for professional sensitivity 132
Screening 132
Recommendations 141

7 Physical examination *142*

Neonatal and 8-week examinations *142*

Screening by physical examination after 8 weeks of age *145*

School entrant medical examination *145*

Physical examination *149*

Recommendations *160*

8 Growth monitoring and nutrition *164*

Requirements for growth monitoring *165*

Benefits of growth monitoring *170*

Weight monitoring *173*

Length and height monitoring *176*

Obesity *179*

Occipito-frontal head circumference (OFC) *184*

Recommendations *186*

Appendix: Regression to the mean *189*

9 Laboratory and radiological screening tests *192*

Neonatal blood-spot-based programmes *192*

Miscellaneous *197*

Urine infections *198*

Other screening programmes *198*

Recommendations *198*

10 Iron deficiency *201*

Definition *201*

Prevalence *202*

Screening *203*

Primary prevention *204*

Recommendations *205*

11 Screening for hearing defects *207*

Permanent childhood hearing impairment (PCHI) *207*

Early diagnosis and intervention for PCHI *211*

Approaches to screening *212*

Recommendations *219*

12 Screening for vision defects *223*

Conditions causing a disabling vision impairment
as the primary problem *223*

Screening for common non-incapicitating vision defects *224*

Pre-school screening for vision defects *229*

Detection of strabismus (squint) *230*

Community screening—evidence and options *230*

Colour vision defects *233*

Vision and 'dyslexia' *234*

Recommendations *234*

13 Identifying children with developmental and behavioural problems *238*

Definition of disablement *240*

Epidemiology *240*

The challenge—identification of developmental disorders and disabilities *241*

Developmental disorders and disabilities—identification and management *244*

How to provide the services needed *266*

Recommendations *268*

14 Children with disabilities and special educational needs *269*

Children with disability *270*

Special educational needs *277*

Recommendations *283*

15 Child protection programme *284*

Child abuse and neglect *284*

Looked after children *296*

Children in private fostering arrangements *307*

Adoption *309*

Summary and recommendations *312*

16 Children in special circumstances *313*

Asylum seekers, refugees, and internationally adopted children *313*

Travellers *318*

Homelessness *320*

Children, young people, and prison *321*

Recommendations *324*

17 Personal Child Health Records and minimum dataset *325*

Personal Child Health Records *325*

Information *331*

18 The universal programme *335*

Why we recommend a universal or core programme *336*

General principles *337*

The objectives of the universal or core programme *337*

Vulnerable children *339*

Primary care for children *340*

Summary of the core programme *340*

Targeting child health promotion programmes *349*

Conclusions *357*

Recommendations *357*

19 Implementing the programme *358*

Appendix: Policy framework, legislation, and policy *366*

Special units *366*

Cross-cutting policies *367*

Education policy *372*

Health policy *374*

Social care policy *378*

Reports *379*

Index *383*

Executive summary of the fourth edition of Health for all children

1 The 2002 programme sets out proposals for preventive health care, health promotion and an effective community-based response to the needs of families, children and young people. It takes account of, and is in line with, Government policies and initiatives. The report does not address issues of hospital or acute care but provides links to other sources of information on these topics.

2 Primary care organizations (PCOs) working in partnership with other agencies will need to ensure that the programme is available and accessible to all families within their boundaries, including socially excluded and hard-to-reach groups.

3 In the light of growing evidence that communities, relationships, and the environment are important determinants of health, investment in community development and social support networks is increasingly important; health professionals should contribute to and sometimes lead in these aspects of health care.

4 PCOs should ensure that allocation of resources between and within areas reflects the greater needs of neighbourhoods that are challenging by reason of deprivation, violence, language barriers, lack of facilities, hostility, etc. Staff recruitment and support should take account of the difficulties of working in such areas.

5 The holistic approach of family medicine is commended and the importance of considering the impact on children of parental mental and physical illness, domestic violence and substance misuse is stressed. Health professionals working with adult patients should enquire about their children and liase closely with paediatric services where needed.

6 Every child and parent should have access to a universal or core programme of preventive pre-school care. The content of this is based on three considerations: the delivery of agreed screening procedures, the evidence in favour of some health promotion procedures, and the need to establish which families have more complex needs.

7 Formal screening should be confined to the evidence-based programmes agreed by the Fetal, Maternal, and Child Health Sub-group of the National

Screening Committee. The agreed screening programmes are given in the table on page 351. Screening activities outside this framework are important in order to ensure continuing refinement of the evidence base, but should be treated as research, reviewed by an ethics committee, time limited, and reported for peer review.

8 There is good evidence to support health promotion activity in a number of areas including prevention of infectious diseases (by immunization and other means), reducing the risk of sudden infant death, supporting breast-feeding, encouraging better dental care, and informing and advising parents about accidental injury.

9 There is as yet no single health promotion measure to reverse the emerging problem of obesity, but the importance of the problem and the need to address it as a public health issue are stressed.

10 There is growing evidence that language acquisition, pre-literacy skills, and behaviour patterns are all amenable to change by appropriate patterns of child management. These insights can be incorporated into programmes like Sure Start but can equally well be provided in non-Sure Start areas.

11 Many illnesses, disorders, and disabling conditions are identified by means other than routine preventive care programmes, but health professionals must respond promptly to parental concerns. Reluctance to carry out appropriate assessments or refer for more expert advice remains an important cause of delays in diagnosis in both primary and secondary care. Clear pathways of care are vital to facilitate prompt and appropriate referrals and need to be developed at local level.

12 Formal universal screening for speech and language delay, global developmental delay, autism, and postnatal depression is not recommended, but staff should elicit and respond to parental concerns. An efficient preliminary assessment or triage process to determine which children may need intervention is vital.

13 The core programme includes antenatal care, newborn examination, agreed screening procedures, support as needed in the first weeks with particular regard to breastfeeding, review at 6–8 weeks, provision of health promotion advice either in writing (where appropriate) or by face-to-face contact, the national immunization programme, weighing when the baby attends for immunization, and reviews at 8 or 12 months, 24 months, and between 3 and 4 years. However, it is expected that staff will take a flexible approach to the latter three reviews according to the family's needs and wishes, and face-to-face contact may not be necessary for all families.

14 The Personal Child Health Record is commended. There should be a basic standardized format for universal use, which should be used to gather a core public health dataset.

15 Children starting school should receive the agreed screening programmes and their pre-school care, immunization record, and access to primary health care schedule should be reviewed.

16 There is an evidence base for the health care of school-age children derived from a range of interview studies with teachers and children designed to establish what they perceive as their main needs. It should include the following: support for children with problems and special needs; participation in Healthy Schools programmes designed to improve the school environment and social ethos, promote emotional literacy,exercise opportunities and healthy eating, and reduce bullying; health care facilities for young people in line with their clearly stated and well-established requirements for privacy and confidentiality.

17 There is an urgent need to secure the provision and the quality of a range of more specialized services to back up those working in primary health care, education, and social services.

18 Access to a child development centre or team and a network of services, including referral to tertiary units when needed, is essential for the assessment of children with possible or established disabilities. There is ample evidence as to what parents expect, in terms of quality, from these services. The care of children with disabilities involves all the statutory agencies and, in many cases, the voluntary sector as well.

19 Emotional and behavioural disorders are common, but service provision is often inadequate and fragmented. A substantial investment involving all statutory agencies is needed, both in preventive programmes at community level and in managing both straightforward and complex problems.

20 There are statutory duties in respect of child protection, looked after children, and adoption procedures. The requirements for staffing are set out in the body of the Report. Child abuse in all its forms is a major but often unrecognized problem, and there is an urgent need for better multi-agency training of all staff and for improved support for those working in this difficult area.

21 There are also statutory duties in respect of liaison work with education authorities with regard to children who have special educational needs. In addition, the development of health promoting policies and programmes

for school age children, in collaboration with education professionals, parents, and young people, requires staff time and expertise.

22 The report stresses the importance of leadership and management of the whole programme. A coordinator is needed to develop and sustain an overview of the health of all children within the district for which the PCO is responsible.

23 It must be clear who is responsible for screening programmes, maintenance and reporting of immunization uptake, introduction of new immunization programmes, health promotion, care pathways for children with health or development problems, socially excluded groups, child protection, looked after children, links with education, staff training, and data management.

24 Since all these activities are interlinked, there is a need for a multi-agency steering group to ensure a focus on desired objectives and outcomes.

25 All staff in contact with children should be appropriately trained and take part in regular continuing professional development.

Chapter 1

Health for all children?

This chapter:

- ◆ Summarizes the evolution of the concepts underpinning preventive child health programmes
- ◆ Describes the origins and definitions of the terms 'child health surveillance' and 'child health promotion'
- ◆ Sets out the changing philosophical, political, and policy context that makes a fourth edition necessary
- ◆ Discusses definitions relevant to the public health of childhood
- ◆ Comments on the importance of children's health in the context of the family and the benefits of family-centred health care
- ◆ Examines the issues of inequalities, poverty, deprivation, and social exclusion
- ◆ Introduces the concept of social capital
- ◆ Discusses needs assessment
- ◆ Reviews statutory duties in respect of child health and care
- ◆ Considers user and carer involvement
- ◆ Defines the term 'children in need' and explains the Framework for Assessment of Children in Need
- ◆ Considers the evidence base for child health promotion.

The fourth edition of *Health for all children* sets out to answer two questions posed on behalf of parents: What health care programmes are available to promote my child's health and development? Which are effective? In the twenty-first century, social, economic, and environmental factors are more important than biological disorders as causes of poor health in children. There is growing evidence that experience and environment in early infancy affect the formation of neural pathways. The contribution of medical care to health gain is correspondingly modest and, for maximum benefit, health care must focus more on prevention. This involves community approaches as well as individual health care, and must take into account the physical and mental health of the adults who interact with children and young people.

Modern primary care and family medicine take a holistic view of health. However, those responsible for advising on, or providing, the delivery of increasingly complex programmes of care need to be familiar not only with a wide range of primary prevention opportunities, but also with the statutory duties imposed by legislation and Government guidance. Furthermore, they will need to make this provision for the whole community for which they are responsible, including the marginalized and socially excluded.

The focus of this book is on community programmes, rather than hospital—based care for acute or complex disorders. The latter is of course vitally important, but health care providers in general have a better understanding of hospital care than of community-based services. Therefore, we have not attempted to address acute or hospital care in our review, but useful links can be found on the *Health for all children* website.

The address of the *Health for all children* (4th edn) *(HFAC4)* website is: www.health-for-all-children.co.uk

This website includes:

- the 'Further reading' list from the third edition of *Health for all children*
- references to articles and other sources referred to in the fourth edition
- links to other relevant websites
- a discussion forum
- details of equipment, growth charts, etc. relevant to paediatric practice

In the text, topics for which further information is available at the time of publication are indicated by a cross-reference to the HFAC4 website.

The first part of this book (Chapters 1–5) describes primary prevention and health promotion, the second section (Chapters 6–13) deals with screening, the third (Chapters 14–16) is devoted to children in special situations, and the fourth (Chapters 17–19) addresses the topic of management and the implications for service provision.

A decade of change

The first and second editions of Health for all children

The first edition was published in 1989. It reviewed the evidence base for the programme known as Child Health Surveillance—a programme of routine child health checks and monitoring in the first 5 years of life. The aims of the programme were described and a new approach was proposed. The second edition in 1992 considered how this more rational programme of care might be delivered. The focus was on the knowledge and skills required rather than on professional labels, an approach that is now adopted in many areas of health care.

An independent review in 1989 by Butler described how the term 'child health surveillance' (CHS) was being used to denote any or all of the following: the oversight of the physical, social, and emotional health and development of children; measurement and recording of physical growth; monitoring of developmental progress; offering and arranging intervention when necessary; prevention of disease by immunization and other means; health education. It could include not only the supervision of the health of the individual child, but also the process of monitoring the health of a whole community of children, by analogy with the public health function of monitoring the incidence of infectious diseases. Butler rightly deplored this multiplicity of definitions and *Health for all children* attempted to clarify these concepts and terms (*see* HFAC4 website).

The third edition

The third edition of *Health for all children*, published in 1996, was a response to evolving professional perceptions of preventive health care. Its message was that preventive health services for children should extend beyond the narrow remit of child health surveillance, with its focus on the detection of abnormalities, to encompass positive efforts to prevent illness and promote good health. Following the suggestion of Butler (1989) we re-defined CHS as 'activities related to secondary prevention, i.e. the detection of defects'. We proposed that CHS should be regarded as just one component of a child health promotion programme.

This change in emphasis recognized the need to modernize the relationship between parents, children, and health professionals to one of partnership rather than supervision, in which parents are empowered to care for their own health and to make use of professional services and expertise according to their needs. The input needed to achieve this aim would vary between families. Emerging evidence on the mechanisms underlying emotional and cognitive development suggested that an increased focus on prevention might pay dividends. We quoted Ireton (*see* HFAC4 website):

> In the future, health professionals, mental health professionals and educators may be able to collaborate to provide continuity of care, education and support to young children in ways that will make screening obsolete. A longitudinal, developmentally oriented care and educational system could be far superior to any cross-sectional screening approach for meeting the needs of young children in general and children with special problems in particular.

The fourth edition—extending the age range and updating the scope of Health for all children

In 1995, the Polnay Report (*see* HFAC4 website) set out recommendations on meeting *The health needs of school age children*. Since then, there has been a rapid evolution of thought and important new work on school health issues has appeared. Care for children who are disadvantaged by social or biological factors should be continuous throughout childhood and it no longer seems sensible to publish policy reviews for pre-school and school-age children as separate documents. Therefore, for the first time, *Health for all children* includes recommendations for children's care from birth to secondary school. A more wide-ranging review of health care for young people is in preparation (*see* HFAC4 website).

The pace of economic, political and scientific change justifies the appearance of this fourth edition just 5 years after the third (*see* box). The Human Rights Act and the UN Convention on the Rights of the Child have already had an impact on attitudes to health care. Confidentiality, consent and participation have been extensively discussed. There is a strong Government commitment to reducing inequalities of health and inequities of access (see below) and to developing health, education, and fiscal policies that address these concerns. Cross-department collaboration—'joined up thinking'—is vital to achieve these aims. Public health issues are the focus of attention—for example, social exclusion, pre-school support schemes, inadequate provision for looked after children, the importance of early adoption, teenage pregnancy, mental health, healthy eating and eating disorders (ranging from anorexia and bulimia to food fads and obesity), cardiovascular disease, and diabetes. Screening programmes are now considered on a national level by a National Screening Committee (*see* HFAC4 website).

This new edition takes further the shift from a defect-detecting model of CHS to a health promotion programme, while continuing to emphasize the importance of excellence in individual health care and of access to appropriate professional expertise as and when needed. The growing interest in how the health of local communities relates to the health and illness of individuals is

- ◆ The Human Rights Act and the UN Convention on the Rights of the Child
- ◆ Devolution—separate health departments in the countries of the UK
- ◆ The NHS Plan
- ◆ Government commitment to reduce inequalities and eliminate child poverty by 2020
- ◆ Increasing public expectations of the NHS
- ◆ Greater emphasis on mental health
- ◆ Greater public access to information via the Internet
- ◆ Increasing readiness to complain and to initiate legal actions
- ◆ Advent of risk-management schemes
- ◆ Concerns about health of refugee children, asylum seekers, children locked up, looked after children
- ◆ Increase in number and scope of systematic reviews and meta—analyses both in scientific and medical literature (Cochrane) and in other areas (Campbell)
- ◆ Publication of consultation document for an overarching strategy— 'Building a strategy for children and young people' (CYPU 2001) which sets out a vision for children and young people, defines a set of principles, stresses the importance of a focus on outcomes, and argues for better delivery of policies and services (see www.cypu.gov.uk)

The public policy context: see the Appendix at the end of the book for details of relevant Government reports and initiatives.

reflected in new material on public health, community development, and 'social capital'. The advent of Sure Start (*see* HFAC4 website) offered the opportunity to focus on primary prevention and the promotion of optimal development rather than on screening and deficit models, as was suggested in the third edition of *Health for all children*.

An increasing emphasis on the promotion of health and on coordinated service provision has implications for planning and commissioning, service delivery, the structure of records and the type of information which should be collected in order to monitor the programme. An exciting and challenging task awaits the newly formed Primary Care Organizations (PCOs).[1] The role 4r

[1] Structures vary across the four countries of the UK. The term 'Primary Care Organization' encompasses all systems intended to organize and manage primary care.

of primary care and general practice in caring for children and young people will increasingly come under scrutiny. See http://bmj.bmjjournals.com/cgi/content/full/330/7489/430.

Since the fourth edition of this book was first published in 2003, there have been a number of government initiatives and publications relevant to child health policy, of which the most significant were 'The National Service Framework for Children, Young People, and Maternity Services' (see page 376); 'Every Child Matters' (see page 371); and 'The Children Act 2004' (see page 376).

The standards set out in the NSF address a wider range of issues and the individual standards are mentioned in the appropriate chapters.

Definitions and concepts

Definition of the terms used in preventive child health care is difficult but is a first step towards establishing the nature of the task and the effectiveness of the activities involved. In particular, the terms 'health promotion' and 'child health surveillance' have been the source of much debate. Child health promotion incorporates a number of activities and concepts.

Health promotion can be defined as 'any planned and informed intervention which is designed to improve physical or mental health or prevent disease, disability and premature death'. Health in this definition is taken to mean a 'positive holistic state in which mental and social well-being are as important as physical well-being'.

Child health promotion (CHP): although the health of children is first and foremost a parental responsibility, society has a vested interest in ensuring that the rights and needs of children are respected. Health in childhood is affected not only by biological factors, but also by the lifestyle and problems of the parents, including unemployment, low income, and poor housing. Individual and community relationships play a major role in health.

Therefore better health is potentially achievable by community-wide interventions in many spheres, such as provision of a healthy social, physical, and work environment, education, and public policies affecting benefits, finance or employment.

Medical approaches to CHP tend to focus on the determinants of disease at the level of the individual. It is aimed at persuading parents to take responsible decisions and make changes to their lifestyle to benefit their children (e.g. stopping smoking). It can appear to 'blame the victims' for their ill health, ignoring the social and economic factors which often prevent people from making appropriate choices. For example, parents may be too poor to buy 'healthy' foods or recommended safety equipment.

The *self-empowerment model* is concerned with 'empowering' people to achieve control over the factors which affect their lives, while recognizing and affirming their personal responsibility for their own health. This is achieved by the development of assertiveness and self-esteem and addressing obstacles to this goal at both individual and community level.

Successful health promotion needs both community-wide action and, at the individual level, a cooperative and respectful approach, with interpersonal skills which need to be developed to a high level.

Disease prevention has three components: primary, secondary, and tertiary.[2] The goal is generally the prevention or amelioration of a particular disease or group of diseases. Prevention programmes are regarded as successful if they reduce the incidence of their target disease.

Primary prevention means the reduction of the number of new cases of a disease, disorder or condition in a population, i.e. reduction of the *incidence*. It includes activities such as immunization, prevention of accidents and child abuse, advice and support for parents ('anticipatory guidance' in the USA literature), dental prophylaxis, etc.

Secondary prevention is aimed at reducing the *prevalence* of disease and other departures from good health by shortening their duration or diminishing their impact through early detection and prompt and effective intervention. It includes screening for conditions which can be treated but not cured (e.g. PKU and its dietary management).

Inevitably, the distinction between primary and secondary prevention is hazy at times, particularly in the area of developmental and psychiatric disorders. We regard *child health surveillance* as a programme of secondary prevention, and it includes *screening* which is just one of the means by which early identification can be achieved (p. 129).

The early identification of defects is of little value unless the parents subsequently experience a well-organized service, with a clear pathway of care from first suspicion of a problem to definitive diagnosis and management. The commissioning of a CHP programme, including screening, must be closely linked to the clinical support services required for effective diagnosis, treatment and care.

Tertiary prevention is aimed at reducing impairments and disabilities (see p. 248 for definitions), minimizing the suffering caused by existing departures from good health, and promoting the child's and parents' adjustment to conditions that cannot be ameliorated.

---

[2] The use of these terms does not imply that primary prevention is the task of primary health care teams or that secondary prevention is the province of specialists.

Health protection refers to measures adopted to safeguard the health of the community as a whole: clean water, good sanitation, safe roads and playgrounds, sound policies in home-building, etc. The term *healthy alliances* refers to collaboration between statutory agencies and voluntary bodies in health protection, community development, and health education.

Health education is defined as 'any activity which promotes health through learning, i.e. some relatively permanent change in an individual's capabilities or dispositions'. It can be directed at individuals, groups, or whole populations. It may incorporate:

- basic biological knowledge of how the human body and mind work, how they can go wrong and what can be done to maintain health, information about child development, interactions within families, acquisition of child-rearing skills, etc.
- consumer information on services and benefits
- personal strategies to cope with stress, loneliness, unemployment, poor housing, etc., and to develop assertiveness, individual strengths, and interests.

The first of these represents what most professionals have understood by health education, but a more modern view incorporates all three elements.

Health education loses its impact if it overloads the parent with too many messages. It may be necessary to *create* interest in topics that are perceived by the parent as irrelevant to their life situation. A 'curriculum' or agenda of parent education may be helpful, but is unlikely to bring about changes in lifestyle and parent practices unless a relationship is developed over a period of time:

> Parent educators do not add information into a void. Parents sort, fit and modify new information according to their assumptions, values and levels of reasoning about parent-child relationships. (Wandersmann)

Advocacy is a long-established tool in public health. It means speaking out on behalf of a child, a family, or an issue (e.g. the need for day nursery provision or legislation on tobacco advertising). It may be undertaken on behalf of individuals or communities, or nationally. It requires a good argument, persistence, and the avoidance of party political bias, together with an awareness of how the political system and the media operate. It is more effective if a group of professionals, together with the voluntary sector, speak with one voice (*see* HFAC4 website).

Community development is the process by which local people define their own health needs and organize to make these needs known to service providers, or take action themselves in order to bring about change. This process may be facilitated by health professionals who can help to generate community interest in health, but it should not be solely dependent on them. For examples of community development projects, *see* the HFAC4 website.

Strengthening local communities and building 'social capital' continues to attract interest as a way of improving children's lives, both in the UK and in the USA. Promoting healthier communities and narrowing health inequalities is a priority for central and local government. 'Choosing health' (DoH, 2004), highlights the leadership role of councils in giving explicit priority to health improvement and narrowing health inequalities. *See* Promoting healthier communities and narrowing health inequalities: a self-assessment tool for local authorities (2004). See also: www.hda.nhs.uk.

Community Interventions to Promote Healthy Social Environments: Early Childhood Development and Family Housing. A Report on Recommendations of the Task Force on Community Preventive Services. Anderson LM, Shinn C, St. Charles, J (2002). www.cdc.gov/mmwr/preview/mmwrhtml/rr5101a1.htm.

Intervention means activity initiated by a professional (or other individual outside the family) intended to deal with a problem affecting health or development. It should take account of the needs and views of the individual and should aim to develop self-reliance rather than create dependence. Some interventions are at the individual level and follow a 'medical' model; examples of these are hospital paediatric services, community paediatric or psychiatric nursing, speech and language therapy, educational assessments, remedial teaching, and social work input. Group and community interventions play an increasingly important role.

Primary care

The **primary health care team (PHCT)** is generally taken to mean the general practitioner, nursing team (which may include, for example, health visitor, practice nurse, district nurse, school nurse), practice manager, and ancillary staff. However, the concept of a PHCT will probably acquire a broader meaning with the shift in management to PCOs. This report uses the term 'primary health care team' to encompass all health professionals who contribute to the primary care of children, although we recognize that the interface between primary and specialist care is itself changing.

PHCTs provide preventive health care programmes, advice, and support. They are usually the first point of contact for acute and non-acute illnesses, disabilities, and behavioural and emotional problems, and liaise with other agencies to support children and families with problems that fall outside the narrow definition of health.

Adult and family health

A major gap in health care can arise where the adult is the index patient, but the team providing adult-oriented health care fails to consider the impact upon children in the family. Ignoring the role of children as carers is just one well-documented example. The potential strength of primary care is the whole-family approach—the impact of adult health, mental health, and disability on children can be assessed, and appropriate intervention and support can be arranged.

Many problems in child health are associated with changing social norms. By the age of 16, one in four children will have experienced the divorce of his or her parents. One in five children live in lone-parent families. Between 1977 and 1997 the proportion of children growing up in no-earner households doubled. One in four children grow up in poor housing conditions.

Therefore, this fourth edition is addressed to the whole health community, rather than just those working in paediatrics and child health. It aims to raise awareness in adult services and promote a more proactive approach. This theme is developed further in Chapters 18 and 19.

Terms and concepts used in public health

This section does not attempt to give a complete overview of public health terminology, but aims only to introduce those terms of relevance to this book.

Public health aims to provide a collective view of health needs and health care of a population. It can be defined as 'the science and art of preventing disease, prolonging life and promoting health through the organized efforts of society' (Table 1.1).

Table 1.1 The elements of public health

- Assessing the health and needs of a population
- Working with local people to identify needs
- Identifying groups most in need of health care and most likely to benefit from health care; identifying health inequalities and working to improve the health of the socially excluded
- Determining the social, economic, and environmental factors that impinge on health
- Planning and implementing programmes that promote and protect health, both within the health sector and with other sectors to address the wider threats to health (e.g. housing, transport, social exclusion)
- Assessing the impact of interventions on the health of the population

Equity: parents find it confusing that they may be offered widely differing services in closely adjacent parts of the UK. Health care should not be dependent on a child's postcode. The principles of equity and evidence-driven policy development underpin the development of national child health programmes. The concept of distributive justice focuses on equality of outcome rather than equality of service provision.

Resource allocation within the National Health Service (NHS) is based upon two fundamental principles. The first principle is that two populations with equal health needs should receive the same access to health care—horizontal equity. The second principle is that populations with greater health needs should receive higher levels of access—vertical equity. These principles are also deemed to apply to individual patients or clients.

The Resource Allocation Working Party (RAWP) proposed a formula based upon the characteristics of the local population. It reflected the greater needs and demands generated by children, the elderly, and populations with generally poorer health. The York Relative Needs Index (RNI) was developed in order to update the RAWP formula, but the principles and basic methods of estimating target-funding levels were unaltered. With the introduction of GP fundholding, concern arose about the equitable allocation of funds to practices and in particular the use of the York RNI formulae at sub-health authority level. More recently, the DETR index has been used. Nevertheless, substantial inequity of resource allocation persists.

For at least 20 years, the NHS has sought to allocate resources to health authorities in an equitable manner (Box). These approaches have a number of limitations. In particular, they are all based upon an analysis of those factors that are associated with **current levels** of service utilization or demand, rather than the **needs** of the population. For example, there will be a tendency for all health visitors to undertake similar volumes of work, irrespective of the underlying needs of the populations they serve. This issue is discussed further under the heading of 'targeting' (Chapter 18).

Inequalities: avoidable adverse health outcomes show a steep **social class gradient** which is associated with undesirable living conditions, stress, and poverty (Table 1.2) Minority ethnic families are more likely to live in poverty (see p. 37). Although morbidity and mortality in childhood have fallen overall, the differential between social class I and social class V has not, and for some

Table 1.2 Evidence for health inequalities in children

Infant mortality	Infant mortality 1993–95 was 77% higher in NS SEC 1.2 than in NS SEC 7
Birth weight	Mean birth weight in the West Midlands showed a difference of 220 g between the least and most disadvantaged area
Nutrition	Breastfeeding rates are much higher in social class 1. Dental disease and iron deficiency are more common in children living in deprived areas
Accidents	There has been a higher rate of decline in death rates from injury in social class 1 in comparison with social class V; inequalities are widening
	Deaths from house fires are 16 times more common in the poorest households
Development and education	Overall, educational attainments are substantially lower in deprived families
Behaviour	Emotional and behavioural problems are nearly four times more common in the families with the lowest incomes
Child protection	Child abuse is reported more often from conditions of social deprivation and poverty.
	Three out of five children in every classroom are estimated to have witnessed domestic violence of some kind

indicators it has widened. Reducing inequalities and abolition of child poverty are important goals of Government.

Reducing inequalities is a definable and measurable aim that involves a range of legislative and policy initiatives, such as increased investment in education, financial benefits, help for parents who experience conflicts between child care and the need to work, pre-school provision, support for families of children with special needs, etc. This policy goal, which we support, requires a refocusing of child health services. *Choosing Health: Making healthy choices easier* 2004. DoH: London.

http://www.dh.gov.uk/PublicationsAndStatistics/PublicationsPolicyAndGuidance/PublicationsPolicyAndGuidanceArticle/fs/en?CONTENT_ID=4094550&chk=aN5Cor and Wanless D. (2004). *Securing Good health for the Whole Population*. HM Treasury: 2004.

Poverty and deprivation

Poverty and deprivation are complex issues. In industrialized countries, the effect of relative poverty may be more important than absolute income (box).

In many studies, the extent of inequality in income and wealth relates more closely than absolute wealth to a number of outcomes, both at macro (state-wide) level and at the level of individual localities. The pressures of consumerism, the high levels of crime and violence that accompany perceived inequalities, and the sense of personal hardship and deprivation engendered by advertising may all play some part in this. However, not all research confirms this (see box below).

... The sense of relative deprivation, of being at a disadvantage in relation to those better off, probably extends far beyond the conventional boundaries of poverty. A shift in emphasis from absolute to relative standards indicates a fall in the importance of the direct physical effects of material circumstances relative to psycho-social influences. The social consequences of people's differing circumstances in terms of stress, self-esteem and social relations may now be one of the most important influences on health.

> R. Wilkinson, Income distribution and life expectancy,
> *British Medical Journal*, **304**, 165 (1992)

By necessities, I understand not only the commodities which are indispensably necessary for the support of life, but whatever the custom of the country renders is indecent for creditable people, even of the lowest order, to be without.

> Adam Smith, *The wealth of nations* (1776)

Health status increases with increasing socioeconomic status in every wealthy society on earth ... the socio-economic gradient of health status. It has remained unchanged since the beginning of the 20th century despite the fact that the principal causes of death have changed completely since 1900 ... societies which minimize the socioeconomic gradient in life expectancy maintain better health status for all social classes than societies which do not ...

Equality is good, not only for the vulnerable but for the privileged too.

> Hertzman, in *Developmental health and the wealth of Nations*,
> Guilford Press, New York 1999.

Health, hierarchy, and social anxiety

Wilkinson suggests that 'the main reasons why populations with narrower income differences tend to have lower mortality rates are to be found in the psychosocial impact of low social status ... where income differences are greater, violence tends to be more common, people are less likely to trust each other and social relations are less cohesive. The growing impression that social cohesion is beneficial to health may be less a reflection of its direct effects, than of its role as a marker for the underlying psychological pain of low social status. Low social status affects patterns of violence, disrespect, shame, poor social relations and depression. In its implications for feelings of inferiority and insecurity, it interacts with other powerful health variables such as poor emotional attachment in early childhood and patterns of friendship and social support.'

R. G. Wilkinson, *Annals of the New York Academy of Sciences*, **896**, 48–63 (1999)

A contrary view on the relative–absolute poverty debate

Recent research from Denmark has suggested that this may not be universally so and the observed effect may be due to other factors such as a lack of high school education. The effect of education inequality may be mediated via lack of material resources, occupational hazards, and certain 'learnt risk behaviour'.

See also HFAC4 website

There is a gradient effect in the relationship between poverty and outcomes, with families close to but just above the arbitrary poverty line showing worse outcomes than those with higher incomes. Examples of inequalities in health within the UK are given in Table 1.2.

4r **Poverty**

The Literacy Trust has a useful database of sources on poverty, young carers, and related matters. See www.literacytrust.org.uk/Databse/excuse.html.

A review of progress in tackling poverty is at www.dwp.gov.uk/publications/dwp/2004/autumnreport/children/target1.asp.

Social exclusion

This refers to 'the inability of our society to keep all groups and individuals within reach of what we expect as a society and the tendency to push vulnerable and difficult individuals into the least popular places' (see box).

Social exclusion

Originally a French concept referring to the difficulties of disabled people in participating fully in society. In the UK the concept was extended to include the disability caused by poverty and disadvantaged circumstances. Disorganized services in run-down housing estates with high unemployment, shifting population, poor schools, inadequate pubic transport, vandalism, crime, etc. greatly reduce a child's chance of employment and stable relationships as an adult. Material resources are a necessary but not sufficient requirement to improving the situation. Poverty and social exclusion are not confined to urban areas, and there are many pockets of deprivation in rural areas. See page 366.

Preventing social exclusion—a report by the Sure Start Unit www.surestart.gov.uk
G. Watt, Policies to tackle social exclusion. *British Medical Journal*, 2001, **323**, 175–6.
See also HFAC4 website

Social capital

Although nearly a century old, this concept has recently been 're-discovered'. It refers to the wealth inherent in social networks of mutual trust and reciprocity. The concept is developed further on p. 31.

Targeting

Reduction of health hazards and promotion of good health for all children involves not only 'traditional' one-to-one professional contacts but also a range of community-based measures. Some of these are aimed at the whole population of children or families, but others should be targeted at localities or specific groups who are considered to be at increased risk or to have exceptional or complex needs.

Identification of these groups is an essential public health task. Some families are difficult to reach with routine services and need special provision, for example children of travelling families, the homeless, armed forces personnel, children who are detained in secure premises for any reason, and asylum seekers. Access to care is made difficult for many families by distance, poor transport, or parental illness or disability. The organization of preventive and primary health care for all such families presents a challenge to existing systems of care and must be addressed (see Chapter 18).

Deciding on the balance between universal and targeted health care programmes needs careful judgment. From a population perspective, seeking modest improvements in the health of the whole population may sometimes be more profitable than targeting a small number of outliers (see Fig. 8.1 for further discussion and example).

Needs assessment

This term is used in two ways: in public health it refers to the needs of a population (for instance, a health district, a locality, or a primary care practice population), whereas in the health care of an individual it implies a review of their current problems and circumstances.

In the course of their work, clinicians gather data on the needs of individual families and these data contribute to the development of the needs profile for populations or segments of a population (e.g. defined by geography, school or category of need).

Determining the needs of a population

This should be approached both from a professional viewpoint, based on measures of ethnicity, morbidity and mortality statistics, linguistic barriers, age distribution, local geography and transport, the gap between available and desirable services, and the ability of the population to benefit from service provision, and from the consumer viewpoint, taking into account local perceptions of the priorities and the concerns of local people as to what influences their health.

Determining health care needs of individuals

Identifying needs for health care and stimulating awareness of health care needs are two key elements of health visiting practice. The UK has a long tradition of universal health visiting for every parent. More recently, there has been increasing interest in targeted services. Both are important. The 'Framework for Assessment' (Department of Health 2000) sets out guidance on how to assess and describe the dimensions of a child's life and circumstances. The Common Assessment Framework is described on page 21.

Statutory duties

Health authorities and trusts have a duty to provide services to local education and social service departments under collaborative arrangements set out in the

Children Act 1989 and the Education Act 1996. The Secretary of State has powers to issue guidance on inter-agency working, for example *Working together to safeguard children* (The Stationary Office, 1999) and *Framework for assessment of children in need and their families* (The Stationery Office, 2000). Although these duties arise from legal obligations, such inter-agency working is an essential requirement for successful clinical work in social paediatrics and in educational medicine. Chapters 14, 15 and 16 develop this theme further.

Interprofessional working

Criticism of poor services or reviews of disasters often point to poor teamwork and communication rather than individual error or incompetence. Professional training often fails in respect of gaining an understanding of teamwork and the role of other professionals, concentrating on 'within-discipline' skills and knowledge. Key elements of successful teamwork are:

- continuity of staffing within the team
- effective communication
- protected time for team meetings
- clear definitions of tasks and objectives, individual responsibility, leadership, and accountability
- written team guidelines
- good and shared record-keeping
- control of workload through allocation, clear referral and discharge criteria, caseload monitoring, and workload monitoring
- knowledge and respect for expertise of other team members
- personal respect
- ability to reach and keep to joint decisions.

User and carer involvement

There is a growing perception that patients and carers are the "experts" in how they feel and what it is like to care for someone with a particular illness or condition... active patient participation in consultation and giving people good information are significant factors in achieving better outcomes of care and patient satisfaction. (The expert patient, Department of Health, 2001)

Involving parents and young people directly in planning meetings has two immediate benefits—it forces professionals to treat parents with respect and to avoid stereotyping, and it ensures that different professional groups avoid jargon and use plain English.

Users and carers should be involved in the definitions of standards set for NHS services locally and the development of NHS policy both locally and nationally. They should be the key people to monitor service provision and ensure the quality of service.

Children and young people have a right under the UN Convention on the Rights of the Child to have their views elicited on 'all matters affecting the child'. They should be involved in consultation both at the planning/commissioning level and in decisions about their own personal health services. Age should not be a bar to their inclusion in the proposed patient forums and the local authority scrutiny panels (*see* HFAC4 website).

> The child's right to express an opinion, and to have that opinion taken into account, in any matter or procedure affecting the child.
> Article 13, UN Convention on the Rights of the Child

4r Children's Rights

The relevant NSF standard is Standard 3 (Core standards): *Child, Young Person, and Family-Centred Services*. Follow the links from www.dh.gov.uk/policyandguidance/healthand social care top.cs/childrenservices

The *Archives of Disease in Childhood* 2005, volume 90 (February edition), carried several articles on the UN Convention and its implications.

Pediatrics devoted a supplement to the topic of equity: 'Toward equity in child health' *in* Supplement to *Pediatrics* Sept 2003; **122** (number 3, part 2 of 2).

4r A useful account of current issues regarding children's rights and comments on the newly established post of children's commissioner can be found at the website at Children's Rights Alliance for England. See www.crae.org.uk/cms/index.

Children's service plans

Since 1996 it has been a legal requirement for local authorities to produce an inter-agency children's service plan (CSP) every 3 years. The CSP should be the vehicle for rationing, coordinating, and securing more coherent and effective planning for vulnerable children. The social services department consults with other bodies such as the health authority, education, leisure services, housing, police, and voluntary groups to assess the need for provision for services for children in need under Part III of the Children Act 1989. A plan must be published setting out the multi-agency strategy that will be put in place.

CSPs have specific functions in respect to:

- planning services for children in need as defined within the Children Act 1989

◆ the current requirement within the Quality Protects Programme (p. 300) to produce annual management action plans associated with the Children's Special Grants

◆ Setting out joint investment plans to improve the health and social case of children.

The Children Act 2004 subsumes many existing planning requirements into a 4r single children and young people's plan (CYPP) that local authorities will be required to have in place by April 2006. Authorities will work with local partners towards the recommendations and targets they set out.

The CYPP will cover all the services available to children in a locality, and so the involvement of local partners in the formulation of the plan is fundamental to its success. As well as including local authority services for children and young people, it will also link to plans for other services, including health services, youth justice, voluntary and community services, Connexions, and drug action for children and young people. See www.everychildmatters.gov.uk/strategy/planningandperformace/

Partnership in action

Partnership in action (Department of Health 1998), describes policies to provide more opportunities for joint working between health and social services. These can be at three levels: strategic planning, service commissioning, and service provision. Proposals include pooled budgets between health and social services to provide an integrated programme of care, lead commissioners, and integrated provision that would enable an individual PCO to provide social care services. The NHS Act 1999 provides the legislative basis to these recommendations.

Inter-professional collaboration has been reviewed in detail following Lord 4r Laming's report on the death of Victoria Climbié and recommendations made:

Review of Education and Training on Inter-agency Working-at www.chssc.salford.ac.uk/scswr/projects/interagency_working.shtml.

Children in need

The Children Act 1989 defines the concept of **children in need** (box). The definitions of children in need and children with special education needs (SEN) provide a series of overlapping groups (Fig. 1.1). Not all children in need will have SEN and not all children with SEN will (technically) meet the Children Act definition of disability. Many terms are now used to describe the effective integration of health, education, and social care for children: joined-up services, partnerships, holistic, seamless. All children require primary health care wherever they fall in the diagram. There must be a universal pro-

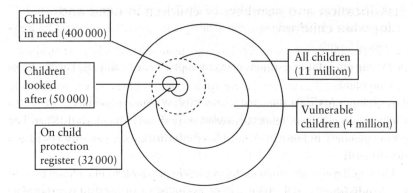

Fig. 1.1 Continuum and subgroups. The diagram, taken from *Framework for assessment of children in need*, describes a continuum from all children, through vulnerable children, through to children in need with the most severely disadvantaged being at the centre of the 'children in need' circle. Of the 11 million child-ren in England, 4 million are vulnerable and 400 000 are in need, including 32 000 children on child protection registers. Children may also move towards the centre or the periphery of the figure depending upon their individual needs, parenting ability and resources, and the presence or absence of effective support. For SEN, 20 per cent of the child population will be included at some time. For special medical needs, 4 per cent of those aged 0–4 years, 6 per cent of those aged 5–15 years, and 7 per cent of those aged 16–19 years will have long-standing illness reducing their functional capacity. Government policy and targets to reduce health inequalities and social exclusion aim to reverse the trend of a growing population of vulnerable children and children in need. The model, which is based upon national figures, can be rescaled to reflect the population of an individual health authority or PCT and the wide variation that exists in the real world between the most deprived and most affluent areas (see Chapter 18 for further discussion).

gramme able to identify vulnerable groups and children in need, ensuring that there is timely referral to, and engagement with, specialized and targeted services.

A child is considered as being **in need** if:

(a) he is unlikely to achieve or maintain, or to have the opportunity of achieving or maintaining, a **reasonable** standard of health or development without the provision for him of services by the local authority

(b) his health or development is likely to be **significantly** impaired, or further impaired, without such provision

(c) he is **disabled**

Classification and numbers of children in need and vulnerable children

Based upon the estimates in Fig. 1.1, average numbers can be calculated for a PCO with a total population of 150 000 and a city with a population of one million (Table 1.3). However, these average figures hide a seven- to eightfold variation in rates between local authorities. Within authorities there is also wide variation in these indices between deprived and affluent wards. Therefore service planners and providers must have information on a locality as well as a district basis.

These groupings, although useful, represent populations of children in need who, individually, will have a wide range of complex and overlapping

Table 1.3 Average numbers of children in need and vulnerable children

	PCO	City
Total population	150 000	1 000 000
Child population (0–18 years)	33 000	220 000
Vulnerable children	12 000	80 000
Children in need	1200	8000
Children looked after	150	1000
Child Protection Register	96	640

difficulties (e.g. special educational needs and social needs) that will require coordinated services from several agencies.

Framework for assessment of children in need

The promotion of children's health involves consideration of their developmental needs, the quality of parental care, and the circumstances in which they grow up. These three dimensions are summarized in Fig. 1.2. They form the basis for assessment of children in need and are equally relevant in routine practice.

The Common Assessment Framework

A Common Assessment Framework (CAF) for Children and Young People is a nationally standardized approach to conducting an overall assessment of the

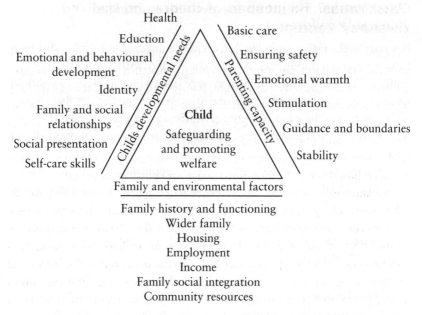

Fig. 1.2 Assessment framework.

A framework . . . which provides a systematic way of analysing, understanding and recording what is happening to children and young people within their families and the wider context of the community in which they live . . . . Clear judgements can be made as to whether the child is in need, whether s(he) is suffering significant harm, what actions must be taken and which services would meet the needs of the child and family. . . . Early intervention is essential to support families before problems . . . escalate into crisis or abuse. (www.doh.gov.uk/quality.htm)

The three dimensions of assessment are summarized in the figure. They were developed as the basis for assessment of children in need (p. 19) and are a useful way of structuring observations of children in routine practice. (Reproduced from *The framework for the assessment of children in need and their families*, Department of Health; Department for Education and Employment; Home Office, 2000. The Stationery Office, London.)

needs of a child or young person and deciding how those needs should be met. It has been developed for use by practitioners in all agencies dealing with children and, ideally, where parental consent is given, the CAF will facilitate greater sharing of information between practitioners. Information will follow the child and will be added to at intervals to form a picture over time.

What works? The need for evidence and the 'best-buy' concept

Like any other health care intervention, health promotion activities can do harm as well as good. The information offered may turn out to be inaccurate or incorrect. Screening tests may perform poorly for a variety of reasons (p. 135). Health information may cause anxiety or guilt to individuals who for various reasons cannot act on the advice given. There is an ethical imperative to ensure that CHP activities are subjected to as robust an evaluation as any other health care intervention. It is important to marshal evidence of effectiveness and to establish how this may be monitored and, where possible, increased.

Our aim has been to adopt an evidence-based approach wherever possible. The exponential growth in research publications, not only in health care but also in many other disciplines, makes it ever more difficult to offer an overview of the literature, although the advent of systematic reviews and meta-analysis has to some extent simplified our task. On the other hand, the increasing sophistication of research methodology is balanced by greater caution in interpreting and generalizing the results of studies from one country to another or even to different parts of the same city.

'Absence of evidence of effect is not the same as evidence of absence of effect.' We must not be paralysed by uncertainty. It will never be possible to make recommendations which are wholly based on scientific considerations (box). Studies on the impact of community-wide projects rarely follow traditional models of medical research and a pragmatic approach to interpretation and generalizability is needed. The value of some activities is supported by persuasive evidence, whereas for others the evidence is insufficient to make any firm judgement. The concerns and preoccupations of parents must be considered and services that are clearly valued by the 'consumer' should receive careful consideration even if evidence of effectiveness is scanty; how-

---

Why the research base in health promotion takes time to develop

+ The effectiveness of health professional interventions is inextricably linked with other disciplines within the health service and other agencies such as the social services, education, and housing departments, the police, the NSPCC, etc.

+ In many cases the important outcome measures can only be determined many years into the future.

◆ Collection of information required to assess and monitor preventive child health services is difficult because of the many geographic sites where the services are delivered (homes, schools, clinics, nurseries, etc.). Problems with computer databases and issues of data protection and confidentiality limit the comparison of data between districts.

◆ Most health promotion involves three levels of input: legislation, local government initiatives, or community pressure to bring about changes in the environment or in products; advertising (written information, TV campaigns, videos, etc.), which provides information and influences behaviour; education at the level of the individual or community-based group. The effects are synergistic and often involve interdependence between professionals and agencies, making it difficult and perhaps even misguided to attempt to measure these separately. The introduction of seatbelt legislation, the change in society attitudes to drunken driving, and the decline in smoking rates provide excellent examples of successful but multifaceted campaigns.

◆ Some of the adverse outcomes which health promotion activities may seek to prevent are rare, so that very large samples are needed to measure effectiveness directly. For example, sudden infant death (SID) is rare in an individual district. It may be necessary to use proxy measures; for example, the number of parents who place their babies to sleep in the supine position can be assessed at local level but the impact on the rate of SID can only be measured in much larger populations.

◆ Health professionals vary in their skill in health promotion, their impact on individual parents, and their ability to maintain enthusiasm outside the research setting. Thus caution is necessary when generalizing from a research study to other situations.

◆ Some alterations in health-related behaviour only occur gradually and may depend on cultural changes or on shifts in the parents' own expectations of health and of the health care system. The time span may be too long for changes to be identified within the scope of a research programme.

◆ 'Quick-fix' solutions may look tempting yet may not necessarily offer the best long-term answer to a problem. For an example, see the discussion on iron deficiency anaemia (p. 201).

◆ Public demand for prevention research is limited, research funding is not easy to obtain, and the level of service required must be defined by professional assessment of need.

ever, when resources are limited, it seems logical to give priority to services of demonstrable effectiveness.

The programme we will recommend at the conclusion of our report should be regarded as a 'best buy' in the light of current evidence. We anticipate that it will continue to be refined and altered in the light of further research and experience.

The need for innovation and experiment

In many districts, there will be one or more services which are not specified in our list of recommendations. *Provided that* (a) the justification for these is clearly articulated, and (b) useful data are being collected, such services can be a valuable 'natural experiment'. Programmes and projects that differ from the nationally agreed policy should either be justified by an alternative interpretation of the literature or treated as research projects; the latter should be peer reviewed and submitted to ethics committee scrutiny in the usual way.

Process and outcome measures

It is important to specify the aims of the CHP programme. Process measures include information on coverage and uptake of services, completion of data returns, attendances at clinics, etc. Outcomes, although more important, are always more difficult to measure. Falls in perinatal, neonatal, and infant mortality rates and in the gradients between social classes for a number of measures (Table 1.2) are legitimate indicators of progress. Proxies likely to be associated with improved outcomes may suffice. Examples include improved maternal mental health, increased immunization uptake rates, reduction in active and passive smoking, and the acquisition of safety equipment such as car seats. Improved educational outcomes might be expected to result from better pre-school and school-age services.

Setting targets helps to concentrate the minds of health care staff and encourage a focus on desired outcomes, but care must be taken to avoid perverse incentives and professionals should not be put in the position where they have to override their common sense and judgement.

Recommendations

1 Primary Care Organizations (PCOs) should plan how to discharge their responsibility for the health care of *all* the children and young people living within their boundaries.

2 The evidence strongly favours a holistic health-promoting approach which crosses agencies and disciplines, rather than a narrow defect-detecting programme.

3 Resources will always be insufficient to do all that is possible; therefore screening, surveillance, and parent support and health promotion activities should, where possible, be prioritized on the basis of evidence of effectiveness.

4 Involvement of users and carers in service planning is important, and the available methodologies are now sufficiently robust to recommend that this should become part of routine practice.

5 There are a number of statutory duties which must be fulfilled and these are likely to be the responsibility of the PCO.

6 A public health overview of children's health care in each PCO will be essential.

Chapter 2

Child health promotion—
focus on parents

This chapter:

◆ Gives an overview of activities involved in promoting child health

◆ Stresses the importance of a holistic approach to working with families

◆ Introduces concepts of social support, social capital, and social networks

◆ Discusses the challenges of working with families in difficult circumstances

◆ Outlines the evidence that social support is beneficial

◆ Considers the impact of various adult health issues on children—parents who have mental illness, are cared for by children, have learning, communication or physical disabilities, have HIV infection, are involved in substance abuse

◆ Summarizes the evidence regarding the characteristics of effective programmes

In this and the next two chapters we consider child health promotion programmes for pre-school children in the light of Government initiatives to reduce inequalities and social exclusion, eliminate poverty, and improve educational outcomes. Chapter 5 discusses the promotion of health in children of school age and young people, and the issue of support for those with additional or special needs is reviewed in Chapter 14. Our review will illustrate and emphasize the considerable level of knowledge and skill required for effective child health programmes in the community (box).

Central to pre-school programmes is the need to assist parents with personal support, information, advice and material resources as appropriate. 'Social support', the specific needs of children whose parents have health problems and 'parenting' have until recently been regarded as nebulous notions not worthy of scientific study, but this attitude has changed dramatically, with growing evidence that support networks and social capital (p. 31) do influence outcomes for children and families and can be changed for the better. Techniques are now available for helping parents to manage their children more effectively, not only in research clinics but in real world settings. Sure Start (see p. 371 for details) is an English programme that aims to bring together these ideas and put them into practice.

> The challenge to community child health professionals is to encompass three different ways of thinking—promoting health and development, identifying defects and disorders, and taking a public health approach to prevention and community development.

In Chapters 3 and 4 we focus on more specific issues. Chapter 3 reviews child development. Parenting programmes offer one way of reducing the incidence of developmental, emotional, and behavioural disorders, and child abuse and neglect (primary prevention), so that the child is able to obtain maximum benefit from education when s/he starts school. It is also important to identify disabilities and disorders as early as possible (secondary prevention) and to provide support and care for children with permanent disabilities (tertiary prevention) (Chapters 6, 13, 14).

Chapter 4 examines opportunities for prevention in pre-school health care—it describes how programmes can minimize risks such as sudden infant death, injuries, and accidents, and promote optimal nutrition and dental care.

Child health promotion—an overview

A wide range of activities are undertaken to promote the health of children (see box) and a variety of skills are needed. Health visitors, school nurses, and other professionals increasingly work in teams, rather than aiming to provide all the necessary expertise in one individual.

Activities undertaken to promote the health of children

- **Resource allocation** Ensuring that each locality and district receives an appropriate share of resources according to their needs
- **Needs assessment** Determining the needs of a community and of individual families—defining the balance between universal and targeted care

- **Social support** Listening, sharing experiences, providing counselling for depression and mood disorders, friendship, introductions to other people in similar circumstances, formation of groups
- **Provision of education** by information (written, verbal, media, video etc), demonstration or role modelling
- **Detection of disorders and health problems** (see Chapter 6)
- **Practical help** Information about benefits and access to legal expertise, crisis assistance, introduction to services, help with transport, interpreting, advocacy; specific health care measures which are difficult for some individuals to access (e.g. home immunization of child where parent is disabled or agoraphobic)
- **Community based projects** (e.g. equipment loan schemes)
- **Community development**

The literature—a focus on health visiting and school nursing

In the UK, health visitors are particularly identified with the health of mothers and pre-school children, and much of the relevant research involves assessment of health visiting practice, both in the UK and overseas. In the North American literature the term 'home visitation' is used; in some countries, the nurse is called an MCH nurse (maternal and child health).

The concepts of the 'public health nurse' and 'skill mix' are of growing importance to the future of health visiting and school nursing. The emphasis on health visiting in the following discussion does not imply that this is the only discipline with an interest in or responsibility for health promoting activities, or that health visitors are the only professional group capable of undertaking these tasks. Nor does it mean that health visiting and home visiting programmes are a panacea for all problems.

Similarly, when we refer to school nurses we do not mean to imply that they have a monopoly of expertise in supporting school-age children and young people.

A holistic approach
Promoting child health by working with families

Effective health promotion involves more than just giving information or offering help. The vast majority of parents want to make a success of bringing up their children and many welcome help and guidance provided that it is given in a sensitive fashion. But parents can also feel inadequate and isolated and are often subjected to inconsistent advice from a variety of sources, yet may feel reticient about asking for information and help.

When compared with the nation as a whole, people who have low incomes or live in areas of deprivation are more likely to suffer depression and to have poor health and unhealthy lifestyles; their babies are more likely to be of low birth weight; their children are at higher risk of illness, sudden unexpected death, neglect, abuse, dental decay, injuries, and educational problems. As the children grow older they are more likely to have unplanned teenage pregnancies, engage in substance misuse, leave school with no qualifications, and develop mental health problems.

Traditional 'medical model' approaches to these problems involve one-to-one interventions based on assumptions about the parents' deficits in knowledge, insight, skill, or motivation. The preoccupation of many parents with their life circumstances and their environment (Fig. 2.1) makes it difficult for them to benefit from professional expertise and advice.

Relationships matter for health. This is true for relationships between partners and family members, between parents and children, and between members of a community. An increasing body of research and experience suggests that relationships and community-wide issues must be addressed if real progress is to be made. Projects that exemplify this are described in the boxes. A wide range

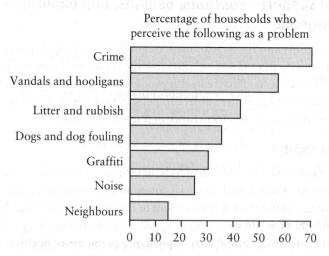

Fig. 2.1 Urban anxieties. Reproduced by permission of The Economist Newspaper, London.

of early intervention, home-visiting programmes, and parent education and support programmes now incorporate these insights into their service delivery.

> A series of community development programmes in the USA, based in Vermont and Missouri, provide evidence of the potential benefits of community development programmes.
>
> *See* HFAC4 website for links

> **The Beacon community regeneration project in Cornwall**
> A project run by two health visitors in the Penwerris area, one of the poorest wards in the UK. The area was seriously deficient in facilities and services. The project involved multi-agency funding bids to improve health and reduce poverty with a particular emphasis on better insulation and heating, since high fuel bills were a priority concern for local people. Other investment improved road safety and children's play areas. Residents played a key role throughout. Substantial improvements have been made in quality of life in these areas as a result.
>
> *See* HFAC4 website for further information

Social support—concepts, benefits, and implications for targeting

Social support and the development of good relationships with individual parents and families is not only worthwhile for its own sake but is also an essential prelude to effective health promotion. Support can be defined as 'information leading the subject to believe that s/he is cared for, loved, esteemed and a member of a network of mutual obligations'.

Social capital

The extent to which an individual feels that s/he is part of a wider community is important. Factors such as social cohesion of a community, the sense of belonging, and the level of involvement in community affairs together make up a concept now known as 'social capital' (box). A growing body of evidence suggests that social capital is as important a predictor of health outcomes within a community as the absolute levels of wealth or poverty (*see* HFAC4 website).

Social capital refers to the institutions, relationships, and norms that shape the quality and quantity of a society's social interactions. Increasing evidence shows that social cohesion is critical for societies to prosper economically and for development to be sustainable. Social capital is not just the sum of the institutions which underpin a society—it is the glue that holds them together (R.D. Putnam (2000). *Bowling alone.* Simon and Schuster, New York).

See HFAC4 website

Social networks

Individuals turn first for support to family and friends, and subsequently to a range of people encountered during everyday life. These together form a social support network, a 'set of interconnected relationships among a group of people who provide enduring patterns of nurturance and reinforcement for efforts to cope with everyday life'. Some networks are informal, some are contrived extended families, and some are created in response to a common life situation or crisis.

Social networks reduce the stress of disadvantage, social isolation and hopelessness, which characterizes many deprived populations and affects every aspect of life, including motivation for care of self and family and the ability to be a 'good enough' parent. The ability of individuals to cope with stress varies considerably (box). In addition to intrinsic factors, such as mental resilience, temperament, and physical health and endurance, external factors play a part in determining which parent will succumb to stress and which will survive. These include (for example) the influence of family, friends, and neighbours, availability of other interested adults to befriend the children, and quality of local schooling. Social phenomena such as reconstituted families, alienation between parents and children, frequent moves of home, and poor transport are widely believed to weaken social networks and reduce the transmission of child care knowledge between generations.

Resilience in the family system can be divided into:

1 The property of the family system that enables it to maintain its established patterns of functioning after being challenged and confronted by risk factors: **elasticity**

2 The family's ability to recover quickly from a misfortune, trauma, or transitional event causing or calling for changes in the family's patterns of functioning: **buoyancy.**

HI McCubbin, MA McCubbin, AI Thompson, SY Han, and CT Allen (1997) *Families under stress: what makes them resilient:* website http://www.cyfer-net.org/research/resilient.html

See HFAC4 website

Those parents who would have the most to gain from social support networks are often the least accessible and amenable to receiving help unless someone (usually a professional) leads them into participation. Social networks require that everyone has something of value to give in return for what he or she receives: 'People solve personal problems, accomplish tasks, develop social competence and address issues through an exchange of resources with members of their community. This exchange of resources . . . can be tangible goods like information or money, or intangible like emotional nurturance . . .'. People who are heavily in debt to their network may cut themselves off from future trans-actions or be cut off: 'A professional may need to restart the process for a bank-rupt member of the network'.

Most individuals are reluctant to disclose their problems and concerns to a stranger unless an empathic trusting relationship exists or can be created. It takes time to develop such relationships. The role of the professional is to identify need, facilitate the development of support networks, and provide support personally for individuals who for various reasons, such as loneliness or depression, are unable to build other relationships.

Counselling is a means to an end, a more formal way of giving support and helping individuals to assess their own priorities (box). It can be defined as 'an interaction in which one person offers another time, attention and respect with the intention of helping that person to explore, discover and clarify ways of living more successfully and to his/her greater wellbeing' (British Association of Counsellors). Good listening, communicating, and note-taking skills are central to any CHP activity with individuals. These skills can be taught and improvements can be measured. In reality, effective counselling is often difficult because parents are distracted by the presence of their children, or professionals are inhibited by the pressure to cover a wide range of health care issues in a short time, or when the concerns of the individual do not coincide with the agenda of the professional, manager, or commissioner/purchaser.

Parental support is determined not only by what potential helpers do, but by the characteristics of the people providing the services and the relationships they develop with parents. The process of support involves a set of tasks or stages, which begin with the development of a mutually trusting relationship, allowing open exploration of the problems or difficulties facing the parent. If you are not trusted, parents will not talk openly, and you will not discover the true nature of their problems and therefore be unable to help them. The relationship is a partnership, which can be powerfully supportive in its own right. If a parent is regarded with esteem by a respected helper (usually perceived as in a relatively powerful position), then he or she is likely to feel valued, to increase in self-esteem, and to consequently be more able to adapt to or manage perceived difficulties more effectively.

The qualities required in the relationship include:

- respect or what Carl Rogers called unconditional positive regard— valuing parents as people and assuming competence and strength, not weakness and incapacity;

- genuineness, which implies attempting to be yourself, honestly and openly, and not being closed and defensive, not hiding behind a professional façade. If you really care, parents will know, and will equally spot pretence with its obvious implications for the helper-parent relationship;

- empathy—the attempt to understand the world from the viewpoint of the person you are trying to help, as opposed to the imposition of the helper's own views;

- humility allows the person who is seeking help to contribute to the process and not to simply be in the hands of someone who is all-knowing and all-powerful.

Training courses to facilitate the development of these models and skills produce considerable improvements in the confidence and competence of a range of professionals to relate to and support parents, and people trained in this way facilitate considerable benefits for parents and for children with problems ranging from intellectual and multiple disabilities to emotional and behavioural adjustment (Hilton Davis 1998).

See HFAC4 website

Quality health visiting

A number of observational and reflective papers offer some insight into the characteristics of effective home visitors. They examine the content and practice of home visiting and together set out some useful insights into what a quality service should offer:

Collinson S, Cowley S (1998). An exploratory study of demand for the health visiting service within a marketing framework. *Journal of Advanced Nursing* **28**:499–507.

Appleton JV (1997). Establishing the validity and reliability of clinical practice guidelines used to identify families requiring increased health visitor support. *Public Health* **111**:107–113.

Cowley S, Houston AM (2003). A structured health needs assessment tool: acceptability and effectiveness for health visiting. *Journal of Advanced Nursing* **43**:82–92.

King L, Appleton JV (1997). Intuition: a critical review of the research and rhetoric. *Journal of Advanced Nursing* **26**:194–202.

Korfmacher J, O'Brien R, Hiatt S, Olds D (1999). Differences in program implementation between nurses and paraprofessionals providing home visits during pregnancy and infancy: a randomized trial. *American Journal of Public Health* **89**:1847–1851.

Knott M, Latter S (1999). Help or hindrance? Single, unsupported mothers' perceptions of health visiting. *Journal of Advanced Nursing* **30**:580–588.

Baggens C (2001). What they talk about: conversations between child health centre nurses and parents. *Journal of Advanced Nursing* **36**:659–667.

Larson CP (1980). Efficacy of prenatal and postpartum home visits on child health and development. *Pediatrics* **66**:191–197.

Davis H, Spurr P (1998). Parent counseling: an evaluation of a community child mental health service. *Journal of Child Psychology and Psychiatry* **39**:365–376.

The challenges of working with deprived and 'socially excluded' populations

Families regarded as having high levels of need because of poverty, disability, illness, membership of minority groups, etc., are diverse, differing in lifestyle, support networks, and beliefs. Some have had so many life disappointments that they are very difficult to engage in any useful professional contact; for example, those who have had no employment for two or even three generations. Others, though poor and underprivileged, hope that their children may have a better life and have the personal capacity to work for this. This applies, for example, to many first-generation immigrants and refugees.

The health care system does not easily adapt to the needs of such families. Poor families may not seek help when it is needed. They may be less able to cope with internal and external pressures and are often preoccupied with problems of money, housing, or work, so that health checks for apparently healthy children may have low priority. Lack of transport and telephones result in missed appointments, which irritates professionals and is often misinterpreted as indifference or neglect. Parents and children are difficult to visit at home because they are out at work or seeking work, they move frequently, and the child may be with a friend, a childminder, or the extended family for a large part of the day.

The families at greatest risk are 'outside the system'; this includes alcohol and drug abusers, victims of domestic violence, many homeless families, and some with unorthodox lifestyles. They do not seek help; they cannot handle the bureaucracy and perceived middle-class orientation of the health care system; they find that public services are largely irrelevant to their lives. Such families are often suspicious of professionals and may see them as inspectors, or as representatives of the police or social services.

Nevertheless, most parents have concerns if their children have 'bad' behaviour, learning difficulties, or poor social skills. They worry about whether their child will make satisfactory progress when s/he starts school and appreciate guidance as to how they can help their child prepare for reading and other school work. If the child is slower than average, anxiety about the possible need for a 'special school' may be an important issue.

4r Hard to reach children and families

This topic is attracting increasing interest in several disciplines. Even in the best Sure Start programmes, engaging all eligible families has proved to be very challenging and some remain hard or impossible to reach. This experience reflects the findings in traditional child health surveillance programmes, where there is a steady decline in coverage of the population as children get older and the decline is steeper in the poorest social groups. While this may partly be due to the fact that even in the most deprived areas there are some more prosperous families who may feel that they do not need such services, the evidence suggests that most of these hard to reach families are in fact among the most needy, with an excess of teenage mothers and of parents with problems such as substance abuse, mental illness, or violence.

USA Head Start data suggest that although early intervention programmes benefit most children, there is a risk that children in the most needy families may perform worse in some programme areas and that early intervention may actually increase inequalities. This may to some extent be because the more capable families in any locality will access and benefit from any available service more effectively, partly because the intervention programme results in resources being unintentionally diverted from supporting the most needy families, and partly because poor families may be overwhelmed by any additional demands. For example *see National Evaluation of Sure Start — Local Evaluation Findings* www.ness.bbk.ac.uk/findings.asp

Several papers discuss the phenomenon. Murray *et al.* described their experiences in a project designed to help women with depression; Barlow *et al.* based their paper on their research into parenting education: Duggan *et al.* reviewed their Hawaii experience and noted that many more parents were lost to follow-up in their early intervention programme than had been anticipated by the staff involved. These parents were particularly those with multiple problems such as alcohol or substance abuse, domestic violence or mental illness. *See*

Murray L, Woolgar M, Murray J *et al* (2003). Self-exclusion from health care in women at high risk for postpartum depression. *Journal of Public Health* **25**:131–7.
Barlow J, Kirkpatrick S, Stewart-Brown S *et al.* Hard-to-Reach or Out-of Reach? Reasons Why Women Refuse to Take Part in Early Interventions. *Children and Society.* 2005. **19**: 199–210.
Duggan A, Fuddy L, Burrell L *et al* (2004). Randomized trial of a statewide home visiting program to prevent child abuse: impact in reducing parental risk factors. *Child Abuse & Neglect* **28**:623–43.

The Head Start experience is reported in *Making a Difference in the Lives of Infants and Toddlers and Their Families: The Impacts of Early Head Start* available at: www.headstartinfo.org/infocenter/ehs_tkitl.htm

A more generic approach was taken in a review of inequalities and this too indicated how programmes intended to reduce inequalities might have the opposite effects: Ceci SJ, Papierno PB. The rhetoric and reality of Gap Closing. *American Psychologist* (2005) **60**:149–60.

Housing problems

For many parents, poor housing is a major preoccupation (box). Inadequate insulation, condensation and damp, inefficient heating systems, and fuel poverty (defined as spending over 10 per cent of income on fuel) contribute to the problem. Health professionals can identify families who would benefit from recent Government initiatives on housing and fuel poverty, putting them in touch with the relevant department of the local authority. High-rise housing is an additional cause of stress for many families. Ill health, in both children and adults, may be associated with cold damp housing.

A systematic review found health gains associated with housing improvements but the size and quality of the studies limited their generalizability. The authors noted that 'the basic human need for shelter makes the relation between poor housing and poor health seem self evident . . . [but] good evidence is lacking on the health gains that result from investment in housing [or] on the mechanisms of interaction of social factors'.

H Thomson, M Petticrew, and D Morrison *British Medical Journal*, **323**, 187–90 (2001).

See HFAC4 website

'New to area'

In some circumstances, parents who move into an unfamiliar area may do so because of unemployment, family break-up, or domestic violence. They may be reluctant to establish new social links, and as a result the child or children may not benefit from the services available. Finding such families and supporting them can be difficult and time-consuming but they are a high-risk group and should be targeted.

'Middle class' parents

Amidst concerns about deprivation, it is easy to overlook the concerns of 'middle-class' parents. Such parents are probably more able to find solutions to their problems with a minimum of professional help, for example by establishing and maintaining contacts with peer groups or by using the Internet. Nevertheless, divorce, financial problems, and ill health can be just as devastating. They may need help with concerns about issues such as child mental health and behaviour or learning and language problems. Even parents who are highly educated are sometimes surprisingly uninformed about child development and the limits of normality.

Meeting the needs of minority ethnic groups

Service provision for all ethnic groups is important if the needs of all children are to be met. The incidence of socio-economic deprivation is higher in minority ethnic groups; over 60 per cent of Pakistani and Bangladeshi communities in the UK live in poverty. Thus for many families in these communities the first and most important health disadvantage is poverty.

It is important to be aware of institutional racism (box). This does not mean that the individual staff are racist, but rather that the structures or operating policies of an organization result in particular sections of a community being disadvantaged. Information and advice must be culturally sensitive and relevant. Staff need to understand the attitudes, customs, and communication styles of the groups with whom they work. In particular, the differences between the prevailing Western culture of individualism and the collectivist world view of many other cultures should be appreciated.

Examples of institutional racism in the NHS

◆ Provision of services and information only in English

◆ The inappropriate use of close family members as interpreters, a practice that may force children or distant relatives to share confidential or distressing information

◆ Cultural and ethnic stereotyping: for example, widespread but often erroneous beliefs about the use of physical punishment or the attitudes of various religions to termination of pregnancy or disability

◆ Unsympathetic counselling when a child with a recessive disorder is born to consanguineous parents

◆ Failure to help parents find their way through the complex maze of services for children with disabilities or chronic health problems

Based on E. Webb, Health care for ethnic minorities, *Current Paediatrics*, **10**, 184–90 (2000).

The individual–collectivist distinction: *see* Bridging cultures in our schools. 2000: website http://www.WestEd.org

See HFAC4 website

Provision of special programmes for conditions such as sickle cell disease is a necessary but not sufficient response to the needs of ethnic groups. Other requirements may include close liaison with, and support of, community groups, link-worker schemes, dieticians with knowledge of weaning and feeding practices in different cultures, translations of written information, local radio health programmes, etc.

The problem of low literacy

Estimates of illiteracy and of problems with reading and writing vary, but perhaps 10 per cent of people may have such difficulties. Many people will be unable to benefit from written material even at a simple level, yet much health promotion literature requires a sophisticated level of reading skill and excellent reading comprehension. Readability scores provide an objective method of assessment. The production of more accessible materials and a review of existing literature, posters, etc. should be a priority. Collaborations with adult education units may be one way to proceed. Reading and spelling difficulties have a substantial genetic component, and so the children of parents with such problems are at significant risk of being affected (*see* HFAC4 website).

Poverty and benefits

Poverty is a major contributor to ill health and many families have difficulty in accessing the benefits system appropriately. Health professionals may need to offer assistance in this area, either directly or by referral to the relevant agency. In some neighbourhoods, providing advice in a health centre may be an effective means of getting information to local people.

Help and support in the home

Examples are given in the box. There are many situations where such help is the only way to ensure that children receive the medical or social care they need.

A Cochrane review of home-based support for socially disadvantaged mothers (Hodnett and Roberts 1997) found that: six trials reported lower injury rates in the visited group. Eight looked at child abuse or neglect, and in four it was lower and in four higher in the visited group. Six trials examined the rate of child immunizations, four finding a lower rate of incomplete immunizations in children of visited mothers. Four trials reported on hospital admissions, and in all four the rate was lower in the visited group.

A non-Cochrane review examined 31 trials, of which seven covered the period before birth (Olds and Kitzman 1993). It concluded that home visiting offers a promising approach to the promotion of child health, and it favoured well-trained professionals over paraprofessionals.

Three Cochrane reviews cover support from caregivers during pregnancy, childbirth, and the postpartum period (Hodnett 1997*a*; Hodnett 1997*b*; Ray and Hodnett 1997). These concluded that offering additional social support for at-risk pregnant women was not associated with improvements in medical outcomes, but there was convincing evidence of improvement in psychosocial outcomes; the evidence on social support and childbirth was persuasive, as was that for the potential of social support to reduce postpartum depression.

Summarized by A. Oakley, 1998, in 'Evolution or Revolution' (*See* HFAC4 website)

A. Oakley *et al.* (2001) The Social Support and Family Study. Look at http://www.ioe.ac.uk/ssru/ra_policy.htm for details of current research.

The most effective interventions:

- involved multiple community agencies and primary care services
- were more intensive with weekly home visits, at least initially, either during pregnancy or after the birth of the child
- had a greater impact on those who would be considered at risk due to social disadvantage.

Review: Public Health Home Visiting-www.Health.Hamilton-went.on.ca

See HFAC4 website

Assessing the benefits of social support and community-wide approaches

The evaluation of programmes that focus on enhancing the strengths of the community as a whole (community development programmes), rather than focusing on individual care, is difficult. The methodologies available for assessing these projects are very different from the classic designs for evaluating single medical interventions.

There are several project reports within the UK suggesting benefits from a community development approach that involves local people. These need to maintain a balance between individual health care and support, and the development of new social networks and 'social capital' (see box on p. 31 for example). Sure Start is a programme that aims to improve educational outcomes by building on local strengths and structures.

Adult health issues and their impact on children

Service provision and support are often poor for children affected by the illness or disability of a parent; for example, the child of a parent with relatively well-controlled epilepsy may develop significant anxiety about his/her parent and school refusal after observing a seizure.

Mental health (Box)

Psychiatric morbidity in mothers (especially long-standing depression, alcoholism, and other minor psychiatric conditions) is significantly associated with presentation of the child as a psychiatric patient, antisocial behaviour disorders, and general levels of performance and achievement. In many cases, however, the child's needs remain unrecognized or present in some other way, for example with physical symptoms. The specific issue of postnatal depression is considered on p. 60. There is little evidence to relate paternal psychiatric illness to child morbidity, although there is an association with criminality in adolescence. This is strongest when associated with marital discord and divorce.

More minor chronic disabling conditions, when associated with marital and social adversity, may have a greater impact on child functioning than the more acute severe mental illness requiring multiple admissions. Similarly, acute psychosis has less of an adverse effect on maternal–infant attachment than depression and chronic schizophrenia, which affect social and emotional development, resulting in persisting emotional and cognitive effects when measured at school age.

Pathways for development of these problems are represented by unavailability of the mother either by physical absence and multiple changes of carer or by emotional absence with lack of affect, preoccupation, and hallucinatory phenomena.

Relatively few cases of abuse/murder are the result of a single act of violence. Thus, vigilance and enquiry into patterns of child care, levels of irritability, and temper control with children may identify worrying patterns of interaction before they have too serious an impact. Mothers with mental illness and their families need intensive support, with identification of risk before birth and extending through childhood, to include the child absent from school while caring for anxious or depressed parents. In the latter situation, the young carers can often also be dealing with their own anxieties and fears that are not being addressed, such as worries about similar patterns of behaviour which they revognise in themselves.

Health professionals caring for adults/parents with mental health issues should be able to make an assessment of risk to the child and liaise closely with named professionals responsible for child protection in their region, particularly when there is to be unsupervised contact with parents who have mental ill health.

Close liaison and joint working between adult and child and adolescent mental health services should assist in providing services for these young people. The primary care team is well placed to recognize the impact of the adult illness on the rest of the family.

- Prevalence: 26–60 per cent of women with serious mental illness live with a child under the age of 16, and 25 per cent live with a child under the age of 5; 10 per cent have a child under 1.

- 25 per cent of all homicides involve children, and in 60 per cent of those, the children are under 5; 22 per cent of deaths in the first year are thought to occur on the first day of life. In general, women are more likely to kill or injure younger infants, but in older children the male partner predominates.

- Acute psychosis forms a small part of the psychopathology of these women. Women with 'less severe' disorders such as depression and anxiety, when combined with youth, personality disorder, substance misuse, and social adversity, are much more part of the profile.

- Mental illness is not a feature of men who injure or kill children. However there is an association with a history of criminality and sociopathic personality disorder. The offender is most often not the natural father but the cohabitee of the mother. Frequently in these circumstances the mother has significant mental health problems and is deemed to have 'failed to protect'.

Children as young carers

Young carers are children or young persons under the age of 18 who provide care assistance or support to another family member. They carry out significant or substantial caring tasks on a regular basis and assume a level of responsibility that would usually be associated with adults. The person receiving care is often a parent, but can be a sibling, grandparent, or other relative who is disabled or has some chronic illness, mental health problem, or other conditions connected with a need for care, support, or supervision. Factors which influence the extent and nature of young carers' tasks and responsibilities include the illness/disability, family structure, gender, religion, income, and availability and quality of professional support services.

Where children and families lack appropriate professional support and adequate income, young carers may experience impaired psycho-social development, including poor educational attendance and performance, and restricted peer networks, friendships, and opportunities. These will have

10 141 children (6.1 per cent) are registered as children in need because of parental illness or disability. A similar number are registered because of socially unacceptable behaviour. In some areas support groups exist for siblings of children with disability or illness.

In the UK, almost 3 million children under the age of 16 (23 per cent of all children) live in households where one family member is hampered in daily activities by a chronic mental or physical disability or illness. Office for National Statistics figures suggest that the number of young carers is around 51 000.

http://www.doh.gov.uk/public/tablecnote.htm:
(Table C—Children supported in their families or independently)
See HFAC4 website

Needs of young carers

- Recognition and respect
- Information about care, medical conditions, practical chores, welfare rights, money and services
- Support and services, time off
- Choice to care as well as to receive services
- Someone to talk to

Outcomes for young carers

- Limited opportunities, horizons, aspirations
- Limited social and leisure activities
- Lack of understanding from peers, restricted friendships
- 'Stigma by association' especially with mental health or substance abuse problems
- Fear of professionals
- 'Silence and secrets'
- Emotional difficulties
- Health problems
- Difficulties in child–adult transitions
- Miss a large amount of school or have other educational problems

implications for their own adulthood. Young carers have rights to assessment and support under legislation (Children Act 1989). Specialist projects to provide these needs are one way of helping these children.

The parent with learning difficulty

Children of parents with learning disability, depending on severity, may have a number of problems. These can be related to the cause of the learning disability. The child may have similar difficulties and may need the appropriate investigations to identify the cause. Many of the issues relate to general care. Even with less obvious disabilities, the difficulties can impact on the child significantly; for example, dyslexic parents may have difficulty in helping their child with homework. The degree of difficulty needs to be assessed to ensure that adequate care and supervision of infants and children are provided—this may require intensive support from primary care teams, such as support from education, social services, and paediatric services to enable home help, after-school activities, group support, etc.

Despite the problems they encountered in their childhood, many of which originated outside the home, most people who grew up with learning-disabled parents report that they maintained a valued relationship with their family and remained close to their mother.

Physical disability

There may be problems with attendance at clinics, school and out-of-school activities (e.g. holiday programmes), and in caring for the parent.

HIV

Children who have a parent with HIV/AIDS fall into two categories: the infected and the affected. Children growing up with a parent who has HIV are likely:

- to have the virus themselves, although with growing antenatal diagnosis and appropriate treatment, this is decreasing
- to not have the support of another parent (the support of a surviving parent is positively associated with the grieving child's ability to cope with the loss of the other parent—HIV/AIDS-affected children often do not have another parent available to them)
- to be orphaned at an early age, although this is now often later than before, with antiretroviral therapy

- to have to cope with recurrent hospital admissions for their lone parent, which may involve periods in care and in caring for other siblings
- to have to cope with substance abuse in that parent.

The needs and care of HIV-affected children and young people are still often obscured by the shadow of their parents' and siblings' illness and policies that *only* address the needs of HIV-infected individuals. The secrecy and stigma that surround HIV and AIDS make it difficult for HIV-affected children and young people to benefit as fully as they might from policies and programmes that provide more generic types of care and assistance.

It is estimated that there were a total of 33 200 adults with HIV infection in the UK at the end of 1999, a third of them undiagnosed. The rate of new diagnoses of HIV infections showed no evidence of falling.

HIV-1 prevalence among mothers in London rose ninefold between 1988 and 2000. The rate in inner London rose to 0.41 per cent, 0.19 per cent in outer London, 0.027 per cent in the rest of England, and 0.047 per cent in Scotland.

A growing proportion of transmission is via sex between men and women; the time when most women are diagnosed is in the child-bearing years (15–30 years). There are an increasing number of children being born to these women. The success of high-risk screening and health interventions is possibly reflected in the lower rates of diagnosis now being recognized in the substance-abuse and gay communities.

Antiretroviral therapy is delaying the onset of AIDS and deaths in many of those treated (deaths fell by two-thirds between 1995 and 1999).

Many women with HIV are electing to have children, and in 2000, there were an estimated 452 births to HIV-infected women in the UK. Transmission rates are now as low as 2.2 per cent where the infection has been diagnosed prior to pregnancy.

British guidelines exist for management of women with HIV in pregnancy (G.P. Taylor, E.C.H. Lyall, D. Mercy, *et al.* British HIV Association guide-lines for prescribing anti-retroviral therapy in pregnancy). Instigation of these measures requires antenatal diagnosis, and currently 30 per cent of women are aware of their HIV status prior to pregnancy. In England, despite national policy initiatives to increase the antenatal detection rate of HIV by offering targeted antenatal testing to women perceived to be at higher risk or living in high-prevalence areas (i.e. London), detection rates remained low throughout most of the 1990s.

National objectives set in 1999 aimed to reduce the number of children acquiring HIV from vertical transmission by 80 per cent by 2002 and targets to achieve this have been set.

All pregnant women should be offered testing for HIV infection, as a routine part of antenatal care, so that antiretroviral therapy can be offered to infected women in the later stages of pregnancy, during delivery, and subsequently to the neonate. Elective Caesarean section is the preferred mode of delivery. Breast feeding should be discouraged.

See HFAC4 website.

No one system, alone, can be responsive to the social, mental health, legal, and support needs of these children. Cross-disciplinary initiatives are needed among agencies that administer child welfare services, income support, AIDS care, and children's mental health services at the national and local levels.

Clinical and support services for people affected by the HIV epidemic should have a family focus. Many affected children, like their parents, are living for longer. Care and support for children exists often within adult agencies or family clinics, but children and teenagers have many unmet needs.

There are examples of good practice, particularly in Southeast England, including multidisciplinary family clinics for both child and parent, after-school youth support clubs for children from families with HIV, in-home care, and support for older teenagers. The role of the GP is important, and perhaps more so in more isolated areas.

Substance misuse

Substance misuse is present in the families of around 20 per cent of child protection cases. Prevalence is likely to grow with falling prices and increased consumption. One million children live with an alcoholic parent, thereby putting the child at increased risk of violence or neglect; 25 per cent of calls to NSPCC over Christmas 1997 were related to alcohol. The effects of substance abuse can be both biological and social. Substance abuse in pregnancy in various combinations has been linked to cognitive and interactional difficulties as well as more severe problems such as small head size and low birth weight. The long term effects of intra-uterine exposure are difficult to separate from the significant effects of drug misuse on family social circumstances and a parent's ability to care for a child.

Range of substances

- Alcohol
- Heroin
- Tranquillizers
- Cannabis
- Cocaine
- Solvents
- Antipsychotics

Drug misuse and its effect on children: key points for health professionals

Users of illicit drugs tend to be young and many have children. Addiction to opiates, most commonly heroin, causes many problems for the child's home environment; addiction to stimulants such as amphetamines and crack cocaine may also produce adverse home circumstances. Associated drinking problems are common.

- Babies born to opiate users tend to be of a lower birth weight and may also have a smaller head circumference. There is a high risk of negative long-term outcomes for infants born addicted

- Increased incidence of antepartum haemorrhage and intra-uterine death

- For parents, financial pressure of obtaining typically £10–£100 daily to buy heroin

- High risk of poverty, criminal activity and imprisonment; chaotic lifestyles, poor nutrition, missed appointments, unsafe individuals in the home, frequent parental absences

- Parental risk of death from overdose, infectious diseases, and other causes

- Many drug-misusing parents received poor parenting and have had high rates of all kinds of childhood abuse themselves

- Children of addicted parents as a group, perform less well academically; they have a high risk of emotional and behavioural problems, poor school attendance, substance misuse in adolescence, and attempted suicide. They are more likely to suffer child abuse in various forms and to be taken into care. Neglect is the most common type of abuse

Heroin addicts entering methadone maintenance programmes rapidly show substantial improvements in the time spent with their family and in the time spent attending to the home—this can stabilize families, improve child care skills, and prevent removal of children from care. Therefore the lack of access for addicted parents to maintenance prescribing services affects children as well as adults.

Harm minimization

- If neglect or abuse is suspected, act immediately according to the local child protection guidelines
- Be sure that the family has sufficient funds to provide adequately for the child's physical needs
- Check that the child is not being left alone whilst the parent is out procuring drugs
- Advise parent(s) on where to access drug treatment services and appropriate referral where necessary
- Advice on testing and vaccination for blood-borne viral infections and referral for parent and child where necessary
- Harm minimization advice regarding injecting and safer sex in order to protect parent and child from contracting transmissible infections

Parenting

- General advice on parenting as the parent may have only very poor role models and few support networks
- Advice on nutrition for parent and child, and consideration of parental drug problems as a possible contributing factor where children fail to thrive
- Advice on the safe storage of drugs away from children, especially methadone mixture which is attractive in appearance and has been responsible for a number of child deaths

- Enquiries to ensure that the child has not missed the routine childhood health reviews and vaccinations
- Attention to ensure that children are not lost to follow-up
- Liaison with other professionals who may be involved with the family so that information may be shared in case of concern

Pre-conception counselling

- Enquiries to ascertain whether a further pregnancy is planned, and contraceptive advice where appropriate
- Where a pregnancy is planned or is a possibility, pre-conception counselling focusing on nutrition and the need to reduce or stop injecting and to keep all illicit drug use to a minimum: referral to drug treatment services at this stage if appropriate
- Should a further pregnancy occur, early diagnosis and referral to specialist services
- Early counselling and testing for blood-borne virus status in pregnant woman and neonate

  Based on J. Keen and L.H. Alison, Sheffield Children's Hospital Trust and Community Health Sheffield, 2001.

Communication difficulties

Children of parents with sensory difficulties have special needs for professional assistance. Some of the important findings from research are summarized in the box.

Hearing impaired parents

- Children of deaf parents should have early investigation of their hearing status and close screening of their speech and language development and appropriate professional support if required. A large proportion of school-age children have language problems. A range of specific emotional difficulties is described.
- Deaf parents may be frustrated when their children have problems interpreting due to undeveloped sign language skills. Most children enjoy being bilingual and describe advantages of their situation.

Sight impairment in parents

◆ Observations of interactions between young, sighted children and blind parents demonstrate strong participation; they were remarkably little affected by the parental disability.

◆ In the school-aged child, helping care for a blind parent may require increased responsibility in terms of shopping, medical visits, etc. Appropriate community support may optimize access for the child to a normal curriculum and after-school activities.

A summary of the evidence—what works in child health promotion?

Although the evidence is incomplete, and involves many different cultures and populations, three important themes emerge from the literature. First, services that are highly rated by parents have certain characteristics in common (box). Second, when these criteria are fulfilled, as in demonstration projects and research studies, the benefits of intervention programmes at the level of individual parents and families are not only statistically significant but also clinically useful—but there is no evidence that programmes of mediocre quality and lesser intensity will deliver similar benefits. Third, professional contacts are not by themselves necessarily beneficial; the quality of what happens in transactions between individuals or groups of clients and professionals is probably crucial.

Characteristics of successful programmes and projects

◆ Services are of a broad spectrum and comprehensive, crossing traditional professional boundaries, and are coherent and easy to use

◆ Both the structure and the individual staff are flexible in their ability to respond to unexpected demands

◆ The staff have both the time and the skill to establish a relationship of respect and trust with families

◆ The child is seen as a member of the family, and the family a part of the community

◆ Projects have enthusiastic committed leadership, clearly specified measurable aims, and focus on families with high levels of need (typically poor, unsupported, and young, or having children with special problems)

> ♦ There is sustained high quality and quantity of input and, importantly, sufficient continuity of input to develop a relationship with the individual client (in many cases this implies commencing a professional relationship during pregnancy rather than after the child is born) (See also page 34)

Recommendations

1 There is good evidence for the importance of social support, social networks and 'social capital' as determinants of the health of individuals.

2 There is persuasive, though indirect, evidence that activities that address issues in the local environment and build on the strengths of local communities are at least as likely to improve health as traditional individual health care approaches.

3 There is good evidence that the inverse care law applies in preventive health care. Resources should be allocated on the basis of needs. Thus some localities and some districts should receive more resources than others.

4 There are sound arguments for providing a universal or core programme of preventive health care and parent support, accessible to every parent. Within this there should be activities to identify problems, provide advice and information, offer support, and facilitate access to health care and other services.

5 Health care activities outside the structure of the core programme should be targeted according to need.

6 Assessment of need should be an individual process, based on negotiation and review of family circumstances, strengths, and weaknesses. The principles should be based on those set out in the *Framework for assessment*. There is evidence that methods of allocating resources on the basis of scoring methods or checklists are not effective—they lack sensitivity and specificity.

7 Some families need more help but are difficult to reach and may not be known to the health services. They include the homeless, travellers, refugees and asylum seekers, people with chronic illness or disability (who may be cared for by their own children), substance abusers, and people with communication problems such as the hearing impaired. Finding these families and building a relationship with them needs more time and extra skills.

Chapter 3

Promoting child development

This chapter:

- ◆ Emphasizes the central role of parents in promoting child development
- ◆ Defines helpful parenting
- ◆ Describes the Sure Start programme
- ◆ Sets out the growing evidence that education for parenthood is effective
- ◆ Considers the primary prevention of behavioural and psychological disorders
- ◆ Reviews the relationship between depression, social isolation and child development
- ◆ Stresses the importance of post-natal depression and mental illness associated with pregnancy and the post-natal period
- ◆ Describes how language acquisition and literacy skills could be encouraged
- ◆ Examines child protection and the prevention of child abuse
- ◆ Reviews the overall effectiveness of primary prevention and intervention programmes
- ◆ Presents a concept of 'school readiness' in terms of an 'outcome measure for community intervention programmes

In the previous chapter we discussed support for parents in the community and the need to strengthen social networks. We stressed the importance of relationships in health and introduced the concept of social capital. Here we consider why and how the emphasis should be shifted from an approach that focuses on the prevention and detection of particular developmental problems and disorders, to incorporate a more holistic view that aims to improve children's chances of success by family support, parent education, developmental interventions and behavioural guidance. In England, the Sure Start programme (box) was an important vehicle by which this approach could be implemented, bringing together insights from research and innovative practice. Sure Start was well resourced by Government funding, but the underlying philosophy is also relevant in areas without Sure Start projects. It will be important to ensure that when the model becomes part of mainstream services, sufficient resources are provided to maintain standards.

Sure Start in England: a community-based approach to child public health

Sure Start was a major Government programme for young children living in poverty. Its aim was to close the gap in outcomes between children growing up in poverty and the wider child population. It was designed following the 1998 Review of Services for Young Children, which noted the extent of child poverty and the absence of any multidisciplinary strategy to meet the needs of young children.

It involved cross-agency partnerships at local level in deprived areas. The partners included statutory and voluntary agencies, community groups and local parents. The aims were to achieve better health, educational results and emotional development; to strengthen communities; to ameliorate the long-term effects of poverty. Families in poverty have fewer places for children to play safely; they are more likely to be the victims of crime and vandalism; transport is often inadequate; they are unlikely to risk wasting money on experiments with new or 'healthy' foods.

Each Sure Start Local Programme covered an average of 750 children under the age of 4. They all included home visiting of new parents; quality play and child care; enhanced health advice. The community-based 'bottom-up' approach aimed to make sure that service developments reflect what local communities want and need. Early programmes were in urban areas but rural programmes followed. For discussion of the impact of Sure Start, see page 73.

(A series of publications setting out the background to the project, and information about a range of interventions for young children, is available from the Sure Start website.)

See HFAC4 website for links and more information

Common childhood concerns, such as language delay, behavioural difficulties, and child neglect and abuse, are often associated with, and in part attributable to, life circumstances interacting with genetic influences, which play an important role in development, behaviour, and temperament. With few exceptions, these problems represent a continuum rather than discrete diagnostic entities. They may occur in isolation, but more often a child has multiple difficulties that reflect a host of family and environmental problems and pressures, compounded by frequent episodes of ill health, especially respiratory disorders and ear infections. These complex relationships have important implications for prevention, identification, investigation, and management, illustrated in the 'Framework for assessment'.

Supporting parents or carers 4r

The relevant NSF standard is Standard 2 (core standards)—*Supporting Parents or Carers*. Follow links from www.dh.gov.uk/policyandguidance/healthand socialcaretopics/childrenservices. *See* also the section on 'Hard to reach' families in chapter 2.

Helpful parenting

Most parents manage well for most of the time but, for many, the enjoyment of their children is clouded by uncertainty and lack of information and support. Child psychological pathology is very common and is a risk factor for adult mental health problems. For many young people, their own experiences of childhood do not offer an ideal model and they may have little opportunity to learn about child development or the maintenance of relationships in families.

Parents who are confident and consistent in their handling are likely to have confident and secure children. Positive parenting practices include warmth, sensitivity, involvement in child's activities, praise, and encouragement. Conversely, poor supervision, low involvement in the child's activities, harsh and inconsistent discipline, parental disharmony, high levels of criticism, rejection, neglect, corporal punishment, and displays of violent temper are associated with adverse outcomes such as later antisocial behaviour. Behavioural problems and difficulties with speech and language acquisition often coexist and are associated with learning difficulties in school (see Chapter 13).

The incidence of emotional and behavioural difficulties (EBD) in pre-school and school-age children is currently a matter of great concern. Attention deficit hyperactivity disorder (ADHD) and conduct problems are increasingly prevalent. The pressures on schools resulting from the educational reforms may result in a greater willingness to label children as 'EBD'. Placement in a special school or exclusion from school may result.

The evidence suggests that, to be effective, prevention and intervention should encourage positive relationships as well as address misbehaviour. These important observations prompt two questions. Can parents be helped to adapt their behaviour accordingly and to facilitate their child's development? And are there ways of doing this that would be achievable in real world settings? (*see* HFAC4 website.)

Education for parenthood

Parent training originated in the USA in the 1960s and was based on two traditions—behavioural theory and play therapy. Despite much research since then and increasing evidence that some programmes have worthwhile benefits, no country yet provides widespread access to parent education programmes.

There are currently several approaches to parent education, differing in their research base and theoretical underpinning and in the balance between individual and group-based work. Examples include the following: personal, social, health and citizenship education in school; antenatal classes which impart largely factual information; support networks as discussed in the previous chapter; non-directive counselling as in the Parent Adviser Model (see box on p. 34) programmes based on concepts of infant attachment, mental health, and emotional literacy; methods that are predominantly behavioural in nature.

Many programmes, both local and national, set out to enhance parents' abilities to manage their children, give them confidence, and build up supportive networks. Parents who take part appear to benefit, but they are largely self-selected. Those who are most in need of this help are also the most likely to drop out of programmes. Parenting programmes will not solve social and economic problems, and policies are needed that address these.

The characteristics of programmes liked by parents are listed in the box. The value of such schemes in reducing the overall prevalence of behavioural and emotional disorder is less clear, since this depends on a large proportion of the population being engaged in these programmes.

Parenting programmes and parent education

Parent education is defined as:

- A range of educational and supportive measures which help parents and prospective parents to understand their own social, emotional, psychological, and physical needs and those of their children and enhances the relationship between them; and which create a supportive network of services within local communities and help families to take advantage of them.

- It may consist of: education about parenthood and family life—education provided before conception, for example in school; preparation for parenthood—often provided in antenatal classes; support for parents—work with parents and child(ren).

(G. Pugh, E. De'Ath, and C. Smith, *Confident parents, confident children* National Children's Bureau, London (1994).)

Parenting programmes in general are more favoured by parents if:

- They allow parents to share experiences
- They make everyone feel included
- They are easily accessible
- They focus on educating parents so that they can make their own choices and decisions
- They are offered before the child is 3 years old
- The programme is led by a parent

(R. Grimshaw and C. McGuire, *Evaluating parenting programmes* National Children's Bureau, London (1998).)

Characteristics of parent training programmes whose effectiveness has been demonstrated in trials

Content

- Structured sequence of topics, introduced in set order over 8–12 weeks
- Subjects include play, praise, incentives, setting limits, and discipline
- Emphasis on promoting sociable self-reliant child behaviour and calm parenting
- Constant reference to parent's own experience and predicament
- Theoretical basis informed by extensive empirical research and made explicit
- Detailed manual available to enable replicability

Delivery

- Collaborative approach acknowledging parents' feelings and beliefs

◆ Difficulties normalized, humour and fun encouraged

◆ Parents supported to practise new approaches during session and through homework

◆ Parent and child seen together in individual family work; just parents in some group programmes

◆ Creche, good-quality refreshments, and transport provided if necessary

◆ Therapists supervised regularly to ensure adherence and to develop skills

(S. Scott, Parent training programmes, in *Child and adolescent psychiatry* (4th edn) (ed. M. Rutter and E. Taylor), Blackwell Science, Oxford (2003).)

See HFAC website

Primary prevention of behavioural and psychological problems

Parent education schemes, home visiting programmes, and programmes like Sure Start all include among their aims the prevention of emotional and behavioural problems and the promotion of optimal development, learning and emotional literacy. The characteristics of programmes, shown to be successful in formal trials are summarized in the box. The skill of the practitioner is crucial. Staff training in working with parents and in accessing local resources will be needed to implement these schemes (*see* HFAC4 website).

There is increasingly detailed evidence on what does and does not work in primary prevention and the promotion of optimal development. This needs to be incorporated into home visiting and Sure Start programmes. The most robust evidence of effectiveness is for behavioural programmes such as those devised by Webster-Stratton and developed in the UK in several centres. The Parent Adviser approach (see box on p. 34) has also been shown to be effective. However, both these programmes have so far been offered mainly to parents whose children are at least 3 years old and already exhibit difficult behaviour so, although successful, they must be regarded as secondary rather than primary prevention unless the skills that parents learn generalize to their subsequent child-rearing practices. Despite these reservations, there is increasing optimism that similar approaches may be valuable with parents of very young children.

Many families whose children present behavioural problems have additional difficulties. These include depression, discordant relationships between partners, lack of social skills, and social isolation. These may need to be addressed in addition to the behavioural difficulties; in other words, a purely behavioural approach is unlikely to be as successful as a more inclusive one.

Targeting the most socially disadvantaged families and those with severe difficulties can be effective, but to have a substantial overall impact on population rates of behavioural and emotional disorder, this targeted approach needs to be accompanied by a total population education programme to raise the knowledge and skills of all parents.

It is unlikely that there will ever be sufficient professional resources to treat all children and adolescents with psychological disorders. The obvious and attractive solution is primary prevention—'the promotion of child mental health through the reduction of symptoms, facilitation of development and reduction of known risk factors' (P. Hill, unpublished).

The cost of conventional professional approaches to primary prevention is likely to be prohibitive. Other methods have been suggested, such as the use of video or TV programmes and the inclusion of child rearing in school curricula.

Attachment behaviour and emotional literacy

Insecure infant–parent attachment is an important predictor of social and emotional problems in later childhood and in adult life, and may lead to similar problems in the next generation. The sensitivity of the parent to the infant's attachment signals is a key factor. There is some evidence that parents who have difficulties with attachment can be helped to respond more appropriately and many parents who have participated in such programmes report both short- and long-term benefits.

'Emotional literacy means the ability to understand one's own emotions, the ability to listen to others and to empathize with their emotions, and the ability to express emotions productively' (Claude Steiner). Thus it implies sensitivity to the needs and rights of others and, hopefully, the acquisition of a moral sense. Preventing violence in children is a related and difficult issue (box). Parents vary widely both in their own emotional literacy and in their ability to develop this characteristic in their children.

Issues in preventing violence in children

- The role of violence on TV, on video, and in computer games
- The relevance of smacking and other forms of physical punishment
- Cruelty to animals as a possible marker of future severe conduct disorder

See HFAC4 website

School-age children

Some of the antecedents of difficult behaviour can be observed in pre-school children. Collaboration between health and educational professionals is needed if preventive efforts in the pre-school years are to be successfully continued in primary school. Nurture groups may be helpful to parents (*see* HFAC4 website). Comprehensive Behaviour Support Plans are being drawn up by Education departments in response to a requirement by the DfES, and these should be multi-agency.

Failure to progress with key skills such as reading is often associated with emotional and behavioural difficulties. This combination of problems has a poor prognosis and the effectiveness of intervention decreases as the child becomes older. Programmes that bring together behavioural approaches and the recent advances in helping children with reading are likely to be a good investment.

Somatizers

There is some evidence that adults who respond to life stresses by exhibiting physical symptoms—the so-called 'somatizers'—learn this pattern of response in childhood, and there may be scope for primary prevention by recognizing this at an early stage and helping parent and child to find more positive ways of coping with stress. The benefits of successful prevention would be considerable, for both the individual and the health service; in addition, there might be beneficial effects on school attendance.

The relationship between social isolation, parental depression, and child development

The general theme of mental illness was discussed in Chapter 2. Here, we consider the important issue of depression and mood disorders, which are common among the mothers of young children and occur in all social classes. There are two forms of maternal depression which may have a hormonal basis. 'Baby blues' is common, but is usually transient and self-limiting. It affects 50 per cent of mothers. Acute puerperal psychosis is rare (1–2 per 1000 births) and needs urgent admission to hospital. Psychiatric disorder is now the leading cause of maternal deaths in the UK (box).

Between these two extremes, 'post-natal depression' affects around 10 per cent of all mothers within 3 months of giving birth. In low-income deprived populations, up to 40 per cent of mothers are depressed and one-sixth have severe psychiatric disturbance. It is uncertain whether these figures much exceed those quoted for young women in general, once socio-economic factors have been controlled for.

- Death from mental illness—suicide, substance abuse, or violence during pregnancy or the postpartum period—was the commonest cause of maternal mortality

- The women who committed suicide were often in stable relationships, were not socially disadvantaged, and many had professional qualifications

- The mode of suicide was often violent

- Previous and current history, and positive family history, of mental health problems were common but not always elicited and their severity was often underestimated

- None of the women who died had been seen by a specialized perinatal mental health service or had access to a mother and baby unit

- Use of the term 'post-natal depression' should be confined to non-psychotic depressive illness of mild to moderate severity with its onset following delivery

Findings from 'Why mothers die'—the confidential enquiry into maternal deaths in the UK, 1997–1999. Available at www.cemd.org.uk

Maternal depression not only affects the mother's quality of life, but has a number of important implications for the child. The adverse effects include an impact on behaviour, cognition, and emotional development. Boys are more at risk than girls. The mother's depression probably affects her interaction with the baby but the effect may operate in the reverse direction as well—a less responsive baby may increase the risk of depression. There may also be an increased risk of childhood accidents, sudden infant death, and child abuse, although the magnitude of the effect and the mechanism are uncertain. There are few prevalence data about father's mental health in relation to childbirth and little is known about the effect of paternal depression on partners or children.

Prevention

Little is known about primary prevention, but there is preliminary evidence that women at risk can be identified antenatally and that intervention at this stage can reduce the incidence of post-natal depression, especially if is recurrent with each pregnancy.

Identification and intervention

The identification of post-natal depression is not always easy and only around 50 per cent of cases are identified unless formal enquiries are made. The

Edinburgh Postnatal Depression Scale (EPDS) is often, but inconsistently, used to facilitate detection of depression. It was designed as a screening instrument, and formal psychiatric interview confirms the diagnosis of depression in only about 50 per cent of cases, while some cases are missed. Very high scores are probably more significant than borderline scores. Some mothers may not always give accurate answers to the EPDS because they do not recognize their symptoms as depression or because of concerns that they may be considered unfit to care for their babies.

Although it is already widespread, formal screening has not been recommended by the National Screening Committee since there are still many uncertainties regarding the overall impact of such a programme. A high degree of professional awareness is important and staff training is vital for the detection and management of depression and for the recognition of warning signs suggestive of non-response to intervention or of deterioration.

Intervention involving regular contacts, with non-directive counselling, by health visitors accelerates recovery. Strengthening of social networks may be as important a factor as individual approaches. Medication is needed in some cases.

4r Screening for postnatal depression

The importance of parental mental illness in general, and depression in particular, is unchallenged, but doubts continue to be expressed about the role of standard screening instruments such as the EPDS. Reasons include concerns about the sensitivity and specificity, a strong suspicion that some parents deliberately offer 'false' answers to the screening question for fear of what the consequences might be if they are diagnosed as depressed, and difficulties in adapting the screening process for parents with different cultural and linguistic backgrounds. *See:*

Shakespeare J, Blake F, Garcia J. A qualitative study of the acceptability of routine screening of postnatal women using the Edinburgh Postnatal Depression Scale. *British Journal of General Practice*, 2003, **53**: 614–619.

For a review from Australia, see Austin M-P, Lumley J. Antenatal screening for postnatal depression: a systematic review. *Acta Psychiatr Scand* 2003: **107**: 10–17.

Grace SL, Evindar A, Stewart DE. The effect of postpartum depression on child cognitive development and behavior: a review and critical analysis of the literature. *Arch Women Ment. Health* 2003; **6**: 263–274.

Loneliness

Loneliness and isolation are important associates of depression. Although factors such as lack of transport, unfriendly neighbours and fear of violence play a part, reasons for loneliness lie more in the parents' psychological state—lack of self-confidence, fear of meeting people, and reluctance to accept or reciprocate help. Social isolation is correlated with child maltreatment:

> People who maltreat children prefer to solve problems on their own. They have few relationships outside the home ... they tend to be transient, at least in urban areas ... and to have a lifelong history of avoiding activities that would bring them into contact with other adults ... Social isolation does not *cause* maltreatment, but it is an indicator of a lifelong pattern of estrangement.

It is perhaps not surprising that programmes designed to promote social contact and reduce isolation do not necessarily have benefits for children in families who already have major problems. For many families, however, a strengthened social network will enhance the parents' self-image and their perception of family interaction:

> Personal networks influence child development in several ways ... These include the sanctioning of parent behaviour and the provision of material and emotional support for the child. Network members also serve as models for parent and child, they stimulate the child directly ... these processes stimulate basic trust, empathy and mastery of the skills essential to relationships.

Increasing self-confidence and self-esteem, widening social networks, and initiating new experiences contribute in the long run to improving parents' health and this may have benefits for children. The role of health professionals in initiating these changes is discussed on p. 33 and the effectiveness of various programmes aiming to achieve these goals is discussed on p. 50.

Fathers

4r

The role of fathers has begun to attract researchers' attention, both as caregivers and from the perspective of depression. Depression and mental illness in fathers has been much less researched as compared to mothers, but there is emerging evidence that fathers' depression does impact on the child, both directly and through reduced support for the mother; conversely, a non-depressed father can to some extent reduce the impact on the child of the mother's depression. *See*:

Featherstone B. Fathers Matter: A Research Review. *Children & Society* 2004 **18**: 312–319: available at: http://www3.interscience.wiley.com/cgi-bin/abstract/109604879/ABSTRACT.

Depressive Symptoms in Parents of Children Under Age 3: Sociodemographic Predictors, Current Correlates, and Associated Parenting Behaviors *Lyons-Ruth, K, Wolfe, R, Lyubchik, A, Steingard, R*. In *Child rearing in America*, Eds. Halfon N, Mclearn K, Schuster M. Cambridge University Press, 2003 (e-books 2004).

Promoting child development and language acquisition

Poverty and educational attainment

The effects of poverty on early educational attainment are well known. This does not mean that poor parents are less interested in their children—only that the pressures of life take their toll. But how does an impoverished environment translate into poor attainments? Poverty, stress, poor diet, and sometimes substance abuse affect the health and growth of the fetus. Adverse experiences and under-nutrition can influence the way neuronal connections form in infancy, and this in turn may translate into skill deficits and unwanted behavioural patterns. Limited opportunities for learning affect the acquisition of concepts and skills.

Language development

There is a natural continuity from spoken language acquisition to reading and writing, and this is recognized in the Early Years Curriculum and in the National Curriculum for English, which has three 'Profile Components'—Speaking and Listening, Reading, and Writing. Learning to talk, to communicate ideas effectively, and to listen to others are fundamental skills in their own right and are the foundation on which literacy is built. Some children have major difficulties with mastering language because of global intellectual deficits, hearing impairment, or neurological disorders. Genetic differences and, much more rarely, single-gene disorders, play a part in some cases. The recognition of these children is discussed in Chapter 13. Here we are concerned with the much larger numbers of children whose language and literacy development could perhaps be enhanced by relatively simple measures (*see* HFAC4 website).

Clinicians have observed for many years that children living in deprived circumstances often display poor language skills. In the early 1970s Bernstein argued that these linguistic deficiencies were more apparent than real and were primarily a social phenomenon. Some linguists went further, proposing that language acquisition was such a robust function that it would be limited only by extreme degrees of deprivation. In the last 5 years the picture has changed considerably. There is now ample evidence that environmental and linguistic deprivation of a degree commonly found in the population does contribute to social class differences in language development and literacy, and that it is possible, at least in principle, to improve the progress and therefore the life chances of these children. There is also emerging comparative evidence on different approaches to teaching early literacy.

Measures of children's development at school entry are strong predictors of later attainments, especially in literacy. Baseline measurement and the literacy and numeracy hours, which are now part of the educational system, will provide opportunities for teachers to focus on how each child is doing and to monitor the 'readiness to learn' of young children, which is an important Sure Start target. The development of children's language in Sure Start areas will be monitored at ages two and four years, using the MCDI and the PEDS (see p. 257 for details of these instruments). These are based on parent report and parent concern, rather than formal screening by testing, and are linked to a range of community initiatives designed to enhance language development. Examples of emerging evidence about ways in which language and literacy could be promoted are given in the box.

Motor development and coordination

It is widely believed that children engage in less physical activity, both in the pre-school years and in school, than in the past and that this has adverse effects on motor and social development, as well as increasing the risks of becoming overweight or obese (p. 184). Although there is an extensive literature on

---

The role of environment—observational and correlational evidence

A mother agreed to tape all her interactions with her 3 pre-schoolchildren over two years. In 500 hours of tape she initiated talk to her three children just 18 times. (Heath)

A typical white middle class child in the USA enters first grade with 1000–1700 hours of one-to-one picture book reading behind them—a corresponding child from a low-income family averages 25 hours. (Adams)

In Israel 60 per cent of kindergarten children in a poor area did not own a single book; children from better neighbourhoods owned an average of 54 books each. (Feitelson and Goldstein)

Children from low-income backgrounds develop language that is different in kind and degree from children in the general population . . . On all measures except syntax, children [in this project] have averaged about one standard deviation below the mean.

NB: Even within social groups there are wide variations in the amount of conversation with young children.

Based on a review by Whitehurst

Examples of studies that focus on developing language and literacy

(For projects addressing overall developmental outcomes see Box on p. 71):

Dialogic reading: 'this is different from typical book reading where the adult reads and the child listens. In dialogic reading, the child learns to become the storyteller—the adult becomes an active listener, asking questions, adding information and prompting the child to increase the sophistication of their descriptions'. In at least six random controlled trials in the USA dialogic reading has been found to have beneficial effects on a range of linguistic measures.

UK projects which involve parents and pre-school children: REAL—Raising Early Achievement in Literacy (Sheffield–Hannon); Bookstart (Wade and Moore); Pears Early Education Partnership (PEEP) in Oxford. Many parents need help with literacy themselves and their participation may be crucial in order to help children.

Media print: several studies start from the assumption that TV viewing is an unavoidable part of modern life and aim to capitalize on the opportunities it offers to develop language and literacy skills.

For reviews of early literacy, see Hannon and Snow *et al.* http://www.nap.edu/readingroom/books/prdyc/ch5.html

The WILSTAAR project aims to promote early communication skills.

See HFAC4 website

dyspraxia (p. 265) and on motor skills among 'special needs' children, little is known about the effectiveness of current methods for enhancing motor skills in the early years among the normal population. In the UK, there is a Government commitment to increase the emphasis on and access to sport and physical activity of all kinds (*see* HFAC4 website).

Child protection—primary prevention of child abuse and neglect

This section considers what can be done with regard to the prevention of child abuse and neglect. A review of services for child protection is given in Chapter 15.

The 1989 Children Act Section 31(2) (Department of Health 1989) defines significant harm as 'injury, ill treatment or avoidable impairment of health and development that is due to a standard of care below that of a reasonable parent'. Health professionals have a duty of care to inform authorities if they believe that a child has suffered or is likely to suffer significant harm. The meanings of 'avoidable impairment', 'injury', and what is 'reasonable' are not defined.

There have been many studies on the risk factors which predict an increased likelihood of child abuse. Reduction in the risk of child abuse and neglect is one of the outcome measures used in research studies on home visitation and health visiting (see below). The distinction between primary and secondary prevention is somewhat blurred in dealing with child protection issues. There is some evidence that primary prevention can be achieved in high-risk families, i.e. those characterized by single-teenager parenthood and poverty; it is as yet inconclusive for other situations.

The causes and antecedents of child maltreatment are complex. The truly psychopathic or mentally ill abuser is relatively uncommon. More often, abuse occurs as a result of multiple factors involving the child, parents, their life situation, and a series of events which lead to abuse—the so-called 'critical path'. With increasing understanding of child abuse, lists of 'risk factors' have been developed (box). Although these may alert professionals and enable a

---

Checklist

1 Parent indifferent, intolerant, or overanxious towards child

2 History of family violence

3 Socio-economic problems such as unemployment

4 Infant premature, low birth weight

5 Parent abused or neglected as child

6 Step-parent or co-habitee present

7 Single or separated parent

8 Mother less than 21 years old at the time of child birth

9 History of mental illness, drug or alcohol addiction

10 Infant separated from mother for greater than 24 hours post-delivery

11 Infant mentally or physically handicapped

12 Less than 18 months between birth of children

13 Infant never breastfed

14 Difficult child behaviour

From Browne (*see* HFAC4 website)

high-risk population to be identified, this 'screening' approach is not sufficiently sensitive or specific to be used as a means of allocating resources to
individual families and it 'labels' families even though the great majority will
never in fact abuse their children. The *Framework for Assessment* offers a more
constructive approach to assessing risk and need (p. 21).

Prevention of child abuse in the majority of families is just one of the aims
of a CHP programme. Parents are very aware of child abuse issues and would
expect to be told if their health visitor or another professional had concerns
about the care of their child. In most instances, honesty is far preferable to a
secretive approach. Topics such as the often unrecognized hazards of shaking a
baby provide a non-threatening and non-stigmatizing way of introducing the
subject in all families and not just in those designated as 'high risk'.

Domestic violence

Violence in the home is very common but until recently it has been regarded
as a taboo topic. Now that the extent of the problem is clear, health professionals must be equipped to deal with it, both for the sake of the adults
involved and also because of the additional risks to children in the household
(see box on p. 294).

Children in refuges for female victims of domestic violence

Children living in refuges have often received poor or no preventive health
care; many have witnessed violence and often been abused themselves.
Previously unidentified developmental and behavioural problems are
commonly found. These families have difficulty in using conventional health
services.

Failure to thrive

The problems of preventing and identifying failure to thrive as a marker of
neglect or abuse are discussed on pp. 174 and 293.

Child sexual abuse

Education programmes for children, aimed at the primary prevention of
child sexual abuse and abduction, are effective under experimental conditions, but their impact in real-life situations is not yet established. Little is
known about ways of preventing young people and adults from becoming
perpetrators. Responsibility for preventing sexual abuse should not be placed
solely on children.

Female genital mutilation

Female genital mutilation (FGM) is a traditional practice in various cultures, mainly of African origin. There are many types of procedure but the more extensive ones cause much pain, disfigurement, and distress. The practice of FGM is an infringement of the rights of the child under the terms of the UN Convention and as such is illegal in the UK and many other countries world-wide. There is a conspiracy of silence brought about by the extreme sensitivity of the subject. The physical and psychological health implications of FGM include an increase in incidence of antenatal, intrapartum, and postnatal problems in circumcised women, poor uptake of cervical cytology by women from practising communities, and continence problems. It is imperative that any work undertaken is done in the spirit of openness, information sharing, and the co-operation of the community (*see* HFAC4 website).

Abuse and neglect in children of illicit drug users

This is an increasing problem (see p. 47).

Child prostitution

Sexual exploitation of children is increasingly recognized as a major problem, particularly among those who have run away from local authority homes. This often occurs in association with other forms of abuse and with drug addiction.

The National Plan for Safeguarding Children from Commercial Sexual Exploitation is published jointly by the Department of Health, the Home Office, and the Devolved Administrations.

See HFAC4 website

Secondary prevention

Secondary prevention is the focus of much child protection work. It involves early recognition of warning signs and appropriate action, as dictated by local and national guidelines. Tertiary prevention such as victim and family coun-selling may also be important. See Chapter 15 for further discussion.

Working with social services

The importance of close liaison between health care professionals, social ser-vices, and education authorities is emphasized in the Children Act (see Chapters 14, 15, and 16).

The effectiveness of primary prevention programmes

Primary prevention programmes could accomplish a great deal through parent support, community development, and early intervention for emerging problems. So far the evidence is based mainly on demonstration projects and research programmes, which are usually better staffed and supported than routine service work. Earlier in this chapter we discussed the evidence that focused programmes can reduce behaviorual problems and enhance language acquisition and pre-literacy skills. More naturalistic experiments and good observational studies are now appearing.

Community-wide programmes which address the underlying problems of families seem more likely to achieve the objectives of raising standards and closing the inequalities gap than services that address individual problems in isolation. A common concern for parents is the trade-off between their wish to care for their child and the need or desire to work, both for financial reasons and to extend their personal horizons (box and page 377).

Good programmes will never be cheap. The need for quality and for long-term commitment suggests that investment must be secure over a number of years. It was encouraging that Sure Start, the Government's flagship programme for early intervention, had substantial and sustained funding.

There are a range of early intervention programmes, designed to promote child development, improve parents' mental health and self-esteem, and reduce the risks of child abuse and accidental injury (box).

Examples of intervention programmes

(*Sure Start* is described on pp. 54 and 371)

Parenting programmes There is good evidence of effectiveness, particularly for programmes using a predominantly (though not exclusively) behavioural approach to behaviour problems in children between 3 and 8 years of age (*see* Chapter 13).

Intensive health visiting programmes The best documented study is the one conducted by Olds in the USA. Intensive home visiting by trained nurses (equivalent to UK health visiting but with a much smaller case load), when targeted to poor unsupported teenage mothers, improved obstetric outcomes, reduced hospitalization and child abuse (for the duration of the programme), and had a positive impact on development, behaviour, home safety, and injury rates. The benefits were marginal when home visiting was undertaken for more prosperous women. Ongoing domestic violence limited the effectiveness of interventions to reduce incidence of child abuse and neglect. A USA review suggested that 'more effective programs employed nurses who began visiting during pregnancy, who visited frequently and long enough to establish a therapeutic alliance with families, and who addressed the systems of behavioural and psychosocial factors that influence maternal and child outcomes. They also targeted families at greater risk for health problems by virtue of the parents' poverty and lack of personal and social resources'. The effectiveness of the programme was said to decline as soon as the level of funding and professional support was reduced.

A UK systematic review (which identified few UK studies) noted improved parenting and home environment, improvement in some behaviour problems, improved intellectual development especially among children with low birth weight or failure to thrive, reduced rate of injury and fewer home hazards, improvements in detection and management of postnatal depression, and improved rates of breastfeeding.

Structured home visiting programmes using non-qualified or paraprofessional staff In general, these have been less intensive and less ambitious in their aims. In a series of studies with populations of poor and deprived families in the USA, supported by the Ford Foundation (Child Survival/Fair Start) the measurable benefits included better utilization of health care facilities, including immunization uptake; however, these may reflect the greater difficulty in accessing health care system in the USA. There were small improvements in developmental scores, but little impact was found on smoking behaviour, uptake and maintenance of breastfeeding, weaning practices, or birth outcomes.

The Bristol Child Development Programme involves approximately 20 000 UK families each year. There are several programme models, including the First Parent Visiting Programme, the Integrated Urban and Rural Models, and the Community Mothers Programme. The programmes are based on monthly home visits to families, either by health visitors or by experienced mothers drawn from local communities. Key features include a strong emphasis on empowering parents to find their own solutions to their child-rearing concerns rather than advising them how to do so, a semistructured approach with a behavioural emphasis, and the provision of information through light-hearted cartoon material. Various evaluation studies have been undertaken during the past 15 years. Further information can be obtained from the Early Childhood Development Unit website (www.ecdc.org.uk).

Homestart was founded in 1973. It is a large voluntary organization in which volunteers offer regular support, friendship, and practical help to young families under stress in their own homes, helping to prevent family crisis and breakdown. Each local scheme is independent and has a paid organizer who recruits volunteers and visits families referred to the scheme to assess their needs. Volunteers are usually mothers themselves and aim to befriend families who are having difficulties, reassure and support them, and help them to make friends and use services more effectively. Homestart complements the statutory services and aims to reduce the need for professional intervention. A detailed description and evaluation has been published but there have been no formal random controlled trials.

Newpin (New Parent Infant Network) is a large voluntary organization in the UK providing help for people with parenting difficulties. It was established in 1980 with the aim of preventing family breakdown. There are currently 10 centres in England providing a 'package' of social involvement, therapy, and training. People are referred to Newpin by a wide range of agencies, or may self-refer. The 'Newpin process' begins with a home visit by a centre co-ordinator. If Newpin is thought to be appropriate, the next step is attachment to a centre via being 'matched' with a volunteer befriender already involved in Newpin. Centres provide a drop-in and a crèche. Training programmes include a Personal Development Programme (PDP), which uses therapy to explore the personal roots of parenting difficulty and to promote self-esteem. Newpin emphasizes the value of a caring community based on a non-hierarchical model of support, in which those who have been helped then go on to help others. Evaluations indicate benefits for some of the women but changes in the children have been more difficult to demonstrate. *See* www.newpin.org.uk

Day care There is still debate as to the adverse emotional and cognitive outcomes of day care. For some children day care can be beneficial. Important factors include high-quality day care, with continuity of carers and placement, and parents' satisfaction with the arrangements. Quality child care is in short supply. The National Childcare Strategy aims to remedy this (p. 370). Developmental risks are still associated with early child care. For practical issues in day care, *see* www.copas.net.au/ccch

The long-term outcomes of early intervention delivered primarily in the educational sector High-quality 'compensatory education' for the children of poor families does not increase IQ, but it does have other long-term benefits. These include higher achievements in school and in the job market, and reduced rates of crime and marital breakdown. In contrast, day nursery provision, where structured approaches to learning cannot so readily be provided, may meet a social need but does little to change either immediate developmental progress or long-term outcomes.

Benefits of early intervention for low birth weight infants The Infant Health and Development Program was a randomized trial of a 36-month intensive developmental intervention programme for infants of very low birth weight (< 1500 g). Cognitive development scores in the intervention group were 9.4 points higher after excluding those with overt brain damage (cerebral palsy). Infants weighing less than 1000 g at birth had lower behaviour problem scores. The benefits were mainly seen in the infants of mothers of low socio-economic status and little advantage was seen in children of better educated mothers. Other reports also indicate that such targeted interventions might be beneficial. UK studies have not confirmed this.

Primary prevention on a community wide scale 4r

There is now good evidence that intensive, structured high-quality early intervention programmes such as those described above have significant and measurable benefits for children and their mothers. Delivering such programmes to whole communities is much more challenging. Without continuous high levels of investment in well trained staff and quality assurance, programmes inevitably degrade. This issue is discussed in:

Taking preventive intervention to scale: the nurse–family partnership. Olds DL, Hill PL, O'Brien R. *Cognitive and behavioural practice*, 2003, **10**: 278–290.

Olds DL et al. Effects of home visiting by paraprofessionals and by nurses. *Pediatrics* **114**: 1560–1568, 2004.

The challenge of maintaining focus and quality has become apparent in England's Sure Start programme. Evaluation of the impact on children in programme areas at ages nine months and three years has shown little impact on families' use or perception of local services and only modest effects on parenting and development. There were some *negative* effects on development and behavioural measures in the children of teenage mothers, workless households and lone parents. These findings suggest that the most needy parents have difficulty in taking advantage of any additional services on offer and may even feel overwhelmed when provided with additional support and facilities that are combined with increased expectations of their parenting ability. Similar observations have been made in the USA Head Start programme.

Each Surestart Local Programme had a substantial degree of local autonomy rather than a fixed schedule of prescribed interventions. Programmes that closely followed the principles of the Surestart initiative were more likely to achieve better outcomes. Better outcomes were also more likely to be achieved by programmes led by health than those managed by other agencies, perhaps because the health visiting network made it easier to establish contact with a larger proportion of local families. It is possible that further beneficial effects of Surestart may emerge at a later date. *See:*

NESS Research Team (2005a). Early Impact of Sure Start Local Programmes on Children and Families. Surestart Report 13. London: DfES. Available at http://www.ness.bbk.ac.uk/documents/activities/impact/1183.pdf

NESS Research Team (2005b). Variation in Sure Start Local Programmes Effectiveness: Early Preliminary Findings. Surestart Report. London: DfES. Available at http://www.ness.bbk.ac.uk/documents/activities/impact/1184.pdf

For a useful review see: Rutter M Is Sure Start an Effective Preventive Intervention? Child and Adolescent Mental Health Volume in press 2006

Transforming the early years in England. Sylva K, Pugh G. *Oxford Review of Education* 2005; **31**: 11–27

The experiences of one Sure Start team were well summarized in:

Weinberger J, Pickstone C, Hannon P. Learning from Sure Start. OUP; Maidenhead, 2005.

Another useful systematic review was commissioned by the HTA. (Dretzke J, Frew E, Davenport C et al. The effectiveness and cost-effectiveness of parent training/education programmes for the treatment conduct disorder, including oppositional disorder, in children. (Health Technol Assess 2005; 9(50). http://www.hta.nhsweb.nhs.uk/fullmono/mon950.pdf)

The desired outcomes of pre-school programmes

Programmes like Sure Start aim to ensure that children are 'ready' for school. School readiness is a controversial topic, and there are many different views. Early formulations of school readiness tended to discriminate against disadvantaged children and absolved the school and community of responsibility for those who were not 'ready' at the appropriate age. Recent creative concepts of school readiness take a different approach (box).

School readiness

Children who start school with adequate social and communication skills, the ability to cope with frustration and stress, and with age-appropriate motor, language, and cognitive development are able to take advantage of learning opportunities offered by school.

Readiness is a relative concept. It needs to take into account the child's family and community background, his/her response to classroom experiences, and the ethos and expectations of the school—thus assessment of how 'ready' a child is can best be assessed over time during the first few months in school, rather than as a single evaluation.

This concept of readiness is attractive in that anonymized measures of school readiness for each cohort of children can be used in community participation projects. Local heads and communities can establish educational and health goals relevant to all the local children and treat their achievement as a collective responsibility. For example, the **Early Development Instrument (EDI)**, created in Canada, is a teacher-completed instrument which measures readiness to learn at school for *populations* of children and is intended to help communities assess their progress in supporting young children and their families.

See: http://www.offordcentre.com/readiness/SRL_project.html

See HFAC4 website

4r

Summary and recommendations

1 The evidence favours a move towards a more holistic approach to child and family health with the aim of reducing the prevalence of language delay, behavioural problems, and child abuse.

2 There is good evidence that parent education programmes with a behavioural focus can be effective, but they also need to address other issues of importance to the family.

3 Sure Start is an innovative programme provided for the most deprived areas but is not universally available. There is good evidence that other programmes incorporating similar methods have long-term benefits. The principles and concepts involved in Sure Start need to be disseminated more widely to all deprived communities. Assessing children in the first year after starting school may offer insight into the quality of their pre-school experiences and the effectiveness of community-wide interventions.

4 Postnatal depression, as well as depression at other times in parents' lives, are common problems. The evidence regarding formal screening is equivocal, but the high prevalence of depression in parents and the associations between depression and adverse child outcomes indicate a need to identify and support depressed parents. The risk of suicide and other death related to mental illness in pregnancy and the post-natal period

needs to be understood by all staff and there must be adequate specialist support for primary care staff.

5 Family support may help to reduce the risk of child abuse but checklists of risk factors for abuse are an unsatisfactory way of targeting resources.

6 Domestic violence is an increasingly important contributor to the distress of children and sometimes is a direct cause of abuse. This topic must be included in planning of training and policy development.

7 There is good evidence that lay workers can make a valuable contribution to parent support, as an additional resource to support quality care rather than a substitute for professionals. They do not pose a threat to professional skills or jobs.

Chapter 4

Child health promotion—opportunities for primary prevention

This chapter reviews:
- Ways of reducing the incidence of infectious diseases (including immunization)
- Reducing the risk of sudden infant death
- Ways of reducing parental smoking
- Unintentional injury prevention
- Nutrition and prevention of dental disease
- Situations requiring specialized services

This chapter considers the opportunities for primary prevention which should be incorporated in a programme of child health promotion.

Reducing the incidence of infectious diseases

Increasing immunization uptake

The Working Party did not undertake a detailed study of immunization, as there are many other reviews available. After clean water and safe sewage disposal this is the most effective of all preventive health care measures.

Maintaining and increasing immunization uptake is a complex matter. Parents are subjected to a barrage of confusing information. The media carry advertising campaigns emphasizing the importance of immunization but also run stories about disasters attributed to vaccines. Professionals are often ambivalent and ill-informed. Familiarity with the diseases immunization is designed to prevent, a knowledge of what the evidence actually shows with regard to effectiveness, risks, and contraindications, a firm commitment to immunization among all primary care staff, and honest acknowledgment of areas of uncertainly are essential in child health promotion; it is the immunization coordinator's job to make sure that this is done.

An immunization uptake of around 80 per cent can often be obtained with relatively little difficulty, but considerable professional effort and skill may be needed to ensure that the last 15 or 20 per cent of children are immunized. Sometimes it may be necessary to immunize a child at home. This can be done by appropriately trained nursing staff.

The roles of the immunization coordinator are well established. The tasks can be accomplished by one or several individuals as long as there are clear lines of responsibility (box). Whereas previously this role was usually the responsibility of health authorities or hospital/ community trusts, it will now rest with PCOs.

Immunization coordinator

- Establish and monitor the information and appointments systems; ensure that efforts are made to reach 'difficult' families.
- Make monthly reports of immunization statistics.
- Ensure continuing education on the subject of immunization at local level.
- Form an advisory group with members from other disciplines including community or public health, nursing, general practice, pharmacy, health promotion, etc.
- Monitor cases and outbreaks of vaccine-preventable infectious disease in collaboration with the consultant in communicable disease control (CCDC).
- Plan campaigns, programmes for the introduction of new vaccines, and programmes for changes in the existing protocol of immunization; maintain readiness (including personnel) to institute mass immunization campaigns at short notice.
- Ensure the maintenance of the 'cold chain' (i.e. ensuring safe refrigerated transport and storage of delicate vaccines, in particular polio vaccine which is inactivated by heat or sunlight).
- With the CCDC, monitor service provision for BCG, tuberculosis contacts, and hepatitis B vaccine coverage as well as for the basic vaccine programme.

- Provide advice in cases where doctors and/or parents are doubtful about immunization or there are contraindications in a particular case. Many districts provide an *immunization advice clinic*.
- Ensure that immunization policy development and training programmes for practice nurses and health visitors are undertaken.
- Provide *training for health visitors* to give immunizations at home for families who are hard to reach.

The concept of the immunization coordinator was introduced by the Department of Health in 1985 (HN/85/10), following a recommendation by the Joint Committee on Vaccination and Immunisation. S/he may be a community paediatrician, public health doctor, nurse, or other person with a special interest and commitment to immunization.

Reproduced from *Health care needs assessment* (2nd edn) by permission of the Radcliffe Press, Abingdon.

The structure of services for the prevention and control of infectious diseases is currently under consideration in the light of the Chief Medical Officer's report (Chief Medical Officer. *Getting ahead of the curve*. London: Department of Health, 2002). Whatever the details, rapid communication and good co-operation between professionals at all levels will be extremely important.

The Chief Medical Officer has re-emphasized the importance of the functions of the immunization co-ordinator in the changing environment 'whatever the arrangements and responsibilities for field officers [of the new National Infection Control and Health Protection Agency], the functions of the immunization co-ordinator must continue, with an identified individual responsible for the programme in each locality.'

Organization is simplified and costs are reduced if immunizations are as far as possible carried out on the same occasion as other preventive care activities, and therefore our recommendations take account of the times at which each immunization should be given (Chapter 18).

Whenever contact takes place with GP, paediatrician, health visitor, practice nurse, or school nurse, the immunization status of the child should be checked and, if possible, any outstanding immunizations given, assuming that there are no contraindications. This may be more difficult in the school setting where vaccines are unlikely to be stored on site.

Most premature babies can be fully immunized using the routine schedule. The date of immunization should be calculated from the child's actual date of birth, not from the expected date of delivery. This may mean that some babies are immunized while they are still in special care or neonatal units. As the evidence is not yet conclusive, it has been suggested that, for babies born at 28 weeks gestation or earlier, a blood test should be done after completing their immunizations to check that they do have adequate protection against Hib and hepatitis B.

Prevention of tuberculosis

Tuberculosis (TB) is still an important problem, particularly among some ethnic groups from areas of high prevalence. BCG vaccine should be given to high-risk infants and children (box), but several local audits suggest that this task is often neglected and lines of responsibility are ill defined.

The definition of high risk is those where there is a close relative or contact of the family receiving treatment for TB; those where a close relative or contact of the family has received treatment for TB within the last 10 years; those likely to be going to stay in a country where TB is endemic; those with parents or grandparents from countries with a high prevalence of tuberculosis. A high prevalence is defined as those with a prevalence 40 or more cases per 100 000 population.

When an adult is found to have active pulmonary TB, contact tracing is mandatory to ensure that any infected child is identified and treated promptly. This needs close liaison between the chest clinic, the contact tracer (usually a health visitor or nurse), and the paediatric department. TB in a child is rarely a risk to others, but it is vital to discover the source of the infection because the (often initially unsuspected) adult source may have infected other young children; if contact tracing is not done promptly, there is a risk that another child from the community will present with miliary TB or TB meningitis, with potentially devastating consequences. The BTS guidelines recommend that close household contacts should be traced *within 2 working days*.

See HFAC4 website and www.nice.org.uk/page.aspx?o=CG033

Hepatitis B vaccine

In the UK, this is given only to high-risk groups, but universal antenatal screening of mothers is recommended. The first dose is usually given in hospital before discharge, but four doses are needed and, as the children

Prevention of vertical transmission of hepatitis B infection

Worldwide, hepatitis-B-related liver disease is an important cause of morbidity and mortality. One of the commonest modes of transmission is from mother to infant, at or around birth ('vertical' transmission).

The administration of hepatitis B immunoglobulin soon after birth to babies of highly infective mothers, and a course of vaccine to all, reduces transmission, by over 90 per cent. Because hepatitis B infection in pregnant women is relatively uncommon in UK (ranging from 0.2 per cent or less in some areas to over 1 per cent in some inner cities) universal neonatal hepatitis B immunization is not recommended. Instead, all pregnant women should be screened for hepatitis B carriage and the babies of those mothers found to be carriers should be immunized.

The at-risk population is disproportionately disadvantaged and the reasons for poor uptake include:

- general lack of awareness of the need for vaccination by professionals and parents
- lack of understanding by parents whose first language is not English
- change of surname (and sometimes misspelling) in the first few months of the baby's life
- great mobility of high-risk families
- unclear allocation of responsibility for the different aspects of the programme
- lack of adequate monitoring and audit of the programme.

In the light of these problems, many areas have looked at ways of improving uptake. Measures suggested include:

- written information for parents and professionals, perhaps a page in the Personal Child Health Record (PCHR)
- the designation of one individual to organize and monitor the programme;
- regular feedback on the success of the programme.

The nature of the problem is such that in areas where there is a relatively high prevalence of hepatitis B carriage, significant resources have to be provided to ensure that all the at-risk infants are protected.

See HFAC4 website

involved may be born into families with a variety of other problems, it is easy to miss the subsequent doses (box).

New vaccines

4r Meningococcal C vaccine has been successful but vaccines against meningococcal B strains are needed. Pneumococcal conjugate vaccine is to be added to the routine schedule; at the same time, boosters of Hib and meningococcal vaccine are to be added.

Prevention of other infectious diseases

The Consultant in Communicable Disease Control and the Environmental Health Officer are the main sources of expertise on these issues, but primary health care teams should take an active role by providing information and advice for their clients. A variety of strategies could be employed to reduce the risk of infectious diseases among children. Examples include better food and kitchen hygiene, close supervision of young children using toilets in nurseries (where hepatitis and *Shigella* diarrhoea are common problems), and prompt management of outbreaks of meningococcal disease. Parents worry about the risk of toxocariasis leading to blindness. Numerically the risk is very small, but dog fouling of play areas is seen as an important problem by parents. Mothers who are planning a further pregnancy need information about safe eating to reduce risks of listeriosis, toxoplasmosis, etc. Headlice are a perennial cause of parental concern (see box).

Guidance on the control of communicable diseases in schools and nurseries is available on the Wired for Health website: (http://www. wiredforhealth.gov.uk/healthy/healcom.html).

For advice about head lice, see:
www.CHC.org/bugbusting/
www.hsph.harvard.edu/headlice.html
www.doh.gov.uk/headlice
www.headlice.org

See HFAC4 website

Prevention of sudden infant death syndrome (SIDS) and sudden unexpected death in infancy (SUDI)

The incidence of SIDS has fallen since the late 1980s, when it was around 1.8 per 1000 live births, and is currently 0.45 per 1000 live births. The fall is largely attributable to the change in sleeping position from prone to supine as a

Table 4.1

Approximately 400 babies die each year in the UK from SIDS
The magnitude of the risk of SIDS is related to the following factors:

Infant sleeping position
Exposure to tobacco smoke
Social class
Age of mother
Birth interval
Infection in pregnancy
Maternal drug addiction
Male sex of infant
Maternal depression
Premature or low birth weight
Multiple births
Congenital defects
Previous sudden infant death (more likely to be due to persisting social or child
  care factors than to genetic links)

Advice to reduce the risk (*see* HFAC4 website)

This is based on guidance published by the Foundation for the Study of Infant Deaths
(FSID) (http://www.sids.org.uk):

◆ Place your baby on the back to sleep (there is an eightfold increase in risk with
  sleeping prone)
◆ Your baby can safely play in the prone position
◆ Side sleeping carries a higher risk than supine (twofold increase)
◆ Cut smoking in pregnancy—fathers too!
◆ Do not let anyone smoke in the same room as your baby
◆ Do not let your baby get too hot or too cold; make sure your baby is appropriately
  clothed for the room temperature; do not let your baby sleep next to a radiator or in
  direct sunlight
◆ Keep baby's head uncovered—place your baby in the 'feet to foot' position to prevent
  from wriggling down under the covers
◆ If your baby is unwell, seek medical advice promptly

The risk of SIDS is lower for babies sharing a room with their parents. The role of bed
sharing is still uncertain but FSID current advice is 'The safest place for your baby to sleep
is in a cot in your bedroom for the first six months. There is a proven risk in bedsharing if
you or your partner smoke (even if you never smoke in bed or in your home), have been
drinking alcohol, take drugs or medication that make you drowsy, or are very tired. Avoid
bedsharing if your baby was born premature or low birth weight, or has a high temperature. If your baby does come into your bed watch out for accidents, use lightweight blan-
kets and keep the baby's head uncovered.'

The role of breast feeding as a protective factor is still uncertain.

Mattresses: 'There is NO evidence to support the theory that toxic gases from mattresses
play a part. It does not matter what kind of mattress you use, or whether it is new, as
long as it is firm, not soft, does not sag, shows no sign of deterioration. Keep it well-aired
and clean. Mattresses with a PVC surface or a removable washable cover are easiest to
keep clean. Ventilated mattresses (with holes) are not necessary. Place your baby with his
feet to the foot of the cot. Never sleep your baby on a pillow, cushion, bean bag, or
water bed, or sleep together with your baby on a sofa.'

---

consequence of the Back to Sleep campaign. Some groups of infants are at particular risk of sudden death (Table 4.1). The prevalence of prone sleeping, exposure to tobacco smoke, and sleeping in inappropriate environments is much higher in deprived families. Infants in these families are also at increased risk of poor growth, developmental delay, and respiratory morbidity. There is an overlap in the factors which predict an increased risk of child abuse and those which predict sudden death. A minority of sudden deaths are probably non-accidental.

SIDS can occur in any social group and prevention messages as outlined in Table 4.1 should be made available to all families. The social groups at highest risk of SIDS are generally also those who are hardest to reach through conventional health service approaches. The identification of families where more health professional support is required should be based on broader considerations of need and risk, rather than being focused solely on the risk of SIDS (see p. 70).

Some infants who die suddenly have undetectable and irremediable disorders, but others die of potentially treatable conditions. Preventing avoidable deaths involves increased parent awareness of the symptoms and signs of illness in babies. Failure to recognize that a baby is ill occurs more often with young poorly educated mothers, particularly if unsupported by, and living away from, their own families.

A check list such as Baby Check might help mothers to identify illness more effectively, but at present there is insufficient evidence to support its routine use in this way. More information is needed on its effectiveness in the community as a whole, and how it will integrate with NHS Direct. Easier access to services and improved professional response to acute illness in babies are clearly important. *See* HFAC4 website.

4r Recent findings on SIDS

A recent study confirmed the increased risk of SIDS associated with parents sleeping on sofas with their infants.

Blair PS et al. Major epidemiological changes in sudden infant death syndrome: a 20-year population-based study in the UK. *Lancet.* Advanced online publication January 18, 2006

It has also been claimed that the use of dummies is associated with a reduced risk of SIDS but this remains controversial:

De-Kun Li, Marian Willinger, Diana B Petitti, Roxana Odouli, Liyan Liu, Howard J Hoffman.

Use of a dummy (pacifier) during sleep and risk of sudden infant death syndrome (SIDS): population based case-control study BMJ 2006; **332**:18–22 (7 January) (and correspondence).

4r   The Foundation for the study of Infant Death have produced an advice card to reinforce advice for patents: www.sids.org.uk/fsid/roomshare.htm

Reducing smoking by parents

Parental smoking is correlated with a number of adverse outcomes for the child, though it may be difficult to determine whether pre- or post-natal exposure is the more important factor. A reduction in smoking during pregnancy is a Sure Start target and would make a major contribution to reducing the incidence of low birth weight, which is itself an important marker of social inequalities. (Persuading mothers to stop smoking in pregnancy is made more difficult by their worries about putting on weight and by a belief among some mothers that smaller babies will mean an easier labour.)

Children inhale smoke from their parents' cigarettes, so-called passive smoking. Passive smoking has adverse effects on children's health, and there are well-established links between smoking and a variety of adverse outcomes. For example, among the babies of mothers who smoke, the risks of sudden infant death, middle-ear disease, meningitis, and admission to hospital for respiratory illnesses are significantly increased. Smoking is an important cause of fires in the home. There may also be long-term effects on the risks of adult diseases such as coronary artery disease and cancer.

The effects of passive smoking are not always made sufficiently clear to parents. While it is important not to take a punitive approach, a child's respiratory or ear, nose, and throat illness (p. 209) offers an ideal opportunity to address the issue. Parents should also be aware of the influence their smoking may have on their children's smoking behaviour later in childhood.

Smoking—a high-risk activity

120 000 deaths per annum in UK from smoking-related diseases.

Stopping smoking

- The chance of successfully stopping smoking is more than doubled if pharmacological aids are used together with advice and counseling.
- Nicotine replacement therapy and bupropion are effective.
- The greater the support for the smoker, the greater the chance of stopping.

For young people

Health promotion measures (e.g. Smokescreen—peer-to-peer project).

Other measures

Tobacco advertising ban; code of practice regarding smoking at work.

See HFAC4 website

For many parents smoking is a social activity, a substitute for personal support, a private pleasure ('something they do for themselves'), or a means of coping with poverty and stress. Primary prevention is the ideal solution. Some health professionals feel that it is sometimes insensitive and intrusive to focus on smoking when it is a response to severe life stresses which cannot easily be removed.

Little is known about how best to reduce parental smoking in the first few months of the baby's life. Most research has focused on attempts to reduce smoking in pregnancy. The latter is important, since 90 per cent of women who smoke in pregnancy are still smoking 5 years later. Two-thirds of women who succeed in stopping smoking while pregnant restart after the baby is born. The evidence in respect of fathers' smoking is less clear, but fathers' smoking is probably important at least to the extent that a mother will find it harder to give up smoking if her partner continues.

The aim of reducing smoking should not be pursued in isolation, but rather in the context of more wide-ranging efforts at health promotion within particular families by creating a good relationship with the parents and promoting self-confidence and self-esteem. Simple advice to stop smoking may not be effective on its own but when given by a general practitioner it has a significant impact. Support groups, telephone help lines, counselling, and medication (nicotine replacement therapy or bupropion) may all contribute. *See* HFAC4 website.

Unintentional injury prevention

This term is preferred to 'accidents' because the latter implies unpredictability and therefore a negative attitude to the possibility of prevention. Unintentional injuries (including poisonings) are the most common cause of death and a cause of considerable morbidity in children between the ages of 1 and 14 years (see Table 4.2). Reducing both the absolute number of injuries and deaths from accidents and the social class gradient are important objectives which need multi-agency collaboration and investment.

The causes of unintentional injury at different ages reflect the child's state of development, the child's changing perception of danger, and the degree of exposure to different hazards at various ages. Prevention strategies must reflect this and need to address the many different ways in which young children can be injured. Table 4.2 summarizes prevention programmes aimed at reducing the risk of particular types of injury, together with evidence for the effectiveness of the strategies suggested and the implications for prevention programmes.

There is a marked social class gradient. Some injuries are up to six times more common in the poorest areas than in the most prosperous, while there is a 16-fold

Local accident data

There are two approaches:

- Surveillance systems that record all injuries.
- Surveillance systems that concentrate on one kind of injury (playgrounds, bicycle injuries, etc).

Overall surveillance systems

There are three systems in existence in the UK at present

- Glasgow, Canadian Hospitals Injury Reporting and Prevention Programme (CHIRRP). Children only
- All Wales Injury Surveillance System. All ages.
- Newcastle: Population-based Injury Surveillance System (PHISSCH). Children only.

With the new Government target to reduce 'serious' injuries (i.e. injuries with a length of hospital stay of 4 days or greater) Hospital Episode Data can be used at the level of PCGs/PCOs.

Surveillance systems recording one type of injury

There have been a number of local surveillance systems recording one type of injury. Examples are:

- Playground injury surveillance.
- Farm injuries.
- STATS19 data collected by the police and local authorities on road traffic injuries. These have been used in a number of national evaluation studies, e.g. the evaluation of 20 mph zones in England—a 70 per cent reduction in child pedestrian injuries and a 48 per cent reduction in child cyclist injuries was found.

The way forward

A&E based surveillance targeted towards specific injuries, and with sufficient local exposure data to pinpoint exposure specific risk, is likely to be the route to follow. The 'black spot approach' is not particularly useful, especially for child pedestrian injuries.

Table 4.2

Injury type	Implications
MVA*—passenger	Children should travel in car seats or restraints—good evidence that they prevent or reduce injury. Legislation combined with programmes to promote car safety results in increased use *but* many children still travel without any restraints. Loan schemes for safety equipment for poorer families were rarely financially viable because equipment was never returned. Effort now devoted to low-cost schemes.
MVA—pedestrian	Educating young children (1–5 age group) unlikely to be effective. Parent education may play a small role—some parents overestimate a young child's capacity for road sense. **Needs: traffic-calming schemes; traffic-free areas, safe play areas; safer journeys to school.** (NB Parents often take their children to school—prompted by fear of abduction as well as anxiety about traffic).
Bicycle injuries	Not common in under-fives but important to encourage safety from the start. There is good evidence on the effectiveness of cycle helmets in reducing frequency and severity of head injury following increases in cycle helmet use. There is some evidence that bicycle training schemes can improve safe riding behaviour. It is likely that the optimum way to reduce cycle injuries to children consists of a combination of designated cycle tracks, cycle proficiency education, and cycle helmet legislation.
Drowning	Site of drowning relates to age: babies who cannot protect themselves when they fall in bath water; toddlers who wander off and drown in accessible water (garden ponds in the UK, drainage ditches in The Netherlands, and domestic swimming pools in Australia and Southern Europe); older children die whilst swimming when unsupervised; some children drown in hotel pools whilst on holiday. No home with children under 5 should have an open garden pond. Fencing domestic pool can prevent drowning. Supervision of swimming and water activity should prevent drowning. In the UK only one child a year dies in municipal pools where there is clear observation of swimming enforced by the Health and Safety Executive, whereas many die in rivers, lakes, and canals where there is no supervision. Lifeguard supervision should be extended to private pools and open water where swimming is common.
Farm injuries	Farm environment is hazardous for young children: animals, machinery, muck heaps, etc. The dominant types of injuries

Table 4.2 *Contd.*

Injury type	Implications
	are falls, crushes, and eye injuries. One child in 50 living on a farm presents with a farm-related accident each year. Legislation prohibits the driving of tractors by children under the age of 13, and riding as passengers on tractors, trailers, or other field implements, but is often ignored. A safe community approach is being tried.
Horse riding accidents	Little data on horse-riding but importance of safe helmets is recognized
Fire and flame	Fires and flames are a significant cause of accidental death in childhood. Most are in conflagrations in private dwellings. Many die from gas and smoke inhalation rather than by direct heat. House fires are 15 times more common in Social Class V than Social Class I. There has been a fall in the number of deaths from the ignition of clothing following flame-proofing regulations and fewer open fires and paraffin stoves. Smoke detectors have an important role in the prevention of conflagrations and the use of wired (rather than battery) alarms should be enforced in both public and private housing. The impact of smoke alarm campaigns in the UK has so far been disappointing. Alarms are often deliberately inactivated by householders because they are set off by cooking or cigarette smoke, and batteries are often not replaced when needed. Other strategies are needed. Some fire brigades are helping families to develop a personal fire-escape plan.
Scalds	Scalds are rarely fatal but are very painful, need prolonged treatment, and may cause permanent scarring. There has been a change in the pattern of scalds but not a fall in the total number. Hot water from teapots has declined, but hot liquids from cups are a major cause due to widespread use of instant coffee and tea bags in the cup rather than in the pot and are difficult to prevent. The incidence of scalds from hot water in kettles and baths has also risen. Most common in under-fives and those living in deprived circumstances. Modification of the child's environment is more likely to be successful than education. Coiled or short flexes (no longer than 80 cm) may help. Bath scalds occur when the child falls in the water. Standards for gas and electricity recommend 60 °C maximum for thermostats, but many households have water temperatures above 60 °C (can cause a partial thickness burn in 10 s). An educational programme to reduce hot-tap water temperatures in homes can produce significant decreases in water temperature; the use of thermostatic mixertaps for the bath set at 43 °C is good practice but expensive. Scalds can be non-accidental but diagnosis is difficult.

Table 4.2 *Contd.*

Injury type	Implications
Suffocation and strangulation	Examples include inhalation of peanuts, sweets, etc., plastic bags over the head, becoming trapped in disused refrigerators, playing games involving 'hanging', etc.
Poisoning	Most common in under-fives and in older children if developmentally delayed. The peak age is between 1 and 4 years. Divided into medicines (prescribed and non-prescribed), household products, and plants. Most children who take poisons do not have serious symptoms. Medicines may be of low toxicity (e.g. the oral contraceptive pill or antibiotics), intermediate toxicity, which may cause symptoms in young children, or potential high toxicity (iron tablets, aspirin, tricyclic antidepressants). Many household products may be relatively non-toxic. However, a few, such as caustic soda, dishwasher powder, chemistry set contents, soldering flux, and paint stripper, may cause serious harm. All prescribable solid dose medication is now placed in child-resistant containers or safety packaging such as opaque unit packaging. In 1985 Department of Trade and Industry regulated for a number of household products to be sold in child-resistant containers. There is good evidence that child-resistant containers and packaging prevent childhood poisoning.
Baby-walker injuries	3.5 injuries per 1000 users per year. Baby walkers have no demonstrable benefit to babies. Use is common across all social groups and is associated with other unsafe practices such as not using stair gates or fireguards. Health professionals should ascertain each family's reasons for walker use and try to find acceptable alternatives, make the family aware of the importance of properly fitted stair gates and fireguards, and help the family to obtain and use such items of safety equipment. There are European Union regulations on baby walkers but many do not comply with them. Many believe that baby walkers should be banned.
Falls	Falls from high-rise flats (windows and balconies) are potentially fatal. Prevention programmes involve window catches, bars or guards, making balconies safe, and providing other safer play areas. Playground injuries—risk reduction by use of safer materials and good design. **Needs: collaboration with local authority—housing department and parks/ playgrounds. To initiate actions, health visitors need access to carpenter/locksmith/fitter**.
Stair gates and fireguards	Although their use is logical and some authorities run loan schemes, there is little evidence of benefit. They may allow parents more peace of mind but could also be a cause of if a child tries to climb over a stair gate. Remember to place at the end of the stairs where the child is, not just at the top

Table 4.2 (contd)

Injury type	Implications
Glass injuries (doors, windows, etc.)	Preventable by use of safety glass, membranes, etc., and by good design at planning stage. Little evidence regarding interventions.
Dog attacks	Little research available in health sector but understanding of applied canine psychology is potentially useful. There are several voluntary sector programmes on dog safety. A child should never be left unsupervised with a dog.
Sunburn and heat stroke	Severe sunburn in early childhood is a risk factor for skin cancer. 'Heat stroke' can occur if children are left in cars in full sun. **Needs: parent education re appropriate use of sunscreens and danger of leaving children to sleep in cars**.
Playground injuries	These are multifactorial and the surface should be considered as well as the equipment. They are uncommon and represent only between 1 and 2 per cent of injuries to children. Injury rates increase over fall heights of 1.5 m. Safety surfaces, both bark and rubber, offer much greater protection than concrete or tarmac, with rubber having a lower injury rate than bark. Significant head injuries are very rare in modern playgrounds with safety surfaces. A number of children sustain arm injuries, including fractures, from falls from equipment onto safety surfaces. Injuries from falls from monkey bars and climbing frames are more common than those from slides and swings. Playground injuries can be prevented by simple measures such as increasing bark depth under equipment and replacing monkey bars.

* MVA, motor vehicle accidents.

Acknowledgements: J. Sibert and E.M.L. Towner.
Health Development Agency, London (2001).

difference for child deaths due to house fires (Table 1.2). Differences in the environment and in social patterns and attitudes underlie this gradient; for example, the degree of independence children are allowed by their parents, the amount of supervision which can be provided on the journey to school, opportunities to play outside the home in safe areas, and differing attitudes to the roles of police, council officers, etc. Where no play facilities exist, young children are often permitted to play in the road outside their home and negotiate road crossings alone before they are old enough to judge the speed of traffic.

Misconceptions about injuries and accidents

There are many misconceptions about accidents and injuries. Parents worry more about the risk of abduction by paedophiles than about a road accident, even though the latter is 20 times more common. Parental worries about safety in general have resulted in a reduction in children's exposure to traffic and by implication a lack of experience of outdoor play and exploration and reduced exercise opportunities (see the section on obesity).

Although parents are often 'blamed' for accidents and their supposed careless-ness is the focus of some prevention strategies, many families, even in the poor-est areas, are well aware of potential hazards to their children and know what action they would like to be taken in order to reduce the risk. Similarly, there are myths about the 'accident-prone' child. Although it is true that boys are more likely to have accidents than girls, the majority of children experiencing serious injury are victims of circumstance rather than of their own impulsive actions.

Strategies for prevention
Nationwide

In addition to education campaigns and legislation focusing on just one type of injury there have been several campaigns aimed at raising general awareness

---

Environmental change and childhood injury prevention

Environmental change can prevent accidents, some examples are:

- **Pedestrian road traffic**: traffic calming
- **Bicycle injury**: cycle helmets (2–6), attention to bicycle design
- **Passengers in cars**: seat belts and car safety seats; car design
- **House fires**: smoke detectors
- **Nightdress fires**: reducing flammability of nightdresses
- **Bath scalds**: thermostat reduction of the temperature of the hot water in domestic systems
- **Drowning in municipal pools**: supervision of swimming pools by Health and Safety regulations has meant that only one child dies per year in England and Wales
- **Drowning in water at home**: fencing domestic swimming pools prevents drowning in Australia
- **Falls from windows**: window guards reduced falls in Children Can't Fly programme in New York

> - **Falls in playground**: attention to playground design—impact-absorbing surfaces, reducing height of equipment
> - **Accidental child poisoning**: reduced following the use of child-resistant containers
> - **Accidental choking**: small part toy safety regulations
> - **Glass injuries**: safety glass
>
> *See* HFAC4 website

of hazards in the home and environment. TV series on safety can reach millions of parents. The Newcastle Project involved a combination of media coverage with a health-visiting programme in which the messages were tailored specifically to the needs of their target audience. Significant benefits were reported.

Community level

A campaign in Falköping, Sweden, involving local policy-makers and the whole community, demonstrated a significant fall in injuries over the study period. The Massachusetts Statewide Child Injury Prevention Campaign (SCIPP) provided five intervention programmes aimed at various types of injury; a significant reduction was shown in only one type (motor vehicle passenger injuries). The difficulties inherent in such campaigns and in demonstrating robust benefits were apparent in this programme:

> . . . future interventions must include the active participation of local public health agencies, a media component to increase the awareness of both the public and professionals, and evaluation over a longer time period.

There have been many initiatives such as equipment loan stores (for stair gates, car seats, etc.), smoke alarms, first aid courses, swimming lessons, etc. (see Table 4.2 for evidence of benefit). First aid courses may not only help adults to deal with the immediate aftermath of an injury, but also heighten awareness of hazards and thereby reduce the number of injuries.

Individual practitioners can contribute in various ways (see box).

Possible roles of the practitioner in injury prevention are:

- As an advocate for children, where there is a strong evidence base
- Promoting positive messages of safety in local media

- Encouraging a safe environment for children during the core CHP programme
- Working with local authorities and non-governmental organizations on safe community activities
- Opportunistic Education
- Supporting national organizations

In 1977, Court and Jackson were instrumental in the formation of the Child Accident Prevention Trust (CAPT) in England which fosters research and action on accidents to children. There are similar groups in Wales (Child Safe Wales—Diogelu Plant Cymru) and Scotland (Child Safe Scotland).

Current status of injury prevention

The prevention of injuries cannot be addressed purely as a health services issue. Multi-agency planning is essential. Research findings from other disciplines and agencies, such as the Transport Research Laboratory and the Community Fire Service, must be incorporated into local policy. Health care staff need further information and training in injury prevention. Suitable materials are available, though their impact has yet to be fully evaluated.

A checklist giving examples of hazards and safety checks based on a developmental perspective might enable health professionals to raise the subject with parents more easily but, as yet, there is no information as to how effective this might be.

Accident and emergency departments offer an ideal opportunity to monitor accidents and injuries in each district. Information systems should be modified where necessary so that the data required can be obtained easily and in an accessible format, allowing local people a say in deciding priorities for action. A home visit by a health visitor or other community worker, following an injury, may reduce the risk of further accidents, provided that the timing is right and the natural sensitivities of the parents are respected.

An Accidental Injury Task Force was established in 2000 with members drawn from Government departments, national agencies, and academic departments. It has set up three expert working groups on children and young adults, older people, and measuring and monitoring. The most important priorities for action to reduce the burden of injuries amongst children and on reducing health inequalities will be identified.

Injury   4r

A useful review examined how injury rates relate to social inequalities: *Injuries in children aged 0–14 years and inequalities*: a report prepared for the Health Development Agency (2005) www.hda.nhs.uk

Nutrition

Breastfeeding

Support for breastfeeding is a priority topic for health promotion. The WHO recommends exclusive breast feeding until 6 months of age. There is evidence that this is nutritionally adequate. However, mothers may introduce complementary feeding for many valid reasons. The UK position is somewhat more flexible but recommends that complementary feeding should not be introduced before 4 months (17 weeks) and preferably delayed until 6 months.

Even in industrialized societies, breastfed infants have a reduced risk of infection, particularly those affecting the ear, respiratory tract, and gastrointestinal tract. The protective effect is particularly marked for low-birth-weight infants. There may also be other benefits: improved cognitive and psychological development, and a reduced risk of childhood obesity and maternal breast cancer. The evidence regarding protection against allergic disease for those genetically at risk and a reduction in risk of SIDS is more controversial.

The reasons for not starting breastfeeding or discontinuing it at an early stage include social limitations, lack of partner and family support, ambivalent attitudes to sexuality and nudity, societal attitudes, lack of privacy or facilities, a need to return to work, distaste, the uncommon risk of unrecognized underfeeding at the breast (which can be associated with hypernatraemic dehydration), the low levels of vitamin K in breast milk, and the association with 'breast milk jaundice' (a benign condition but one that may cause anxiety (see p. 196)).

In 2000, the proportion of women who started to breastfeed was 71% in England and Wales, 63% in Scotland, and 54% in Northern Ireland. However, overall, only 45% of those who start continue to 4 months. The majority of those who stop before 4 months would have liked to continue for longer. Many of these women experience feelings of guilt and distress.

When monitoring the level of breastfeeding in a community it is important to distinguish between intention to breastfeed, initiation, continuation to fixed points in time (e.g. end of first week, at the time of Guthrie testing, and at immunization visits), and overall duration. Different strategies are likely to have differing impacts on each of these.

Breastfeeding

4r NICE will be publishing an Effective Action on breastfeeding in the summer of 2006.

Some mothers and babies have problems establishing breastfeeding and this can result in significant weight loss, but neither the poor intake nor the weight loss are always clinically obvious, and underfed babies may fall asleep rather than crying. Cases of hypernatraemic dehydration associated with weight loss of more than 20 per cent have been reported.

Most midwives weigh babies from time to time, but there are no definitive guidelines or evidence as to what weighing regimen might best meet the two aims of safety for the baby while minimizing anxiety for the mother. Some midwives are reluctant to weigh babies at all because they believe that it worries the mother and may lead to her giving up breastfeeding.

Some authorities take the opposite view and argue that weighing substantially decreases the risk of dehydration and poor weight gain. Those who support regular weighing suggest the following:

- an accurate birthweight
- a weight at 3–4 days (the point of maximum weight loss, which should not be more than 10 per cent of the birth weight)
- a weight at 7 days (when the baby should have started to gain)
- weight at 10–12 days (the baby should be back to birth weight).

Notes: (1) In the early days of life record age in hours, not non-specific hospital 'days'.

(2) The weighing referred to is a single weight, not a formal test weighing to measure the intake of an individual feed—this is *not* advised as a routine procedure.

See HFAC4 website

Intention to breastfeed

Women make decisions about breastfeeding early in pregnancy or even before they become pregnant, influenced by cultural attitudes, social background, and education, and this limits the scope and timescale for intervention in pregnancy to increase the number of women who intend to breastfeed. Information about the benefits of breastfeeding could be provided in school as part of personal, social and health education, but very little is known about the effectiveness of this

Table 4.3   The 'Baby Friendly' initiative

UNICEF will designate a hospital as 'Baby Friendly' if it follows the 10 steps to breastfeeding

1 Have a written breastfeeding policy routinely communicated to all health staff

2 Train all health staff in skills to implement this policy

3 Inform all pregnant women about the benefits and management of breastfeeding

4 Help mothers initiate breastfeeding within half an hour of birth

5 Show mothers how to breastfeed, and how to maintain lactation, even if they should be separated from their infants

6 Give newborn infants no food or drink other than breast milk, unless *medically* indicated.

7 Practice rooming-in (allow mothers and infants to remain together) 24 hours a day

8 Encourage breastfeeding on demand

9 Give no artificial teats or pacifiers (also called dummies or soothers) to breastfeeding infants

10 Foster the establishment of breastfeeding support groups and refer mothers to them on discharge from the hospital or clinic

April 2006 there were 43 accredited hospitals and seven community facilities in the UK.
See HFAC4 website

approach. Nevertheless, there has recently been a more positive attitude by health professionals to the benefits of breastfeeding, coupled with consistent advice and support. Improved breastfeeding rates in some areas suggest that this is paying dividends.

Establishing lactation

Many women who plan to breastfeed do not persevere in establishing feeding, fail to maintain it after leaving hospital, or give up after a few weeks. Women who intend to breastfeed benefit from positive attitudes and policies in the maternity unit (the 'Baby Friendly' initiative is described in Table 4.3), encouragement and support in problem solving, increased frequency of feeding, discouraging of 'supplementary' feeding, and showing mothers how to express milk. There should be no breast milk substitutes in the free discharge packs offered in maternity units.

Maintenance

Maintenance of breastfeeding is enhanced by lactation counsellors and peer support which may be more effective than the advice of professionals. The attitude and support of the father is also an important factor.

4r Breastfeeding–current topics

There is growing evidence that both the initiation and the maintenance of breastfeeding can be influenced by various interventions, contrary to earlier defeatist views that women make firm decisions, based on their cultural and social background, long before they are ever pregnant. Useful links to breastfeeding sites: http://omni.ac.uk/browse/mesh/D001942.html

Systematic review to evaluate the effectiveness of interventions to initiate breastfeeding. Fairbank L, O'Meara S, Renfrew MJ *et al*. Health Technology Assessment 2000; **4**: 25. http://www.ncchta.org/execsumm/summ425.htm

The effectiveness of public health interventions to promote the duration of breastfeeding *Systematic review*, 2005. www.publichealth.nice.org.uk/page.aspx?o=511625

The debate about the role of weighing to detect excessive weight loss in the first two weeks of breast feeding is unresolved but there are new data that provide up to date centiles for the extent of weight loss, combined with proposals, as yet unproven, as to how best to identify babies at high risk of severe dehydration with dangerous hypernatraemia. see:

Macdonald P D, Ross S R M, Grant L, Young D. Neonatal weight loss in breast and formula fed infants. Archives of Disease in Childhood: Fetal and Neonatal Edition 2003;88:F472–6

The new centiles are in:

Sachs M, Oddie S. Breastfeeding in the balance. *MIDIRS Midwifery Digest Sept* 2002, **12**(3), 296–300.

Growth charts for breastfed infants have been published but have not been adopted for routine use. (N.B.: The WHO has published growth charts for fully breast fed babies, see p.174). Cole TJ, Paul AA, Whitehead RG. Weight reference charts for British long-term breastfed infants. *Acta Pediatr* 2002 **91** 1296–1300

The issue of tongue tie and frenulotomy has attracted considerable attention recently. The hypothesis is that a tight or short frenulum prevents the infant latching on to the breast effectively, thereby making breast feeding painful. There are some strongly held opinions but few hard data and the topic calls for further research. *See* discussion in the *Systematic reviews* (2005) referenced above. See also: Hall D, Renfrew M. Tongue-tie: Commom problem or old wives' tale? *Arch Dis Child*, Dec 2005; **90** 1211–1215

Division of ankyloglossia (tongue tie) for breastfeeding—guidance http://www.nice.org.uk/page.aspx?o=284322

Evidence has been presented (but challenged by other authors) that breast feeding for the early weeks of life may offer some protection against later cardiovascular risk factors including obesity: see Early origins of cardiovascular disease: is there a unifying hypothesis? Singhal A, Lucas A. *Lancet* 2004; **363**: 1642–45.

Vitamin K

Current advice about the use of vitamin K is summarized in the box. Every member of staff involved with maternity and newborn care should adhere to the local protocol, and multiple policies in one district should not be tolerated.

Vitamin K prophylaxis

- Newborn infants have very low levels of vitamin K which is needed for normal clotting. The aim of prophylactic treatment is to avoid vitamin-K-dependent bleeding (VKDB). There is a higher risk of early VKDB in babies who are preterm, are not feeding or absorbing feeds, had an instrumental delivery, are ill, or whose mothers were on medication (e.g. anticonvulsants that may increase the risk of bleeding in the newborn). Late VKDB is more likely in babies with liver disease or with other bleeding disorders.

- Deficiency of vitamin K can lead to haemorrhage at a variety of sites. Bleeding into the brain, though rare, is the most serious. This can occur at any time in the first few months of life. It is important to recognize without delay those babies who are at high risk of bleeding, namely those with signs of liver disease (see p. 196), unexplained bruising, or minor bleeding from skin, nose, or mouth.

- All babies should receive one dose of vitamin K at birth. Babies fed on feeds labelled 'infant formula'* will receive sufficient vitamin K, but babies who are entirely or mainly breastfed should receive effective long-term prophylaxis. Roche Konakion MM is licensed for oral and parenteral use.

- For many years vitamin K was given prophylactically at birth by intramuscular (IM) injection. However, in 1992 a case–control study suggested a link between IM (but not oral) administration of vitamin K at birth and an increased risk of cancer in childhood. The finding has not been confirmed in several other studies in the UK, other European countries, and North America; nevertheless, it was thought prudent to seek alternative means of prophylaxis, pending the results of further research. No one oral regimen has been shown to be ideal, but most involve administration of at least three doses of oral vitamin K. However, many health professionals have been uneasy about taking responsibility for giving oral vitamin K. Various arrangements have been made to overcome this.

- There is a risk that the further doses needed after the baby has left hospital might be forgotten. If serious bleeding were to result, leading to death or permanent disability, the parent might well bring a legal action against the trust concerned unless the importance of this prophylaxis had been stressed to the parents.

- The Department of Health produces a leaflet for parents, setting out recommendations (*Vitamin K—information for parents-to-be*, www.doh.gov.uk/pdfs/vitamink.pdf). Each district or trust must develop its own policy for normal and high-risk babies. *If oral preparations are used, a mechanism MUST be in place to ensure that babies of breastfeeding mothers receive ALL the doses specified in the policy, and there must be a means of monitoring the implementation of this policy.* Staff MUST record the formulation, dose, route, and date of all vitamin K administration.

* A product labelled 'infant formula' must by law contain nutrients sufficient to meet all the nutritional needs of an infant for the first 4 to 6 months of life. Other products not so labelled do not necessarily meet these standards.

Other nutritional supplements

Frank rickets is now uncommon but a significant number of cases still occur. Low 25-hydroxy-vitamin D in Asian toddlers remains a real problem and often coexists with low iron levels. The current recommendations for vitamin supplements are summarized in the box. The question of iron deficiency is considered in Chapter 10.

Children of vegetarian or vegan parents, and those who need unusual diets for medical reasons, may develop nutritional deficiencies and specialized advice may be needed from a State Registered Dietician, who should be familiar with the cultural attitudes of ethnic minority families. Eating disorders, obesity, and 'failure to thrive' are discussed in the section on weight monitoring (Chapter 8).

Dental and oral disease (see HFAC4 website)

The most common oral diseases in young children—dental caries (tooth decay), periodontal (gum) disease, and dental erosion—are largely preventable.

Vitamin supplements

- *All* children over the age of 1 year should take a multivitamin supplement.
- All *breastfed babies* and *babies in high-risk groups* (Asian children and Caribbean children on exclusion diets) should start the supplement before age 6 months.
- *All* pregnant and lactating women should take vitamin D supplements.
- The uptake of supplements is low. Families on low incomes should be aware that they are available free of charge at health centres.

Nutrition   4r

The Government is planning to reform the Welfare Foods scheme and draft regulations are currently out for consultation: *Healthy start – consultation of food regulations*. (2005). See: www.dh.gov.uk/Consultations/ClosedConsultations/ClosedConsultationsArticle/fs/en?CONTENT_ID=4109303&chk=NJPRJI

See HFAC4 website

Dental caries

The main dental disease affecting children, and the one that will probably have the greatest impact on their dental health throughout adult life, remains tooth decay. National and local studies have clearly demonstrated a decline in caries prevalence during the past two to three decades; however, recent surveys reveal a bottoming out of improvements in the oral health of young children, whilst improvements in older children continue. The decline has ceased in 5-years-olds, and since 1989 local surveys in most parts of Britain have reported higher decay levels in this age group. There is much variability between districts (*see* HFAC4 website).

The 1993 national survey of children's dental health revealed the following.

- Five-year-old children have, on average, two teeth affected by dental caries, and almost half (45%) of this age-group has experienced the disease.
- There is much untreated decay; 40 per cent of 5-year-olds nationally were shown to have active tooth decay.
- Young children who attend the dentist 'only when they had trouble with their teeth' had higher numbers of diseased teeth than those who attended for check-ups, whether six-monthly or less frequently.

• Wide geographical, ethnic, and social class variations in disease levels exist and there appears to be greater polarization of dental caries experience in 5-year-olds. A greater proportion of this age group have untreated decay. Asian children have more decayed teeth than white children and fewer are registered with a dentist. Availability of orthodontic treatment is patchy, with long waiting lists in many places.

• Dental registrations in the 3 to 5-year-old age group average only 60 per cent in England, Wales, and Scotland.

The Government objective (as of September 2000) was that by 2003 the average DMF index (total number of decayed, missing, and filled teeth) in 5-year-olds should not exceed 1, and that 70 per cent of 5-year-olds should have no experience of tooth decay. Many locally based projects involving health visitors with additional training, health promotion specialists, members of local ethnic communities, and additional incentives for dentists are being implemented. A distance learning pack is being developed for use among minority ethnic communities. Data from the children's Dental Health Survey 2003 showed that 40% of 5 year old children had evidence of dental decay-no change from 1993- and DMF was 1.5 (www.statistics.gov.uk/children/dentalhealth).

Nutritional advice

Sugars (non-milk extrinsic sugars) are the most important dietary factor in the cause of dental caries. They are most harmful if eaten or drunk frequently. Prolonged breastfeeding or bottle feeding beyond the age of 1 year is thought to increase the risk of tooth decay. Good weaning practices contribute to dental health, and parents should be encouraged to wean their children onto food and drink which are, as far as possible, free from non-milk extrinsic sugars.

Fluoride

Fluoride in water at 1 part per million (ppm) has been shown to be the most effective method of reducing tooth decay. However, only a minority (10–15 per cent of the UK) receive fluoridated water. Where it is not available, alternatives include the use of fluoride drops or tablets. Their use is recommended from the age of 6 months for children at high risk of dental disease. Dentists can identify those individuals who would most benefit from fluoride and offer it on prescription. Health visitors need advice from their local dental services as to the optimum policy for children who are not registered with a dentist. Active campaigning continues to encourage fluoridation of water supplies.

Medicines

Children taking frequent or regular sugar-based medicines are shown to have increased levels of dental decay. Sugar-containing medicines remain those which are prescribed more frequently by doctors, requested over the counter by parents, and recommended by pharmacists. The use of either solid preparations or sugar-free formulations is preferable for good dental health.

Periodontal (gum) disease

Just over a quarter of 5-year-olds have unhealthy gums due to poor cleaning habits. Effective brushing of teeth and gums using a children's (low-dose) fluoride tooth paste should commence once teeth appear. A small pea-sized blob of paste is all that is required for children up to 6 years of age to prevent unnecessary ingestion of fluoride. Children require parental assistance with brushing until at least 6 to 7 years of age.

Tooth erosion

Nationally, over half of 5-year-olds have experienced dental erosion, i.e. the progressive loss of tooth enamel and dentine resulting from chemical action on the teeth, other than that caused by bacteria. This is related to increased consumption of acidic drinks either as pure fruit juices or as carbonated beverages.

Traumatic damage to teeth

Trauma resulting in loss of or damage to teeth is an important dental problem, best addressed by other measures to reduce unintentional injuries in playgrounds etc.

Primary prevention strategies

The advice given in Table 4.4 should be available to all parents and should be reinforced by staff of the primary health care team. Parents should be reminded that dental advice and treatment, available through the NHS, are free for all children.

Secondary and tertiary prevention strategies

A detailed evidence-based review is available in the SIGN guideline (*see* HFAC4 website for links).

Dental

A good example of a region-wide study on dental health, with analysis and recommendations, is available: The Dental Health of Five-Year-Old Children in the Northern & Yorkshire Region 1999/2000. Northern and Yorkshire Public Health Observatory. www.nypho.org.uk

Decline in obvious decay in children's permanent teeth. ONS 2003. http://www.statistics.gov.uk/downloads/theme_health/cdh_preliminary_findings.pdf

Table 4.4 Prevention of dental disease

1 Encourage parents in the following practices.

- Avoid the use of sugared dummies and juices on a dinky feeder or night comforter
- Wean babies onto a diet which is free from non-milk extrinsic sugars as far as possible
- Avoid using sugar or biscuits in bottles of milk
- Discourage the use of a bottle after 12 months
- Discourage mothers from giving a bottle in bed at night
- Advise Moslem mothers about acceptable weaning foods so that they do not resort only to sweet products
- Restrict the intake of any sugary food and drinks to mealtimes
- Read labels carefully and beware of 'hidden sugars' in food and drink, even in commercially prepared baby foods
- Restrict the intake of acidic drinks (carbonated drinks or pure fruit juices) to mealtimes and dilute any fruit juices with water;
- Brush children's teeth, once they appear, using a small toothbrush with a children's fluoride paste (500 ppm fluoride concentration)—no more than a small pea-sized blob of tooth paste is required;
- Commence early, and regular, dental visits. Six months of age is the ideal time to seek advice from a dentist on a child's need for fluoride supplements. *There is a strong social class gradient in the number of 2-year-olds registered with a dentist.*

2 Prescribe and promote the use of sugar-free medicines.When medicines are needed, particularly long-term, sugary formulations should be avoided. Where possible, solid forms or the equivalent sugar-free formulations should be used.

3 Refer children with suspected or overt dental disease to a dentist and encourage mothers also to register with a dentist.

4 Children with congenital heart disease and a 'heart card' should be reviewed by a dentists because of their risk of endocarditis.

See HFAC4 website

Special situations (*see* HFAC4 website)

Some interventions are designed for special groups. Examples include the following.

- CONI (Care of Next Infant)—a programme of support and care for parents who have lost a previous infant through cot death. Though no claims are made that this reduces the risk of the next infant dying, parents value the advice and support they receive.

- Similar support could be offered to parents whose infants has suffered an apparent life-threatening event (previously called near-miss cot death) or to those suffering exceptional anxiety about their infant for other reasons, such as extreme prematurity, oxygen dependency, or tracheostomy.
- Projects to help parents under stress or in need of personal support and development are reviewed in Chapter 3.
- Assistance in terms of support and developmental guidance to parents of very-low-birth-weight infants is reviewed on p. 71.
- Specialized advice and guidance for parents of children with special needs (i.e. disabled, chronically sick) is reviewed in Chapters 13 and 14.

Recommendations

1 Every PCO should appoint an immunization coordinator or otherwise ensure that all the functions associated with this role are fully discharged.

2 Control of tuberculosis and hepatitis B are often neglected and call for special measures as they do not fit easily into the routine programmes of immunization.

3 PCOs should be aware of the guidance on control of communic-able diseases in schools.

4 PCOs should establish a policy to ensure that all parents are informed about reducing the risks of sudden infant death. This should include help with smoking cessation and reducing passive smoking.

5 PCOs should establish a policy in conjunction with the local authority to reduce injuries and accidents, and should consider (and if necessary improve) sources of data available locally.

6 PCOs should have a policy to encourage breastfeeding and should consider the development of Baby Friendly initiatives and voluntary sector support for breastfeeding mothers.

7 PCOs should ensure that it has, and enforces, a policy for vitamin K administration, in collaboration with all adjacent trusts and maternity units.

8 PCOs should ensure that they have in place a policy for reducing dental disease and facilitating early registration with a dentist.

9 Focused initiatives to support parents with particular needs should be encouraged.

Chapter 5

Health promotion and health care for school-age children and young people

This chapter reviews:

- ◆ The changing needs of health care for school-age children
- ◆ A needs-based approach
- ◆ The views of children and young people about their concerns and the service they want
- ◆ Starting school—preparation for school and reception into school
- ◆ Special medical needs of children in school
- ◆ Emotional and behavioural problems
- ◆ Bullying
- ◆ The need for confidential advice and support
- ◆ The National Healthy Schools Standard and other Government initiatives—health promotion in school
- ◆ Profiles
- ◆ Prevention of unwanted pregnancy and support for young mothers

In this chapter we review the health care needs of school-age children and young people. The evidence base for this chapter is more varied than that offered for preschool children in the previous chapters. Much of it is qualitative in nature, but the convergence of the themes that emerge from various studies is reassuring. The HFAC4 website provides a reference list and links to the main sources.

The statutory duties of the NHS with respect to education are described in Chapter 14. In the early years of the school health service, resources were directed mainly towards the identification of defects and disorders by periodic medical examinations. The place of these in current practice is discussed in Chapter 14. We believe that the focus should now be shifted away from sterile debate about screening, or the functions of school nurses and the school health service, towards a radical rethink of what children need and how it can best be provided. Therefore we have approached the issue from the perspective of the consumers—children and young people, parents and teachers. The latter are education professionals but when confronted with definite or possible health problems they are not necessarily more expert than parents and may seek similar advice, support, and reassurance.

From a commissioning point of view, the service should be directed at the needs of school-age children, rather than being seen simply as a 'school health service' (*see* HFAC4 website). Health needs may be met in many other settings than schools—clubs, internet cafes, parents' evening workshop sessions. As in other aspects of child health services, equity of outcome is the aim rather than equity of input (p. 11). Needs differ from place to place and from school to school. Children in the independent education sector should not be forgotten, and we see no justification for excluding them from consideration although their needs may be different or met in different ways. Traditionally, the school health service has often not been funded to have an input to independent schools. This should be reviewed.

Many of the issues that seem important for children and young people are to do with health in the wider sense, calling for public health initiatives or multi-agency interventions. In contrast, others are very private matters and need confidential one-to-one consultations.

Children's views (*see* HFAC4 website)

The UN Convention on the Rights of the Child established the importance of listening to and working with children and young people and calls on health care providers to take note of children's views. There is now substantial information as to what young people think and want with regard to health and health care.

Children in London listed their top five health preoccupations as violence and safe streets, child abuse, drugs, bullying, and racism. A survey by the Home Office found that young people listed the following as their main needs: (a) accessible confidential health services; (b) greater involvement of young people in planning services; (c) health education that reflects their experiences, especially about drugs and alcohol; (d) specialized advice centres for those with drug problems.

Children and young people acquire attitudes to health care and obtain much of their information from their peer group. There is growing evidence that peer-to-peer education programmes are an effective way of promoting the health of young people, and effective schemes increasingly incorporate ways of actively involving them rather than simply providing them with information. Community programmes to address important health issues among young people can be effective but often fail through lack of planning or insufficient resources.

Starting school

Preparation for school

The changing roles and importance of preschool programmes are discussed in Chapters 2 and 3, where we consider a range of activities and issues such as nursery school, Sure Start, pre-literacy schemes, identification of children with problems, and transfer of information about children with health or developmental problems to the education authority where indicated, as part of statutory duties, and to the child's school.

Broadly speaking, the objectives of preschool programmes are to promote the health and development of children with particular reference to development of language and preliteracy skills, emotional literacy, and the ability to concentrate and work with others, and to identify as far as possible those children who are likely to need additional support to cope with mainstream school or who may need placement in a special school, so that appropriate measures can be put in place.

4r Pre-school services

Children's centers

Government policy is to bring together pre-school provision in Children's Centres, applying the lessons learned from Sure Start, and to provide a comprehensive multi-agency service that includes child care, family support, and some aspects of health care. Similarly, there are proposals for Extended Schools that will offer comprehensive services for school age children. The impact of these changes on community child health services and on general practice remains to be determined. Children's Centres: www.standards.dfes.gov.uk/primary/faqs/foundation_stage/1162267/ Extended schools: www.teachernet.gov.uk/wholeschool/extendedschools/

Early education is an important and effective means of improving children's chances when they start school. Research findings stress the importance of a structured approach and high quality professionally trained staff: The Effective

Provision of Pre-School Education [EPPE] Project: A Longitudinal Study funded by the DfES (1997–2003) http://k1.ioe.ac.uk/schools/ecpe/eppe/eppe/eppepdfs/bera1.pdf

A health care programme at school entry

Increasing numbers of children start some form of schooling well before the age of 5 years, but as long as this remains the age for statutory schooling it will offer the best opportunity of ensuring maximum coverage of the child population. Therefore the following discussion refers primarily to children aged around 5 years. There are many models of service provision at the time of school entry (p. 148), but little evidence on which to base any comparative analysis. Evaluation of benefits depends primarily on defining the aims and objectives. These might include the following.

- Public health aims—profiling the health of children in the local population; using these data to contribute to local and national profiles; ensuring that staff are identified to deliver catch-up or new immunization programmes.

- Building a relationship between parents, school, and school health staff so that parents understand how to access help and advice when they need it.

- Providing information for parents who may have a limited knowledge of health issues related to school-age children. They may appreciate information about what local health services can offer and about issues such as nutrition, exercise and activity, dental care, vision and hearing tests, emotional and behavioural worries, age-appropriate sex and relationship education, safety, and infections.

- Delivering health promotion, depending on the needs of the school and the local population. A wide range of topics might be introduced.

- Offering individual health reviews and delivering individual screening programmes. This topic is discussed in more detail in Chapter 6.

It follows that a review of the health and health care of individual children at school entry could:

- ensure that all children entering school have received an appropriate programme of preventive health care (including immunization) and deal with any omissions

- ensure that all children have access to primary health care and dental care

- identify any physical, developmental, or emotional problems that had previously been missed or not treated and initiate relevant intervention

- provide information about specific health issues for children, parents, and school staff.

Health in school

We have approached this topic taking into account what children and young people tell us that they need and want (see Table 5.1). There is explicit Government recognition of the links between health and education and a commitment to improving the health of school-age children, involving for example investment in staff, buildings, and facilities, opportunities for sports and games, healthy eating policies developed with children themselves, and the free fruit scheme (p. 182) (*see* HFAC4 website).

Consent and confidentiality have been reviewed in several reports (*see* HFAC4 website). The school nursing service can play a pivotal role in addressing the health needs of school-age children in ways that respect their privacy.

Special medical needs of school-age children (*see* HFAC4 website)

Advances in neonatal care, cancer treatments, and management of chronic illnesses mean that more children are surviving into adulthood, and some of these have long-term health needs and/or disabilities. The number of children with complex medical and nursing care needs attending main stream schools is increasing as the principles of inclusive education are adopted. In addition, many more children will have short-term or less severe conditions, which may require medication.

The Department for Education and Skills has produced guidance for schools entitled *Supporting pupils with medical needs* to facilitate policy development on medication in schools and support for individual children with medical needs (see box).

Supporting pupils with medical needs

The employer, usually the school governing body or the local education authority, is responsible under the Health and Safety at Work Act 1974 for ensuring that the school has a health and safety policy. This should include procedures for supporting pupils with medical needs, including managing medication and the action to be taken in a medical emergency. The head is responsible for developing detailed procedures and ensuring that individual teachers receive proper training and support where necessary. The school health personnel and community paediatric nurses can provide expertise and should be involved in drawing up the procedures. While it is acknowledged that parents or guardians have prime responsibility for their child's health, the school health service and community paediatric nurses can provide expert support and advice to pupils, parents and school staff. They are also able to liase with primary, community, secondary, and tertiary health services where necessary.

Table 5.1

Safeguarding the health and welfare of children

♦ Children with health problems may need support in school, including both those with relatively minor disorders such as mild asthma or more serious disorders such as attention-deficit hyperactivity disorder and those with Special Needs or Statements.

♦ Special educational needs coordinators (SENCOs) and teachers need to be fully informed about these children's problems.

♦ All children want to be able to participate as fully as possible in school activities, including outings and journeys.

♦ Children need to be identified when there are emerging emotional and behavioural disorders and problems, learning disabilities, and possible physical illness.

♦ Children want to be protected from bullying of all kinds, racism, etc.

♦ Infectious diseases—ranging from head lice, warts, verrucas, and fungal infections to serious conditions such as shigellosis, hepatitis, tuberculosis, and meningitis—must be prevented and sometimes managed within the school environment. The consultant in communicable disease control is responsible overall for these matters but may need the support of locally based health professionals.

A confidante for children and young people

♦ Children experiencing stress, anxiety, depression, bereavement, abuse, violence in the home, etc. want confidential support, advice, and intervention.

♦ Young people want a health service that offers them private and personal advice on issues such as eating disorders, obesity, menstrual problems, sexual health, skin problems like acne, migraine, alcohol and drug problems, etc.

Health promotion

♦ Children and young people are generally well informed about healthy lifestyles but want an environment that facilitates the positive promotion of health—for example, Healthy Schools programmes incorporating measures to support mental health ('emotional literacy'), good nutrition, exercise and physical activity, avoidance of harmful behaviours, sleep.

♦ Preparation and support for transitions—from primary to secondary school and leaving school.

Extended child and family support

♦ Early intervention for conflicts between parents, child, and school, and for pupils at risk of dropping out of school.

♦ Special additional support for children known to be at very high risk—looked after children, homeless children, excluded pupils, pregnant schoolgirls, etc.

This table is based on the work of Lightfoot and Bines who classified the tasks of school nursing in this way.

Managing absence

School health staff and community paediatric nurses should be involved in the development of school absence policies, and can be a valuable source of support and expertise in individual cases. School absence may be due to acute or chronic illness, or to hospital attendance for treatment or investigation, or it may be a 'non-treatment absence' related to parental anxiety. Managing absence may involve:

- liaison with hospital paediatric departments and hospital schools
- communication between health and education services
- home visiting
- liaison with home tuition service
- determination of fitness to attend school.

Losing the thread, published by Present (previously the National Association for the Education of Sick Children), describes very well the educational experiences and needs ('keeping up not catching up') of children who have health-related absences from school, the need to maintain contact with school and peers ('out of sight, out of mind'), and the difficulties experienced on return to school after a prolonged absence (*see* HFAC4 website).

Every effort should be made to maintain and support individual children in school. This may require the facility to fast track decisions on allocation of responsibility for equipment or services between the health authority, trusts, and the local education authority. Advance planning is needed where building modifications (e.g. wheelchair access or special toilets) may be required. Simple measures such as timetabling classes to ground-floor rooms can greatly increase access to lessons.

Targets

The targets for a well-organized school service for pupils with medical needs are summarized in the box.

Medication

With the exception of asthma, few children really need to take regular medication in school. Many drug regimens can be adapted so that it is not necessary to take a dose while at school. Children who require medication during the school day may include those who are receiving long-term medicine for a chronic condition and those who are well but need to complete a course of medicine for an acute condition. They should be encouraged to take responsibility for its administration. Discussion between pupil, parents, and teaching

Health and safety policy

◆ Each school should have a health and safety policy which includes procedures for dealing with medication for pupils.

◆ Each provider of school nursing services should have a senior nurse able to assess the level of nursing support and equipment needed to support children with complex health needs in school.

Health care plans

◆ Each child and young person with a significant and chronic condition should have a health care plan drawn up in cooperation with the pupil, his/her parents, and relevant clinical staff. The plan should include details of the pupil's condition, any special requirements re diet or activity, medication and any side effects, emergency contact numbers, and the role the school health service and community nursing team should play. The plan should be reviewed and updated at least once a term. The same principles of health improvement should apply to this group of children as apply to others.

◆ Each child who has complex nursing or medical needs should have details of any necessary equipment and instructions for his/her use set out in the care plan.

◆ Those people working with such children should be able to demonstrate their competence in using the equipment.

◆ Health care plans should be confidential and shared only on a need to know basis.

staff should facilitate this. The school nurse and the community nursing team can be a source of support, advice and, where necessary, training to teaching staff. Teachers need reassurance on the safety and effectiveness of the prescribed medication. They administer medication on a voluntary basis and cannot be compelled to do so. Most teachers will agree to do so through goodwill, and it is then the responsibility of the health services to ensure that they receive appropriate advice and instruction, including correct storage with refrigeration if necessary, and easy access to the medication when required.

Some children are prescribed emergency anticonvulsants for administration via the rectum. This raises issues such as privacy for the individual child and teachers' concerns about possible allegations of abuse. Buccal or intranasal midazolam is an excellent alternative for many children.

Many children will need medication, usually via an inhaler, for control of the symptoms of asthma. It is important that teaching and welfare staff are familiar with the use of inhalers, which can vary for each pupil. The timing of such medication should be clearly detailed in the care plan; for example, some may need it before undertaking physical activity. Each child must have easy access to his/her own inhaler.

Responsibility for non-prescription drugs lies with the parents, who may negotiate their use at school with the school staff. An example would be paracetamol for period pain or headaches, including migraine.

Anaphylactic shock and cardiovascular collapse

A very few children, known to be at risk of anaphylactic reaction to certain substances, are prescribed medication to be delivered by injection or inhaler in the rare event of a severe reaction.

Anaphylaxis is a life-threatening condition and it is important that prescribed medication is given and expert help summoned as soon as collapse occurs. With modern delivery systems administration of the drug is not difficult. School staff need to feel confident with the procedure involved, and school health service staff have a duty to educate and train them. Any child needing such intervention should have this condition clearly documented in his/her care plan, including symptoms and signs of anaphylaxis, method of administration, and how to ensure that medication for treatment is accessible and in date. However, there is a growing consensus that the diagnosis of life-threatening allergy, particularly to peanuts, is being made far too readily. It is advisable to review children's histories carefully in such cases to avoid unnecessary anxiety and restrictions (*see* HFAC4 website).

4r   Recently an important and authorative review, *Managing Medicines in Schools and Early Years Settings*, was published by the DfES (2005). *See* www.surestart.gov.uk/–doc/P0001793.pdf

---

Good practice

In Birmingham a school nurse leads the 'Administration of Medicines in Schools Project'. In developing care plans for individual pupils, the ambulance service has been included. Using computer technology, the ambulance service holds records of individual children's needs in the event of an emergency. This ensures that the child's name and school are matched, and if ambulance crews are called, they can respond already briefed and equipped to deal with the specific needs of the child.

Very rarely a child may collapse due to respiratory or cardiac pathology. The school's health and safety policies should cover action required in such an eventuality. The school health service can provide training in basic life support skills to school staff.

Emotional health and well being

Up to 20 per cent of children are said to experience psychological problems at any one time, and so promotion of mental health is an important area. Young people, parents, and teachers need to know what services are available locally to support children with emotional and behavioural difficulties and their families. The provision of child and adolescent mental health services is discussed further in Chapter 13.

Bullying and racism

Bullying and racism are major concerns for many children and young people. There is ample evidence that anti-bullying policies implemented with enthusiasm and sustained over time can substantially reduce this problem (Fig. 5.1). Schools must take the lead on this, but health services can play a supporting role. In addition health professionals need to appreciate how often bullying underlies poor school attendance, physical symptoms, depression, and even suicide attempts.

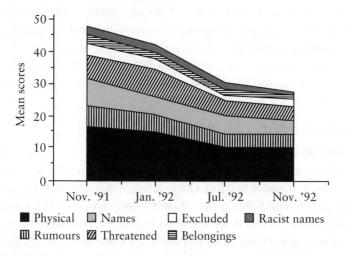

Fig. 5.1 Bullying—an active anti-bullying policy in school resulted in a fall in the various forms of bullying over a 12-month period. (Reproduced from P.K. Smith and S. Sharp (1994), *School bullying*, Routledge, London.)

Confidential advice and support

Teachers may not be in a position to keep confidential information to themselves, nor do they feel equipped and able to give advice on delicate matters, particularly where sexual health is concerned. Children and young people may prefer to talk to health professionals and they need to know that they can rely on their confidentiality being protected (*see* HFAC4 website).

The school nurse is well placed to offer advice and support. For younger children this service would have to be provided within the school setting. However, older children may be reluctant to visit the 'medical room' in school because even being observed entering or leaving may result in loss of privacy. For this reason, various forms of drop-in clinic away from the school are becoming popular in densely populated urban areas, though they are more difficult to provide in rural areas (see box). There is good evidence of their popularity, though of course extensive use does not necessarily guarantee improved health outcomes (*see* HFAC4 website). Services of this kind have the disadvantage that the full personal and family history will not necessarily be available to the 'drop-in' clinic as it would be to the primary health care team. There is concern that errors might be made if the individual's background and their medication history are not known, though this risk may be more theoretical than real.

Good practice

A primary care service is offered in accomodation within the school grounds in a practice in Cornwall, overcoming many of the difficulties about access to records.

See HFAC4 website.

Health promotion in schools

Some health promotion programmes focus on single issues such as drugs, alcohol, diet, exercise, smoking, or sexual behaviour, while others aim to create a climate in which healthy living in a more holistic sense is facilitated. The evidence suggests that most young people are increasingly well informed about health-related topics, but that it is much easier to increase knowledge than to change attitudes and behaviour. A more holistic approach may enable children and young people to feel secure and valued, experience increased self-esteem, interact positively with their peers, respond more effectively to pressures over risky behaviours, and make healthy choices.

The National Healthy School Programme (see box) aims to put these concepts into action. Programmes vary in effectiveness. The commitment of staff and the head teacher is crucial. Many issues that arise in sessions devoted to personal, social, and health education and to citizenship call for some knowledge of medical subjects and some, like sexuality, are very personal and not easy for teachers to handle. School nurses and other health professionals have an important role, but the extent of their involvement depends very much on the resources and time available. They may be invited to lead the programme and to help to construct the education plan. Guidance can be offered on such areas as diet and school food, exercise, drinking water, and safety. Teachers may value help in responding to group and individual questions after classroom sessions and guiding young people to appropriate sources of further information and advice. If drop-in clinics are provided as part of the same programme, young people have the added benefit of knowing the professionals that they are likely to meet in the clinic.

Nutritional issues are often raised. The National Fruit Scheme, breakfast clubs, and school meals are important in the context of obesity prevention (see Chapter 8). Inadequate drinking-water supplies are a surprisingly common concern; children should have access to drinking water rather than being encouraged to buy fizzy or sweet drinks. Breakfast clubs not only provide nutritional benefits but promote punctual arrival at the start of the day and provide new experiences for parents (*see* HFAC4 website).

The National Healthy School Standard (formerly known as the National Healthy Schools Scheme) is part of the National Healthy School Programme. It was proposed in the Green Paper *Our healthier nation* in 1998. In this paper, the Government identified the school as a setting to improve the health of children. A healthy school is in a key position to improve children's health and educational achievement, with the support of other agencies. The Standard provides a framework on which to develop a whole school and community approach to health-related issues that impact on learning and educational attainment. Health professionals play a part by highlighting health needs and contributing to programme development and delivery.

See Appendix (page 375) and HFAC4 website

An Australian study showed the benefits of changing the ethos of the whole 4r
school: Bond L, Patton G, Glover S, *et al*. The Gatehouse Project: can a

multilevel school intervention affect emotional wellbeing and health risk behaviours? *Journal of Epidemiology Community Health* 2004; **58**:997–1003. Available at www.blackwell-synergy.com

Promoting emotional health and wellbeing through the National Healthy School Standard (2004). www.wiredforhealth.gov.uk

Findings from the National School Readiness Indicators Initiative: A 17 State Partnership (2005). http://www.gettingready.org/matriarch/

For useful papers and links on early literacy *see* www.literacytrust.org.uk

Public health focus

School nurses are called upon to strengthen the public health aspects of their role in order to improve health outcomes and address health inequalities.

Key elements of public health for school nurses

- Assessing the health needs of a population (e.g. school health profiling, audit, activity data)
- Planning and implementing programmes that promote and protect health (e.g. immunization, screening, health promotion campaigns)
- Working with other sectors to address the wider threats to health such as housing, transport, crime reduction, and social exclusion
- Identifying health inequalities and taking action to address these (e.g. inclusion projects, targeting services, for example for vulnerable children and young people)
- Working with children and families to identify needs and using a community development approach to deliver health improvement (e.g. Healthy Schools, peer-led projects, school nutrition action groups)

Health profiles

In some districts detailed data are gathered on a range of health measures to construct a profile for the district (see box and HFAC4 website). This is a valuable exercise if there is a commitment to act on the results, but in the absence of this it may be perceived as a demoralizing waste of professional time.

Vulnerable children and young people

A number of initiatives have been developed to reduce the disadvantages of children and young people deemed to be vulnerable.

Good practice

The health profile brings together a range of data from the majority of services working with school age children in the Huddersfield area to identify local need and provide evidence for areas of concern. This is then used by school nurses to negotiate for appropriate services to be made available. These services are delivered in partnership between agencies working from an evidence-based public health programme. The profiles highlight not only general areas of need, but also pockets of deprivation within areas of affluence, and also identify specific health needs such as teenage pregnancy hot spots or areas with a high level of substance misuse. The material produced also contributes to the Health Improvement Plan process and to the Healthy School Standard. This multi-agency project has been running for 3 years and the number of users of the information it collates is steadily increasing.

In Wandsworth a multi-agency school health profile is being developed through the Healthy Schools programme. The profiling tool to date is structured around the key themes of the National Healthy School Standard. Profile findings will inform local health plans and service delivery and have the additional aim of supporting schools in achieving and maintaining Healthy School status. They also facilitate an assessment of school facilities (e.g. drinking water and social and sporting activities).

Conflicts between families and schools are common and it is important to resolve these amicably wherever possible. School based health professionals, who are perceived as neutral, can often be helpful in this regard. There is at least one example of a school nurse employed jointly by a local authority and local health service to deal with children out of school for various reasons (box). Ensuring that young people at high risk are not lost from the educational system is an important task in which health professionals may sometimes play a vital role.

The Government's Quality Protects programme, launched in April 1999 and extended to March 2004, targets vulnerable children of all ages. It aims to ensure that children looked after gain maximum life-chance benefits from educational opportunities, health care, and social care. Many areas have appointed a nurse, employed either by a health trust or social services, to lead the health component of the work. The outcomes of Quality Protects rely strongly on multi-agency communication and cooperation. A designated doctor, usually a community paediatrician, may also be appointed to focus on this group of children.

Every year a number of children and young people, some of them unaccompanied, come to the UK as refugees or asylum seekers. They may have experienced severe trauma and come to the UK leaving a great deal behind. Language and culture are both barriers, and health services should endeavour to meet the health needs of these children. Health workers have been appointed in some areas to focus on the needs of the homeless and/or asylum seekers and refugees. Health professionals should endeavour to use this specialized resource effectively. Interpreting services should be utilized whenever possible and primary health care needs should be addressed. This is not always easy because of lack of historical information regarding interventions such as immunization.

Good practice

Social inclusion initiatives from the Department for Education and Skills have highlighted the increasing numbers of excluded pupils. In Devon a project aims to help pupils aged 5 to 11 with challenging behaviour who may be, or have been, excluded from school. In Devon 480 children were excluded from school because of behavioural problems, and this project provided an innovative opportunity for two school nurses to act as a link coordinator for them and their families. Both practitioners work with named schools which were identified by the steering group. Initial work involved identifying personal training needs, which are ongoing, a process for assessment and intervention, and developing evaluation tools. By working with school staff nurses identify individual children with challenging behaviour and whole-school issues which affect that behaviour, and vice versa, liase with other agencies and health colleagues to also identify such children, and assess and plan appropriate interventions.

See HFAC4 website

Young mothers and teenage pregnancy

Teenage pregnancy is often both a cause and a consequence of social exclusion. Since the publication in 1999 of *Teenage pregnancy—a report by the Social Exclusion Unit*, a body of evidence of practice has been developing in this area.

The UK has the highest rate of teenage births in Western Europe, six times the Dutch rate. Rates within the UK vary between the different countries.

Scale and trends of teenage pregnancy

4r

In 2003 in England:

- Almost 98 600 teenagers (under 20 years) became pregnant.
- 58 900 went on to give birth
- 7300 conceptions were to under-16s resulting in 3700 births
- Around 58 per cent of conceptions to under 16s ended in abortion
- An additional cause for concern is the rising incidence of sexually transmitted infections

---

Northern Ireland and England have teenage birth rates of around 30 per 1000 women; Wales has a higher rate of 37.7 per 1000. Over a third of all births are now outside marriage, but for teenagers the proportion is nearly 90 per cent. A significant number of young women conceive more than once in their teens. Around 87 000 children in England today have a teenage mother.

Social exclusion

The risk of teenage parenthood is greatest for young people who have grown up in poverty and disadvantage or those with poor educational standards. The Sure Start programme coordinates help for those families most in need to ensure that their children have the best possible start in life. It has recently been extended to cover 500 projects by 2003. In addition, Sure Start Plus programmes are being set up in 20 areas with a high incidence of teenage pregnancies. Through Sure Start and other targeted health promotion programmes, improved outcomes for teenage mothers, fathers and their children are anticipated.

The health consequences

Some obstetric risks, such as anaemia, toxaemia, eclampsia, hypertension, and difficult labour, are greater for young pregnant women. Biologically there is no reason why a teenage pregnancy should not have a good outcome. However, because of their circumstances, teenage mothers tend not to have well-managed pregnancies.

- Babies of teenage mothers are 25 per cent more likely to weigh less than 2500 g.

- The infant mortality rate for babies of teenage mothers is 60 per cent higher than for babies of older mothers.
- Mortality rates for both infants and children in the 1- to 3-year age group are highest for mothers under 20.
- Post-natal depression is three times as common amongst teenage parents, with four out of ten mothers affected.
- Teenage mothers are half as likely as older mothers to breastfeed.
- Children of teenage mothers are more likely to suffer accidents, and twice as likely to be admitted to hospital as a result of an accident or gastroenteritis.

Service considerations for prevention and management of unwanted teenage pregnancy

1 The law on under-age contraception is clear. Under 16-year olds:

- have a right to confidentiality for their discussions with medical practitioners (child protection procedures cover issues of possible abuse)
- should not fear being reported to their parents just for consulting a doctor or nurse
- can obtain contraceptive treatment without parental consent if certain conditions are met (*see* HFAC website).

2 Each child and young person has a right to receive appropriate education on personal, health, and social education as part of the normal school curriculum. While adult-run programmes may increase knowledge, peer education can be more effective in changing behaviour.

3 The young mother and father, if he is still involved, should have speedy access to counselling to enable them to make decisions on the future of the pregnancy. This should be through the primary care or family planning services.

4 A teenage mother needs easy access to antenatal services which have been tailored to meet her particular circumstances. Teenagers can have somewhat chaotic lifestyles and this needs to be taken into account. She should have a named midwife to whom she can refer and who will support her in drawing up her birth plan.

5 She should be in control of issues of confidentiality relating to her pregnancy.

6 Consideration needs to be given to the possibility of sexual abuse, and local procedures on referral to social services should be considered. There may also be conflict with parents which could lead to homelessness, and this may also require social work support.

7 Parentcraft education needs to be tailored to the reality of a young person's life, should include the father where possible, and should be delivered by specially trained midwives and health visitors. Some pregnant teenagers may need specialist advice on their lifestyle, including nutrition, smoking, and drug taking.

8 The young woman should be encouraged to continue with her education. Pregnancy is not an illness, and there is no reason why a young woman should not attend school or college with time off for attendance at antenatal and parentcraft sessions. The school nurse can be a source of information and support.

9 Teenage mothers have a higher incidence of depression both before and after the birth of their baby and so should be assessed by a relevant professional and treated as appropriate.

10 Each teenage mother will need to be supported through the benefits system to enable her to maximize her income.

11 Teenage mothers, in or about to leave care, face the additional problem of lack of consistent adult support. Increasingly, these very young mothers are being offered foster care or other suitable supported accommodation as an alternative to living alone in their own flat. Once the baby is born, care must be taken to continue to meet the individual health and social care needs of both mother and baby.

12 Following the birth of the baby some teenage mothers, depending on their circumstances, will require extra support for both themselves and their baby. This will normally be offered within primary care. The health visitor should identify the health needs of mother, father, and baby through the health care plan and offer services as required.

Service objectives

1 Each school should have a personal, social, health, and citizenship education (PSHCE) programme and every pupil should have access to it. School nurses should be involved in the development and delivery of these programmes.

2 Each primary care organization should have a local strategy group for teenage pregnancy, which must include midwifery services and child protection advisors. Antenatal services for this age group should be tailored to meet their special needs.

3 Health visitors and midwives who have received specialist training should develop parenting and antenatal education for teenage mothers which, where feasible, is delivered separately from that for more mature parents.

4 Each teenage mother should have an allocated key worker within 2 weeks of confirmation of the pregnancy. The professional background of this person will be dependent on the particular needs of the client and local resources.

5 Looked-after young people who become pregnant must have the full support of their named social worker throughout their pregn-ancy. Once the baby is born it should have access to its own social worker.

6 Each pregnant woman and postnatal mother should be assessed for depression, and offered support and treatment as required.

7 Every teenager should have easy access to appropriate sexual health services, where their views are sought in developing the service.

Management at the strategic level

Each local authority is required to nominate a coordinator with the task of both preventing teenage pregnancy and supporting pregnant teenagers. The coordinator works with the local education authority, social services, and local voluntary organisations. Tasks include:

+ geographical profiling of teenage pregnancy
+ audit of services (e.g. health promotion, contraception)
+ links to other local plans (e.g. Quality Protects, Health and Education Action Zones, Early Years Development and Childcare Plans, SureStart, Excellence in Cities)
+ identifying opportunities for teenagers to improve self-esteem and confidence.

Targets

The Government has launched a national campaign with the aim of halving the rate of conception among under-18-year-olds by 2010 (*see* HFAC4 website). A cross-departmental ministerial task force, chaired by the Minister for Public Health, has been set up, with a Department of Health unit overseeing implementation. Local implementation will be through performance management of Health Improvement Programmes.

Good practice

Teenage Pregnancy Support Group, St George's Hospital
(started 1989)
Clients are cared for by one consultant and the same midwife throughout their pregnancy. Parenthood education helps the teenage mothers, and

fathers if possible, to make informed decisions about the future and to maintain a positive approach towards their pregnancy.

Newpin Teenage Mums' Project, Peckham (started 1996)
This project works with young mothers and their children to change the effects of adverse family circumstances, to provide opportunities for positive parenting, to raise levels of self-esteem, and to increase the educational and employment opportunities available to young mothers.

See HFAC4 website

Recommendations

Starting school

Our review of the evidence on health promotion and on screening (Chapter 6) does not offer a complete answer for policy-makers. Practical considerations suggest that the best approach might be as follows.

1 *Detection of physical disorders*   This is the role of pre-school health care. The primary care trust should ensure that all children living within their area of responsibility have access to primary care facilities.

2 *Formal screening*   Measurement of height and weight and screening for visual impairment and hearing loss are recommended (see Chapters 8, 11, and 12).

3 *Reduce duplication by sharing information*   Professionals should (with parents' permission) share relevant information about children's health with the school health service and, when appropriate, with school staff.

4 *Prosperous localities*   Send written information about school health issues and services to parents and invite them to contact the school nurse if necessary. The school nurse should meet the children as a group and introduce herself.

5 *Less prosperous localities and socially excluded groups*   A minimum aim is to identify children not in contact with a primary health care service and ensure that they receive whatever additional health checks and immunizations are needed (see Chapters 4 and 18).

6 *Added value from baseline assessment*   A mechanism should be developed whereby teachers can use a standardized baseline assessment method to identify children who need more detailed assessment (see also Chapter 7).

Children and young people in school

1 Health care and health promotion in schools and for school age children have many facets. No single discipline or model of care can cater for all issues. A team approach to school health that includes school nurses, other specialized nurses, dieticians, therapists, doctors, and mental health professionals is needed.

2 There are important counselling and support functions to be fulfilled and, because many concerns of young people incorporate complex health issues, a health professional is often needed for this role.

3 Education services need to lead and support work on the National Healthy Schools Standard and Health Promotion but there is an important contribution to be made by health professionals.

4 The drop-in clinic concept and related opportunities to promote health have demonstrated their worth, and the service should be extended in collaboration with general practice, reproductive medicine, relevant specialist departments, and health promotion teams.

5 A senior nurse, in each area, should be identified to take responsibility for ensuring that adequate levels of suitably qualified staff, necessary equipment, and provision are available to allow children with complex health care needs to take full advantage of their education. The school health service should include staff able to care for children with special needs.

6 There should be a named school nurse and doctor for each school and each school nurse should have access to a wider team of health support such as community children's nurses, paediatricians, and therapists.

7 It should be the duty of the school health service and/or the community nursing service to provide the necessary instruction and training to support school staff.

8 School nursing services should continue to develop their public health focus, building on partnerships with other non-health agencies such as education, social services, youth offending teams, and Connexions.

9 Service reviews and planning should involve users—children, young people, parents, and education services.

10 The health needs of independent school populations and provision to address these should be reviewed.

Chapter 6

Secondary prevention: early detection and the role of screening

This chapter:

- ◆ Asks whether early detection matters
- ◆ Suggests how early detection can be achieved
- ◆ Considers the role of professional help in the early detection of problems
- ◆ Introduces the topic of screening
- ◆ Comments on the need for professional sensitivity
- ◆ Defines screening
- ◆ Sets out the criteria for screening programmes and screening tests
- ◆ Describes and explains recent changes in attitudes to screening
- ◆ Explains how existing potential screening programmes have been evaluated

Even though there has been a continuing change in emphasis from defect detection to prevention, inevitably much of this report will focus on the former. Nevertheless, we wish to emphasize again that the detection of defects is only one of the aims of a child health promotion programme and is by no means the most important. Screening programmes have often been set up in the past without a proper evaluation of the benefits and harms. This is changing, as will be described.

Does early detection matter?

It is not possible to give a precise definition of 'early' but the word implies that defects are found at the earliest stage of the disease or disability that is reasonably possible, rather than waiting until they are inescapably obvious. We believe that early detection is desirable on a number of grounds.

Parents value early diagnosis

The most compelling reason for early diagnosis is that parents want it. There is both research evidence and a weight of clinical opinion in favour of this view. Parents feel that they have a right to know of any concerns about a child's development at the earliest possible stage. Early diagnosis, if accompanied by adequate counselling, facilitates adaptation and adjustment to the problems created by disability, even when the underlying disorder is not amenable to specific treatment.

It is interesting to consider why parents should value early detection so highly, even when it does not result in any effective treatment or in relevant genetic counselling. The reason is probably to do with the 'loss of the perfect child' which is distressing when a serious defect is discovered at birth, but is even more so as the child grows older; the longer the parents believe him/her to be normal, the more devastating the discovery that s/he is not.

For some conditions, parents may have taken their children repeatedly to health professionals before a definitive diagnosis is made. This causes distress to the parents and may jeopardize the relationship between the parents and health professionals. Early detection would reduce this problem.

Improved outcome

In a few disorders, there is no doubt that detection and treatment at the pre-symptomatic stage improve outcome. Examples include phenylketonuria and hypothyroidism. There are also disorders where it is theoretically possible that early detection and treatment improve outcome, but the evidence is equivocal. A good example is cystic fibrosis. Sometimes early diagnosis has no direct effect on the child but permits genetic counselling which may prevent the birth of another child with the same disorder. An example is Duchenne muscular dystrophy.

Improved quality of life for child and family

There are many disorders in which early diagnosis does not improve outcome in the sense of significantly altering the severity of the disability. Nevertheless, appropriate intervention enables the child and family to cope with disability more effectively by reducing parental frustration and isolation, providing services, and helping the child to make the most effective use of any functions and abilities that are preserved. For example, in the case of cerebral palsy, early physiotherapy can prevent or delay the progression of postural deformities and contractures.

Access to educational and social services

Education authorities need to know about children with special needs in order to offer pre-school teaching and to enable them to fulfil their responsibilities under the Education Acts of 1981, 1993 and 1996. Similarly, Social Services have certain obligations under the 1989 Children Act. Furthermore, parents may be entitled to financial bene-fits in some situations.

No legal duty has been imposed on the NHS to *detect* children with special needs. However, there is a legal requirement to inform the local education authority about children with special educational needs (see Chapter 14 for more details).

How early detection is achieved

A large proportion of serious problems are found in one of five ways:

- at the neonatal and 6–8-week examinations
- follow-up of infants and children who have suffered various forms of trauma or illness affecting the nervous system
- close observation of children with a strong family history of a particular disorder
- detection by parents and relatives
- detection by midwives, playgroup leaders, nursery nurses and teachers, health visitors, and GPs in the course of their regular work
- opportunistic detection.

Neonatal and 6–8 examinations

The neonatal examination and the examination performed at 6–8 weeks of age reveal a significant number of abnormalities, for example dysmorphic conditions such as Down's syndrome, congenital heart disease, instability of the hips, and anomalies of the eye.

Neurological illnesses

Infants who have suffered illnesses or insults with the potential to cause neuro-logical damage are normally seen regularly in a specialist clinic. A significant proportion of the severely disabled children known to any child development team are identified by a paediatrician as being actually or potentially disabled as soon as the neurological insult occurs. Examples include premature infants whose imaging studies show persisting brain abnormalities, full-term babies who have suffered hypoxic–ischaemic encephalopathy, neonatal meningitis, or severe hypoglycemia, and infants and children who have had meningitis, encephalitis, head injury, or encephalopathy. Thus many of the disabled infants in any district can be identified and offered early intervention if a well-organized follow-up clinic is available.

We are not advocating a return to the concept of an 'at-risk' register by which risk factors are recorded with a view to alerting community staff to the possibility of developmental problems. This approach to detection of defects was introduced at a time when (i) resources were very limited and (ii) undue emphasis was placed on perinatal factors in the aetiology of developmental disorders and defects. It fell into disrepute for two reasons: firstly, it was imposs-ible to obtain consistent reporting and recording of the relevant risk factors; secondly many children found to have serious handicapping conditions had no antecedent risk factors.

Close observation of children with a family history of a disorder

Some conditions have a genetic component. Thus when there is a close relation with such a disorder, a child may be specifically monitored for the problem. Examples include instability of the hip and disorders of vision and hearing.

The role of parents and relatives

Parents, sometimes with the aid of relatives and friends, are often the first to suspect that their child has a disability. They use their own knowledge, based on experience, the media, or books and magazines, and make comparisons with the babies of their friends and relatives before deciding that their child may not be developing normally. When they report these suspicions to a health professional they must be taken seriously and often prove to be correct.

The parents are often the first to detect visual impairment, cerebral palsy, muscular dystrophy, severe mental handicap, sensorineural deafness, and autism. They may not understand the significance of their observations but they are very efficient at detecting that something is amiss. When they seek help, anxious parents must receive a sympathetic hearing. It is vital that all staff respect and respond to parental worries and do not give out inappropriate reassurance.

Playgroup leaders and nursery nurses

These play an increasingly important role in child care, particularly with the introduction of schemes such as Sure Start in deprived areas and the move to earlier attendance of children at school or some form of child care. They become expert at identifying the child whose health or development requires further evaluation. The value of their contribution should be acknowledged and their skills enhanced by further training and feedback.

Opportunistic detection

Some defects and conditions are first suspected in the course of a consultation or contact arranged for some other reason. This might be described as 'opportunistic detection'. All contacts can also be used as an opportunity to provide health promotion.

All parents need help sometimes—the role of professional advice

Parents have a key role in the detection of defects, but they seldom decide instantaneously that their child might have some abnormality of health or development. The conclusion is reached gradually after discussion and observation. Nor do they always know how to make the best use of health, educational, or social services.

Formation of a constructive relationship between professional and family has several benefits. Firstly, it facilitates primary prevention by providing guidance on health and development. Secondly, such a relationship makes it easier for the parents to seek advice when they have anxieties about their child. Contact with a professional who has a knowledge of child development enables them to clarify and crystallize their worries and decide whether and when they wish to obtain more expert advice. Such decisions are not taken lightly. Although most parents are grateful for assessment and support, they are also very anxious about what the outcome will be.

Therefore a routine review of the child's progress can be valuable in some circumstances, even if the parents have not sought advice or expressed concerns. It also helps them to observe their child's progress more objectively and to identify possible problems themselves. Professionals should develop the skill of holding 'structured conversations' about health, development, and behaviour (see box on p. 258). Sometimes, for a variety of reasons, parents may fail to recognize or understand the significance of symptoms of illness or developmental abnormalities, which might seem obvious to other people. The reasons for their lack of awareness are often complex and are not related solely to social background or education. Parents may seek to rationalize their observations of problems such as slow language development on many grounds, for example normal variation, unusual family history, or adverse life experiences. The opportunity to review these problems without having to request a formal appointment may be much appreciated. On the other hand, parents value the reassurance given when a health professional pronounces that all is well with their child.

The role of formal screening programmes

Some defects are unlikely to be recognized even by the most astute parent and can only be detected by health professionals if a specific search is made. Examples include dislocation of the hip before the child starts to walk, high-frequency hearing loss prior to the age when speech normally begins, some congenital heart defects, and congenital cataracts. The detection of such defects might be achieved by the use of specific screening tests. This is discussed below.

The need for professional sensitivity

When a problem has been overlooked by parents, its identification by professionals in the course of screening or routine reviews is often welcomed. There may also be less positive responses, though these may be concealed. Parents may have been actively denying the possibility of there being anything wrong with the child to protect themselves or their partners against a distressing experience; this may happen particularly at times when they are having to deal with several other sources of stress and anxiety. Alternatively, parents may feel guilt that they had failed to identify the problem or act upon it until it was pointed out to them. As some disorders have a genetic component, this can add to feelings of guilt.

These phenomena are not a reason for withholding information or failing to be honest about one's suspicions, but they do highlight the need for professional skill, sensitivity, and follow-up support and guidance when seeing children.

Screening

Definition

Screening was defined by the American Commission on Chronic Illness in 1957 as 'the presumptive identification of unrecognized disease or defect by the application of tests, examinations and other procedures, which can be applied rapidly. Screening tests sort out apparently well persons who may have a disease from those who probably do not. A screening test is not intended to be diagnostic'.

In essence a screening procedure (which may be a test or questionnaire) is applied to a population who have no manifestations of a disorder to separate out those at higher risk from those at lower risk. The former then proceed to have a definitive diagnostic test. No screening test is 100 per cent perfect in that 'cases' are missed ('false negative'), people without the disorder are falsely labelled as having it ('false positive'), and some may be harmed by the procedure.

Criteria for screening programmes and tests

The concept of screening is attractive. It makes good sense to identify disease or disorder at a pre-symptomatic stage in order to correct it before too much damage is done. Recognizing that the number of diseases for which screening might in theory be possible is almost unlimited, Wilson and Yungner devised a set of criteria by which screening programmes could be evaluated (Table 6.1). These have been modified by the UK National Screening Committee (NSC).

Table 6.1 Wilson and Jungner's criteria for screening programmes

1 The condition to be sought should be an important public health problem *as judged by the potential for health achievable by early diagnosis*
2 There should be an accepted treatment *or other beneficial intervention for* patients with recognized *or occult* disease
3 Facilities for diagnosis and treatment should be available *and shown to be working effectively for classic cases of the condition in question*
4 There should be a latent or early symptomatic stage *and the extent to which this can be recognized by parents and professionals should be known*
5 There should be a suitable test or examination: it should be simple, valid for the condition in question, reasonably priced, repeatable in different trials or circumstances, sensitive and specific; the test should be acceptable to *the majority of* the population
6 The natural history of the condition *and of conditions which may mimic it* should be understood
7 There should be an agreed definition of what is meant by a case of the target disorder, and *also an agreement as to (i) which other conditions are likely to be detected by the screening programme and (ii) whether their detection will be an advantage or a disadvantage*
8 Treatment at the early, latent, or presymptomatic phase should favourably influence prognosis, *or improve outcome for the family as a whole*
9 The cost of screening should be economically balanced in relation to expenditure on the care and treatment of persons with the disorder and to medical care as a whole
10 Case finding *may need to be* a continuous process and not a once and for all project, *but there should be explicit justification for repeated screening procedures or stages*

Modifications proposed to increase relevance for paediatric practice are shown in italics.

Cochrane and Holland described the characteristics of the ideal screening test as follows.

1 Simple, quick and easy to interpret; capable of being performed by para-medics or other personnel.

2 Acceptable to the public, since participation in screening programmes is voluntary.

3 Accurate, i.e. gives a true measurement of the attribute under investigation.

4 Repeatable: this involves the components of observer variability (both within and between tests), subject variability, and test variability.

5 Sensitive: this is the ability of a test to give a positive finding when the individual screened has the disease or abnormality under investigation.

6 Specific: this is the ability of the test to give a negative finding when the individual does not have the disease or abnormality under investigation.

Rose added the concept of 'yield' which was defined as the number of *new* previously unsuspected cases detected per 100 individuals screened. Haggard pointed out that the yield of a screening test declines as case-finding by other means becomes increasingly effective (Fig. 6.1) and coined the term 'incremental yield'.

Formal and opportunistic screening

Formal screening programmes aimed at the whole population are one of the means by which early detection is accomplished, but are not the only method nor necessarily the most important. Opportunistic screening is similar to formal screening except that the initial contact is initiated by the parents for some other purpose and the professional uses the contact to carry out one or more screening tests or proced-ures. In contrast with formal screening programmes, opportunistic screening does not incorporate the requirement to seek out all the children in the population so that they can be screened. However, the health professional still has a responsibility to ensure that the procedure satisfies the basic criteria for a screening test.

Recent changes in attitudes to screening

Research on screening programmes has expanded rapidly in the last few years. There are several reasons for this.

Potential harm

It has been recognized that some screening activities are not merely useless but are potentially harmful because of the unnecessary worry, referrals, and

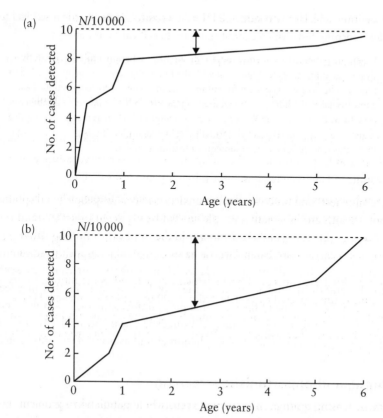

Fig. 6.1 The concept of incremental yield. The diagram refers to detection of hearing loss but could be adapted to any screening programme. It shows the cumulative detection of cases over time. There will usually be a steady trickle of cases detected independent of any screening programme and this is represented by a gradually rising curve during the intervals between screening tests. The incremental yield is the number of new (i.e. previously unrecognized) cases detected *at each successive stage* of the identification programme. In this example, ten cases of congenital hearing loss per 10 000 live births are assumed.

(a) It is assumed that 50 per cent of all cases are found by a neonatal screening test, that 50 per cent of the remainder are found by a screening test at age 7–8 months, and that parents identify a few cases without professional input at random times. The number of cases which remain to be detected after the neonatal screen decreases steadily. The benefits of a screen after 1 year of age (e.g. at 2½) are inevitably small.

(b) It is assumed that there is no neonatal screen and a test at 7–8 months which performs poorly. In this situation, a test at age 2½ has a higher yield. (Redrawn from M. Haggard (1993). *Research in the development of effective services for hearing impaired people*. Nuffield Provincial Hospitals Trust, London, by permission of the author and Nuffield Hospitals Trust.)

procedures which may result (see HFAC4 website). Indeed, it is unethical to offer screening tests which cannot stand up to critical examination:

> When the patient seeks medical advice the doctor's position, ethically, is relatively simple: he undertakes to do his best with the knowledge and resources available to him ... The position is quite different in screening, when a doctor or public health authority takes the initiative in investigating the possibility of illness or disability in persons who have not complained of signs or symptoms. There is then a presumptive undertaking, not merely that abnormality will be identified if it is present, but that those affected will benefit from subsequent treatment or care.

Anxiety

Screening tests and procedures cause anxiety and change people's perceptions about health and normality. People cannot be expected to understand the concept of screening and are seldom told the implications of a positive test before it is carried out. Parents whose babies have had false-positive screening tests show increased anxiety levels which may persist for weeks or even months after the definitive test shows the baby to be normal. Yet they may feel obliged to particip-ate in the screening programme, sometimes against their own better judgement, because of concerns about potential regrets if a problem should be 'missed'. This phenomenon has been called 'anticipated decision regret'.

Litigation

The increasing readiness of patients to resort to litigation when problems are 'missed' by screening highlights the legal hazards of offering screening tests which are not sufficiently robust to perform the tasks expected of them. Although all professionals resist the idea that their activities should be governed by the fear of litigation, this is an issue that can no longer be ignored. There are already a number of cases in which legal proceedings have been brought because a condition was missed at a screening test. Examples include dislocation of the hip, hypothyroidism, spina bifida occulta, and congenital hearing loss. To offer a screening test or procedure which is insufficiently reliable to detect the target disorder is not only unethical (see above) but also hazardous from the legal point of view.

The need for information

More information must be provided about existing screening programmes and any new screening technique must be evaluated not only on the basis of its performance but also from the ethical viewpoint. It should be considered unethical to offer any screening proced-ure whose validity and potential for causing distress have not been assessed. Parents must have full information in a form that is suitable for their cultural, social and educational background. They must be given the opportunity to 'opt out' of tests whose purpose they do not understand or accept. The personal child health record is an ideal vehicle for the transmission of information about screening tests in general, but separate materials are necessary for individual tests.

Genetic implications

Increasing numbers of inherited, or potentially inherited, conditions are being screened for and this raises a number of important questions (see box).

Genetic screening—unanswered questions

- Should children ever be screened for conditions which have no implications for childhood and are untreatable (e.g. Alzheimer's disease)?

- At what stage should a child/young person be informed of a genetic condition which may have implications for his/her reproductive behaviour?

- At what stage should a young person be informed of a genetic condition which will/may impact on his/her adult health, but for which there is no treatment?

- What is the best policy regarding carriers? Some screening tests may not only allow the differentiation of those without a condition from those with it, but may also identify asymptomatic carriers. Even if this has no implications for the health of the individual, it may be relevant when they come to have children.

All these issues must be resolved before embarking on such programmes. It is very important that counselling is in place for parents when the carrier state is identified and also when the children/young people reach an age when they also wish to know and understand what it means to them.

Method of evaluation of screening tests

In 1996, the NSC was set up to look at all existing and potential screening programmes. There was considerable variation around the UK in terms of what screening programmes were in place and how these were conducted, and this was an attempt to introduce order into the situation. In 1998, Child Health and Antenatal Subgroups were set up. In 2005 these groups were combined to form the Fetal, Maternal and Child Health Group (FMCH group). Each existing test has been evaluated and some new ones considered against criteria drawn up by the NSC (box).

4r **NSC criteria for appraising the viability, effectiveness and appropriateness of a screening programme**

Ideally all the following criteria should be met before screening for a condition is initiated:

The condition

1 The condition should be an important health problem.

2 The epidemiology and natural history of the condition, including development from latent to declared disease, should be adequately understood and there should be a detectable risk factor, disease marker, latent period or early symptomatic stage.

3 All the cost-effective primary prevention interventions should have been implemented as far as practicable.

4 If the carriers of a mutation are identified as a result of screening, the natural history of people with this status should be understood, including the psychological implications.

The test

5 There should be a simple, safe, precise, and validated screening test.

6 The distribution of test values in the target population should be known and a suitable cut-off level defined and agreed.

7 The test should be acceptable to the population.

8 There should be an agreed policy on the further diagnostic investigation of individuals with a positive test result, and on the choices available to those individuals.

9 If the test is for mutations, the criteria used to select the subset of mutations to be covered by screening, if all possible mutations are not being tested, should be clearly set out.

The treatment

10 There should be an effective treatment or intervention for patients identified through early detection, with evidence of early treatment leading to better outcomes than late treatment.

11 There should be agreed evidence-based policies covering which individuals should be offered treatment and the appropriate treatment to be offered.

12 Clinical management of the condition and patient outcomes should be optimized in all health care providers prior to participation in a screening.

The screening programme

13 There should be evidence from high quality randomized controlled trials that the screening programme is effective in reducing mortality or morbidity.

   Where screening is aimed solely at providing information to allow the person being screened to make an 'informed choice' (e.g. Down's syndrome, cystic fibrosis carrier screening), there must be evidence from high quality trials that the test accurately measures risk. The information that is provided about the test and its outcome must be of value and readily understood by the individual being screened.

14 There should be evidence that the complete screening programme (test, diagnostic procedures, treatment/intervention) is clinically, socially, and ethically acceptable to health professionals and the public.

15 The benefit from the screening programme should outweigh the physical and psychological harm (caused by the test, diagnostic procedures, and treatment).

16 The opportunity cost of the screening programme (including testing, diagnosis and treatment, administration, training, and quality assurance) should be economically balanced in relation to expenditure on medical care as a whole (i.e. value for money).

17 There should be a plan for managing and monitoring the screening programme, and an agreed set of quality assurance standards.

18 Adequate staffing and facilities for testing, diagnosis, treatment, and programme management should be available prior to the commencement of the screening programme.

19 All other options for managing the condition should have been considered (e.g. improving treatment, providing other services), to ensure that no more cost-effective intervention could be introduced, or current interventions increased within the resource available.

20 Evidence-based information, explaining the consequences of testing, investigation, and treatment, should be made available to potential participants to assist them in making an informed choice.

21 Public pressure for widening the eligibility criteria for reducing the screening interval, and for increasing the sensitivity of the testing process, should be anticipated. Decisions about these parameters should be scientifically justifiable to the public.

22 If screening is for a mutation, the programme should be acceptable to people identified as carriers and to other family members.

In many respects, it is more difficult to assess a test which has been in routine use for a long time, but this is not a reason for omitting the exercise. A particular problem was the well-recognized fact that many of the activities examined do not meet the strict criteria for screening tests, yet cogent arguments are often adduced for their continued usefulness in the evaluation and care of apparently healthy children.

General principles for the management of screening programmes

Planning and purchasing

Early detection programmes cannot work in isolation. The implications for other aspects of the child's care must always be considered. For instance, screening for hearing loss has major implications for the ear, nose, and throat service; growth monitoring generates additional referrals for paediatric endocrine clinics; and reviews of developmental and language abilities result in an increased demand for educational advice and assessment. Unless these services are involved in the planning and monitoring of the early detection programme, the benefits will be limited and the potential to do harm, by increasing anxiety and raising expectations that are not fulfilled, will be increased.

Monitoring and supervision

It is important to ensure that early detection services, and in particular screening programmes, work effectively. Responsibility for child health promotion and for individual screening programmes should be clearly defined (Chapter 19). We suggest the nomination of a local PCO-aligned Child Health Promotion Coordinator. This function may form part of the portfolio of duties of the Director of Public Health but may be delegated to another professional. Aspects which may need to be monitored are summarized in the box.

Features that should be monitored in a screening programme

1 Sensitivity of test—this may not be possible on a local level as most conditions are uncommon. Instead, 'missed' cases should be carefully investigated for any possible lessons to be learnt. National registers will help monitoring

2 Specificity of test

3 Positive predictive value of test

4 Timeliness of test, diagnosis, and treatment—what is the interval between performance of test, provision of result, and, if positive, time to referral for diagnostic test and, where appropriate, initiation of management?

5 Training of staff—not only initial training, but continuing

6 Understanding and satisfaction of consumers with the programme

Referral

We shall also suggest some guidelines regarding referral of children who 'fail' screening tests, although we have not attempted to specify precise referral pathways since the route of referral depends on local resources. It is essential that staff know when, where, and how to refer a child who 'fails' a screening test. If this information is not easily available, there is a danger that the child may be subjected to repeated tests which fail to produce a definitive diagnosis, or else is lost to follow-up and never receives appropriate treatment.

Recommendations

1 Early detection of some disorders is important, but screening tests should not be introduced on a piecemeal basis.

2 Screening tests should only be introduced when the full screening programme is in place.

3 Parents should be made aware of the benefits and limitations of screening tests so that they can make informed decisions about whether to participate.

4 Many of the national programmes, e.g. newborn bloodspot screening, hearing, and sickle & thalassaemia programmes, have nationally produced leaflets. These should be used whenever possible. 4r

5 Each PCO should have a Child Health Promotion Coordinator.

6 The Coordinator should be responsible for professional training and monitoring programmes.

Chapter 7

Physical examination

This chapter covers:

◆ The neonatal and 6–8 week examinations

◆ The school entrant examination

◆ Screening by physical examination for

- developmental dysplasia of the hip (DDH) (previously known as congenital dislocation of the hip)

- heart disease including hypertrophic cardiomyopathy (HCM)

- hypertension

- asthma, and

- undescended testes and other genital abnormalities

In this chapter we review the role of physical examination as an entity and then examine individual screening procedures in more detail.

4r   Also see the National Screening Committee's Fetal, Maternal and Child Health sub-group, which provides information on its website: http://www.nsc.nhs.ut/ ch-screen/child_ind.htm. Useful resources on a number of screening issues can be found at: http://libraries.nelh.nhs.uk/screening.

Neonatal and 8-week examinations

The neonate

A thorough physical examination of every neonate is now universally accepted as good practice and the whole examination can be regarded as a screening procedure with a number of individual components. Some, but not all, of these satisfy the formal criteria for a good screening programme.

The yield of the neonatal examination is high. It is accepted and expected by parents and there seems little doubt that they value the reassurance of normality at this time.

The precise timing of the examination is probably not critical, but the current practice of most paediatricians is that this examination should take place within the first 24 hours of life. While this seems logical both clinically and in logistic terms, and we recommend this as a desirable target, there is no evidence that this is indeed the optimal time and further research is needed to clarify the point.

There is some concern as to how the examination can be accomplished in cases where the mother and baby are discharged from hospital within a few hours of birth, or the delivery is the sole responsibility of a midwife. This has prompted several studies on the role of midwives or nurse practitioners, with appropriate training, in routine examination of the newborn (*see* HFAC4 website). The data suggest that a good standard can be achieved and that parents value information and discussion about the pregnancy and birth, and advice on child care, as much as the examination itself. Thus the newborn examination can be a health-promoting exercise rather than being purely a process of 'screening' for defects.

The health promotion aims of the newborn examination(s) and follow-up in the first days of life are:

- to review any problems arising or suspected from antenatal screening, the family history, or the events of labour
- to discuss matters such as baby care, feeding, vitamin K, hepatitis B and BCG vaccines, reducing the risk of SIDS, and any other matters relevant to the infant
- to identify parents who might have major problems with their infant (e.g. recognizing and managing depression, domestic violence, substance abuse, learning difficulties, or mental health problems)
- to explain problems such as jaundice that might not be observable in the newborn but could be significant a few days or weeks later
- to convey information about local networks and services, confidentiality, and data-handling, and access to the members of a primary health care team
- to inform all families how they can request and negotiate additional help, advice, and support as needed.

A review of current UK experience with the role of neonatal nurse practi- 4r tioners, including examination of the newborn has been published:

Hall DMB, Wilkinson A. The Ashington Experiment. Archives of Disease in childhood (Fetal and neonatal edition) -2005; **90**: F195-200.

Guidance on examination of the newborn is being developed by the National Screening Committee.

A second examination

We do not recommend a second physical examination in the first week of life unless there are specific concerns. Several studies show that the yield of significant findings is very small. However, health care staff should be alert to the problems which emerge in the first few days and weeks of life but are not identifiable by even the most expert newborn examination. Examples include congenital heart disease, metabolic disorders, and progressive jaundice.

Two months

An examination at around 2 months of age is generally thought to be useful, with a smaller but significant yield of abnormalities, and we support its continuation. At 8 weeks of age, the baby should be showing a range of behaviours including smiling and visual following; heart murmurs may be more readily detectable, and testes are more likely to be descended. Measurement of weight and head circumference, and a full physical examination are required.

This examination coincides with the first vaccine dose in the current UK schedule of immunization. For those mothers and GPs who so wish, and can allocate sufficient time, it can be combined with a postnatal examination, at which physical health, contraception, social support, depression, etc. can be discussed as appropriate. If this is to be the case, a conveyor-belt approach, with the mother and baby going to many professionals one after the other, should be avoided. One way of doing this is for either the health visitor or the GP to undertake the immunizations that are due.

There are arguments for an earlier examination—outcomes for DDH and cataracts may be better if they are detected and treated before 6 weeks, and the same may also be true for jaundice due to biliary atresia. However, if this examination were to be brought forward, parents might be less likely to attend again for immunization at 8 weeks. A decline in immunization rates has potentially serious public health consequences compared with the modest and (currently) largely theoretical reduction in good outcomes for treatment of DDH and cataract.

Therefore we recommend that the current approach be continued. The examination should still be planned for 6–8 weeks. In current practice, however, it is often delayed until 11 weeks or later for various reasons. The aim should be to *complete* this examination in *all* babies *by* 8 weeks of age. In view of concerns about delays in treatment of cataract, biliary atresia, or DDH, any baby in whom there is suspicion of the problems listed, resulting from a check at 6–8 weeks, must be referred as a matter of urgency.

The difficulty in timing could be overcome if midwives or health visitors examined the baby at home. While this is achievable, particularly if more midwives are trained to undertake examination of the newborn, it would need a substantial change in working practices.

Screening by physical examination after 8 weeks of age

Although the neonatal and 8-week examinations are widely believed to be worthwhile, the evidence base is still weak and the precise content and nature of the procedures used need further study. There is little evidence for or against physical examinations for screening purposes beyond the age of 8 weeks. On historical grounds, the main contender for a further universal physical examination is at the start of compulsory schooling, which in the UK is around the age of 5 years.

School entrant medical examination

The school health service, which was established in 1908, introduced periodic medical inspections (PMIs) with the aim of detecting previously unrecognized disorders and abnormalities. The dramatic decline of many diseases, coupled with free universal access to health care since the advent of the NHS, have greatly reduced the probability that a child will start school with an undiagnosed serious medical disorder. In most districts the traditional PMI has been discontinued. However, neither the introduction of PMIs nor their gradual withdrawal over the past two decades rested on a secure evidence base (box).

Evaluation of reports on the benefits of universal physical examination is difficult because:

- few authors report the specific aims of their programme, their referral criteria, or the follow-up and interventions offered

- very few reports provide the necessary information for evaluation—there are data on the problems identified by the various procedures and on the costs, but virtually none on how many children ultimately benefited from the exercise and to what extent

- the published reports are often impossible to generalize because of differences in local culture, demography, and attitudes (which vary even between adjacent schools, let alone between districts), and small but possibly crucial differences in the way these various approaches were implemented

---

Identification of physical disorders

Some physical disorders are overlooked because they are asymptomatic or the signs are subtle, non-existent, or readily misinterpreted as benign. Nevertheless, a review of the possible target disorders, taking into account their prevalence and clinical significance, the likely yield, and the benefits of detection and treatment, suggests that, with three exceptions, a search for previously overlooked organic disorders does not fulfill the strict criteria for screening programmes that would justify offering every apparently healthy child a full physical examination at school entry.

The exceptions are screening for growth disorders and for hearing and vision problems, which may fulfil the criteria for screening programmes. These are discussed in Chapters 8, 11, and 12 respectively.

Identification of emotional and developmental problems

Most children with serious disabilities are identified in the pre-school years. However, no pre-school system will identify all children with autism spectrum disorders, or those with developmental language disorders, dyspraxia, dyslexia, etc. Emotional and behavioural problems often remain undetected or untreated prior to school entry. There are several reasons for this,

♦ Coverage of pre-school surveillance is generally incomplete, even in health care systems with a strong commitment to, and high uptake of, health checks.

♦ The most needy families tend to make the least use of pre-school health care, particularly for behavioural and developmental disorders.

♦ Parents may not wish to take up offers of investigation or referral because they do not believe or cannot accept the possibility that their child might have a disabling condition.

♦ The existence or severity of some disorders only becomes apparent when new demands are made on the child at school.

These reasons apply whether or not there is an extensive programme of formal pre-school developmental screening and whatever developmental screening method is used. Therefore there is a case for developmental screening at school entry to identify these previously 'missed' diagnoses. A neurodevelopmental examination can identify a substantial proportion of the children likely to fail in school and bring these to the teachers' attention. The Working Party does not recommend this, because there is no evidence that implementing such a policy on a public health scale is beneficial.

General considerations in formulating policy

Here we summarize points made to the Working Party in the consultation process, which we believe are germane to policy development.

◆ Many of the health problems 'identified' at school medical examinations have already been identified and referred, or are being monitored.

◆ The primary health care team, who usually get to know a child over several years, are much better placed to recognize the child who merits a full medical evaluation than any school-based professional could be. Nevertheless, in some areas primary care is under severe pressure and children may not receive high-quality pre-school care.

◆ Some children miss out on health care (e.g. newly arrived refugees, homeless children, looked-after children, etc.). In this group of children, a serious physical disorder, such as heart disease, or a disabling condition may be identified for the first time at school entry and this may be important to both child and teacher.

◆ Few professionals consider it acceptable to perform a physical examination of a child at school without parental permission in writing. Some will only examine a child with the parent present. This policy inevitably means that the most needy children are likely to be those who are not examined— another example of the inverse care law.

Therefore a case can still be made for a process of health appraisal for all children, and the most obvious time to do this would be when the child reaches the age of 5 and starts compulsory schooling. However, in most populations of children the yield of new, important, and treatable findings is now very low, and other approaches have been tried, usually initiated by school nurses. The options include a health questionnaire, a health interview, and various combinations of these applied universally or selectively.

Health questionnaire

A questionnaire on its own is of dubious value for the following reasons.

◆ Coverage is often poor with the lowest response rates among parents with social problems or reading difficulties.

◆ Some parents are reluctant to disclose information, which they may feel is highly personal, to someone they have never met, and are unsure whether their replies will be confidential to the nurse or made available to the teaching staff.

- It cannot reveal disorders when the parent has not recognized any problem.
- It ignores the additional aims of a school health service, of providing information that is relevant to parents and children's needs.
- Analysis of questionnaires is time consuming, so that savings over other methods are modest.

Health interview

A health interview may include a physical evaluation undertaken by a nurse. It offers the opportunity for all parents to meet the school nurse; previously undetected health problems can be identified and previously recognized ones referred to the appropriate agency; information can be provided on a range of health issues. There are published data on the yield of new problems but no data on health gain.

There are many ways of carrying out these interviews. Some school nurses claim improved use of time by using a preliminary questionnaire or by meeting parents in groups. Group meetings have potential benefits both in resource terms and in giving parents the opportunity to make new friends, which may be very important for some. However, parents are unlikely to disclose confidential personal matters in this situation.

Selective methods

Various selective approaches are used in some districts. The school nurse selects those children who ought to have a paediatric examination or some other referral by a combination of questionnaire and record reviews, face-to-face contact, and discussion with teachers. There are no data to support the effectiveness of this approach, nor does it appear to offer significant cost savings over a more universal method.

Using the knowledge of teachers to identify problems

The doubts expressed about identification of developmental, behavioural, and learning problems by health professionals do not mean that this task is unimportant, only that other approaches may be more practical. Teachers get to know their children in the first year of primary school and they are required to review each child as part of a 'baseline assessment' process.

4r When *baseline assessment* was introduced, 91 different schemes were in use. Teachers are now undertaking a standard Foundation Stage Profile Assessment at the end of the Foundation Stage (reception year). More work is needed on the performance & psychometric properties of this process. See: Foundation Stage Profile Assessment http://www. qca.org.uk/163.html

An Evalution of the Use of Accredited Baseline Assessment Schemes in England. Geoff Lindsay, Ann Lewis, *British Educational Research Journal*, 29(2), 2003, 149–167

Adoption of a single standardized instrument for this assessment could allow several goals to be achieved simultaneously, including the vital one of recognizing which children should be individually reviewed in more depth. The disadvantage of delaying baseline assessment until the end of the reception year may be offset if schools continue to use their current on-entry schemes, building further assessment and review into the reception year, culminating at the end of foundation statutory scheme.

Even after school entry, some children experience long delays before the nature of their difficulties is appreciated and they receive the help they need. They or their parents may be blamed of accused of being lazy, valuable time is wasted, and the child is caught up in a cycle of failure and low self-esteem. Lack of teacher continuity in some areas, because of staffing problems, can exacerbate this. An efficient process is needed by which teachers can identify such children earlier and access expert multidisciplinary assessment for them.

The best-buy policy for school entrants

Our review reveals little evidence base for any firm recommendations regarding health and developmental screening at school entry. The health-promoting functions of school health services in general, and the opportunities at school entry in particular, are discussed in Chapter 5.

The benefits, in screening terms, of any form of universal health appraisal at school entry for children who have had access to and made use of primary health care in the pre-school years, and have been to pre-school facilities where any serious developmental problems are likely to be detected, are probably small in relation to the cost. This may not be true for certain populations of children who have had little or no pre-school care or educational opportunity. It could be argued that the best investment of resources for these children would be in ensuring that they receive the same quality of primary care as other children; within this setting, the whole range of acute and chronic health issues could be addressed. *Identification* of such children is a challenge which may best be met by the school health service at school entry, as this may be the first time that some children have been accessible to any health care system since infancy.

Physical examination

In this section, we shall consider individual physical examination procedures which may be used for screening purposes.

Developmental dysplasia of the hip (DDH)

Definition

The term 'developmental dysplasia of the hip' encompasses a spectrum of conditions in which the head of the femur is, or may be, partly or completely displaced from the acetabulum. It includes dislocation, subluxation, and instability; in addition, it may subsume dysplasia of the acetabulum. This term is now preferred to congenital dislocation of the hip (CDH) as it encompasses a broader range of related conditions and recognizes the importance of the relationships between dysplasia of varying degrees and the stability of the joint. However, dysplasia can exist without CDH and its natural history is not clearly understood. Therefore screening should be targeted at hip instability rather than dysplasia.

Causes

The cause of DDH is not known but genetic factors are important. It is more common in girls. The following factors are associated with an increased risk of DDH: family history in a close relative, breech presentation, abnormalities of the feet, torticollis, oligohydramnios, and tight swaddling. The first four of these are generally used in identifying a high-risk group for screening purposes (see below).

Incidence

Before neonatal screening was introduced the incidence in Northern European populations of DDH requiring surgery was 0.8–1.6 per 1000, with a mean from a number of studies of around 1.25 per 1000. When the Ortolani and Barlow screening tests for DDH were introduced, the incidence of neonatal hip instability was reported to be between 2.5 and 20 per 1000, i.e. up to 16 times higher.

Early detection

Early detection is important. Some hips are irreducible at birth and will come to surgery however promptly the diagnosis is made. In most cases, however, the hip is unstable but reducible. Early detection of these is thought to be worthwhile because conservative treatment, commencing within the first 6–8 weeks of life, is often successful, produces better results, and may avoid the need for surgery. Some infants will respond to conservative treatment if started at any time in the first 6 months, but the probability of success decreases with age and the risk of avascular necrosis rises. Thus there is a degree of urgency about the diagnosis and prompt referral of suspect cases is mandatory.

Universal screening for DDH

This was first recommended in 1969, but subsequent research raised doubts about its effectiveness and the topic was reviewed in detail in 1986. Much new work has been published since then, but there is still controversy over the role and effectiveness of screening. The aim of a screening programme for DDH is to ensure normal development and function of the hip by the end of the adolescent growth period.

Management of hip instability

Splintage is usually recommended in the belief that this will avoid the need for surgery later on. However, since the rate of neonatal hip instability is up to 16 times higher than that for DDH in unscreened populations, it is obvious that many babies must be splinted unne-cessarily. This has disadvantages in cost, both to the health service and to the family, and in the risk of complications such as avascular necrosis of the femoral head and pressure sores.

In some centres the introduction of neonatal screening is said to have resulted in a substantial fall in the number of babies needing surgery, but in others the rate remains unchanged. The reasons for the discrepancy probably include differences in the age(s) at which screening is performed and the skill and training of those doing the examination. Some research reports suffer from incomplete case ascertainment and it is difficult to ensure that all late cases have been identified since no single data source provides a complete list of all children requiring treatment for DDH.

The screening tests

Clinical examination detects dislocation, subluxation, and instability; ultrasound can also detect dysplasia. Evaluation of DDH screening is complicated by lack of a definitive diagnostic test and uncertainty about the natural history.

1. The simplest method of screening is the use of a **checklist of risk factors**. Breech presentation, family history in any relative, foot deformity, and torticollis are thought to be the most useful. A screening policy based only on these high risk factors will miss many cases.

2. Clinical examination of every baby using the **Ortolani and Barlow manoeuvres** can be performed up to the age of 6–8 weeks. Any baby with a hip which is subluxable or dislocated must be referred, but there is no agreement as to whether 'clicking' hips are significant. Nor is there any clear evidence as to when this examination should be performed or how many times it should be repeated. Instability identified at the neonatal clinical examination may be clinically undetectable at 2 weeks but ultrasound may reveal that the hip is still dislocated. Conversely, an ultrasound examination later in the

first week may reveal dislocation in a significant number of babies who have been passed by an expert examiner as clinically normal in the first 24 hours.

3. *Limited abduction and asymmetric skin creases* are found in many cases and are sometimes identified first by the parents. These signs should be sought whenever the hips are examined, though they are rarely present in the neonatal period and are more important after 6–8 weeks of age. The literature lacks any operational definition of 'limited abduction' or any appraisal of the likely referral rates if this physical sign were to be sought more actively. Some babies have asymmetry for other reasons, and abduction may be difficult to assess in active or restless babies. Because of these limitations, together with the uncertainties about early treatment mentioned previously, assessment of these signs does not fulfil strict criteria for a screening test. We do not recommend further routine examination of the hips after the 8-week check. However, we do recommend inclusion in the Personal Child Health Record (PCHR) of details of signs and symptoms that should alert parents and professionals to the possibility of DDH. Only those properly qualified should 'reassure' a parent who is worried about the possibility of DDH.

4. The first time an ambulant child is seen they should be observed walking. Any child thought to have a limp or the gait abnormality associated with bilateral DDH must be referred.

5. Appraisal of *screening by ultrasound scanning* of the hip is complicated by the existence of two methods: the Graf static approach and the Clarke–Harcke dynamic method. Ultrasound scanning of the hip has been used (a) as a primary screen for all babies or (b) as a selective primary screen for babies with risk factors. Options (a) and (b) are designed to make sure that cases are not missed. The third option (c) is as a secondary screen to decide which babies with risk factors or physical signs need splintage, i.e. to reduce 'over-treatment'. Option (a), if performed in the neonate before discharge, would result in considerable over-diagnosis of unstable hips which would resolve spontaneously. However, if it were deferred until 2 weeks, it would present considerable logistic problems and incur high costs which cannot currently be justified as there is no clear evidence of benefit. A popular option at present is a combination of (b) and (c). However, even in the most expert hands, some babies are probably splinted unnecessarily, some cases are still missed, and some who are splinted still require surgery. It is not yet certain that those cases considered *not* to need treatment as a result of the ultrasound findings will invariably have a good outcome, and this is the subject of a current research programme.

Screening policy and recommendations

The 1986 Expert Working Party pointed out that 'it is impossible to detect every CDH at birth ... and there must be continuing surveillance until the child is seen to be walking normally'. They recommended that (a) all infants should have an examination for CDH within 24 hours of birth, at the time of discharge from the hospital or within 10 days of birth, at 6 weeks of age, at 6–9 months, and at 15–21 months, and (b) the gait should be reviewed at 24–30 months and again at pre-school or school entry examination.

Having reviewed all the evidence we support the recommendations of the National Screening Committee as follows.

* All babies should be examined using *Ortolani and Barlow manoeuvres* 4r within 72 hours of birth. All babies with an abnormality on examination should have an ultrasound examination of the hips performed and be seen by an expert in the management of DDH.
* All babies with risk factors (breech presentation, family history, abnormalities of the lower limbs, and torticollis) should have an ultrasound examination of the hips.
* All babies should have a second physical examination by the time they are 8 weeks old.
* The PCHR should contain details of signs and symptoms that would alert parents to the possibility of DDH.
* At any age, when DDH is suspected, referral should be to someone with the appropriate expertise.

Practical aspects
It is clear from our review that training is vital if DDH screening is to be effective. However, the more people who carry out these procedures, the more difficult it is to ensure a high standard of training and monitoring. The burden of extra work on the ultrasound service may be such that screening of some at-risk groups will have to be phased in. The target should be to screen all those with an abnormal Barlow or Ortolani test, a breech presentation, or a family history. As facilities expand, those with other risk factors can also be screened.

Children with neurological disease
Acquired hip disorders are common in children with movement disorders such as cerebral palsy, but these should be identified by regular monitoring in a specialist clinic and not by neonatal screening.

Heart disease
The birth prevalence of congenital heart disease (CHD) in the UK is said to be 8 per 1000. The birth prevalence of CHD diagnosed in infancy is 6.5 per 1000

live births. Acquired heart disease in childhood is uncommon. The main causes are Kawasaki disease and myocarditis. Rheumatic heart disease is very rare in the Western world.

Early detection
Early detection of CHD is desirable for four reasons.

1 Deterioration may be rapid and catastrophic, and the outcome may be better if the infant is investigated before this occurs.

2 If the diagnosis is missed in the first few weeks of life because the infant is asymptomatic, the defect may not present until irreversible changes have occurred (e.g. pulmonary hypertension in children with left to right shunt).

3 Even defects that are trivial in haemodynamic terms may predispose to endocarditis if antibiotic prophylaxis is not recommended for dental and other procedures.

4 Missed diagnoses of heart disease distress parents, even if the delay does not result in any harm to the baby.

Identification—special situations and high-risk groups
A small but significant and increasing number of defects are detected by antenatal ultrasound screening. With routine ultrasound examination, it is possible to detect those conditions which do not have two equal-sized ventricles (single ventricle, hypoplastic left heart, pulmonary valve atresia with intact septum) at 17–18 weeks.

Patent ductus arteriosus (PDA) is very common in premature infants. Most close spontaneously or with treatment, but a few persist beyond the neonatal period and may not be detected until later.

Loud murmurs in an asymptomatic infant may be due to a small ventricular septal defect (VSD), which is benign, but may also be due to valvular stenosis, which needs prompt referral.

Children with Down's syndrome constitute a special case. Approximately 40 per cent have CHD, not always accompanied by significant murmurs or other obvious physical signs in infancy. In cases where there is a substantial left-to-right shunt, the progression to irreversible pulmonary hypertension is unusually rapid. A normal ECG does not exclude CHD. Parents must not be wrongly assured that their child has a normal heart. The Down's Syndrome Medical Interest Group (DSMIG) has a protocol for cardiac investigation of babies with Down's Syndrome (*see* HFAC4 website).

There is also an increased incidence of CHD in a wide variety of other dysmorphic syndromes and in association with malformations, and all such children should be checked with particular care. Children suspected of having Marfan's syndrome need cardiological review.

Parents who have had CHD themselves or a previous child with CHD have an increased risk of a further affected child. They should be offered genetic counselling and fetal echocardiography, preferably at a specialist centre.

Hypertrophic cardiomyopathy (HCM) is transmitted by a dominant gene. Decisions about the management of the offspring of people with this condition should be made by a cardiologist with experience of managing the disorder and of counselling affected individuals and their families. Neonatal screening is unlikely to be helpful. Screening for HCM in any young person embarking on intensive physical activity (such as athletics training) has been suggested, but it is rare (0.2 per 1000) and screening is unlikely to be beneficial or cost-effective (*see* HFAC4 website).

Routine examination of all children for CHD

Routine examination of the neonate may reveal cyanosis, respiratory distress, or tachypnoea. The incidence of murmurs in the neonate has not been reliably established (see box). Even in the most expert hands, many serious defects, such as interrupted aortic arch, coarctation, etc., may be undetectable by physical examination in the first few days of life. Professionals and parents need to be aware that *normal findings in the newborn infant do not guarantee that the cardiovascular system is normal and that serious heart conditions can present at any time in the first few weeks of life.*

The reported incidence of murmurs in the newborn varies from 0.9 to 74 per cent depending on the study. A careful study by Ainsworth *et al.* (*see* HFAC4 website) found a murmur in 0.6 per cent of 7204 neonates examined. Of the 46 babies studied, 25 had a cardiac malformation; 32 babies with no abnormal cardiac signs at birth presented later in infancy with a cardiac malformation.

Infants with serious CHD may present with failure to thrive, tachypnoea (particularly if it interferes with feeding), persistent recession, chest infection, sweating, cyanosis, or any combination of these. (Tachypnoea cannot be defined precisely, but in babies under 6 months of age a respiratory rate persistently above 55 in an infant is suspicious and, over the age of 4 weeks, the rate should not exceed 30 when the infant is asleep.)

4r   Screening for congenital heart disease using pulse oximetry has been
      proposed in the USA and is currently under review in the UK. It is not yet
      clear how much additional benefit would result when compared with
      conventional clinical examination, See Koppel RI, Druschel CM, Carter, T,
      et al. Effectiveness of pulse oximetry screening for congenital heart disease in
      asymptomatic newborns. *Pediatrics* 2003:111(3); 451–5. http://pediatrics.
      aappublications.org/cgi/content/full/111/3/451?ck=nck

      Knowles R, Griebsch I, Dezateux C, Brown J, Bull C, Wren C. Newborn
      screening for congenital heart defects: a systematic review and cost effective-
      ness analysis. *Health Technol Assess* 2005; 9(44).

Examination of infants at 6–8 weeks of age

The cardiovascular system (CVS) should be examined during the review
carried out at between 6 and 8 weeks of age. It is important that this is
thorough and it must include more than simply auscultation for murmurs. The symptoms and signs of CHD listed above should be sought
with care.

Further examinations

The Working Party considered whether examination of the CVS at any time
after the 6–8 week review would be of sufficient value to be regarded as a
screening test. Conditions which might remain asymptomatic for many years
include atrial septal defects (ASDs) and isolated coarctation of the aorta. The
physical signs of small ASDs are subtle and would probably be very difficult
for a non-specialist to detect at a routine 'screening' examination.

Most patients with coarctation are either symptomatic early in life or
present later with hypertension (see p. 157). The majority have abnormal
femoral pulses and many have a murmur medial to the left scapula. However,
we are not aware of any large-scale systematic study of examining femoral
pulses in a community setting and therefore do not think that this can be
regarded as a screening test. It is good practice to check the femoral or
dorsalis pedis pulses as part of a clinical examination, although they can be
difficult to feel in toddlers and will not invariably be impalpable even when
coarctation is present. In a child with symptoms or signs compatible with
cardiac disease, absence of the femoral pulses is significant. On present
evidence, 'missing' coarctation in a primary care setting should not be
construed as negligent.

The Working Party does not consider that any further routine examination
of the CVS after the 6–8 week check meets the stand-ards required for a
screening procedure.

Innocent murmurs

After the first few weeks of life, the most common problem in routine auscultation of the heart is the difficulty experienced by non-specialist staff in distinguishing innocent from pathological murmurs. Innocent murmurs are very
common, occurring in 50 per cent or more of children. They are more often
present and prominent in the febrile child. The diagnosis of an innocent murmur in the neonate is more difficult and usually requires the exclusion of CHD.

The characteristics of innocent murmurs include a low intensity, a musical
quality, localization to a small area of the precordium, and, most important,
absence of any other symptoms or signs referable to the CVS. In this situation,
there need not be undue concern about overlooking organic heart disease.
Conditions which might present with a soft murmur and no other findings
include a small ASD, mild pulmonary stenosis, a prolapsing mitral valve, and a
bicuspid aortic valve. These lesions are unlikely to be of haemodynamic significance. The risk of endocarditis is very small, and antibiotic prophylaxis to cover
dental extractions would only be advised for bicuspid aortic valves.

Referral

In the early weeks of life infants with symptoms and signs suggestive of CHD
need prompt referral for paediatric assessment as they can deteriorate
rapidly.

It is more difficult to suggest guidance on the referral of older infants and
children with murmurs of uncertain significance in the absence of other signs.
Nevertheless, where there is genuine doubt, expert consultation is preferable to
leaving parents in a state of uncertainty. Referral to a paediatrician is probably
the best option, although the advice of a paediatric cardiologist will still be
required on occasions. Echocardiography is helpful in expert hands, but defects
in small infants may easily be overlooked by non-specialist staff.

Primary prevention

There is so far very little scope for primary prevention of CHD. With the decline
of rheumatic heart disease in the Western world, the most common cause of
acquired heart disease in children in the UK is now Kawasaki disease. This is not
preventable, though early treatment of suspected Kawasaki disease may reduce
the incidence of cardiac complications. CHD prevention is considered on p. 110.

Hypertension

Screening for asymptomatic elevation of blood pressure could be
justified on two grounds.

1 It would allow detection of secondary hypertension due to coarctation of the aorta, endocrine disorders, or silent renal disease, for example, at a stage before the child presents with serious symptoms such as encephalopathy or vision disturbances. However, the incidence of symptomatic hypertension is less than 0.1 per cent (one in 1000).

2 A screening programme would also detect children with mild elevations of blood pressure who have an increased risk of developing essential hypertension in adult life. They could be advised to make appropriate changes in diet, weight, and lifestyle. There is as yet no evidence that such advice would be either acceptable or effective.

The main argument against screening is that there is no clear distinction between normal and elevated readings, and therefore an arbitrary cut-off point for referral has to be selected. Many children with mild elevations of blood pressure must be identified and investigated in order to detect the few cases of secondary hypertension. Since the former group cannot be offered any simple treatment programme of proven effectiveness, there is at present a substantial risk that the harm done by producing anxiety may exceed any possible benefits.

In an American study on community screening the examination of 10 000 children did not yield a single case of secondary hypertension and no case with primary or essential hypertension was found in which it was thought justifiable to embark on drug treatment. The authors of the study, and subsequently the USA Task Force on screening, concluded that screening for hypertension in childhood could not be recommended. (However, it should be noted that children in the USA are examined more frequently by their personal physician than is the case in the UK and therefore hypertension might be diagnosed at an earlier stage even without a screening programme.)

More recently, the USA Task Force proposed that children whose initial reading is above the 95th centile should be re-examined and considered for treatment, but four out of five such children will on subsequent readings be found to have a blood pressure within the normal range. The more frequently children are examined, the more likely it is that at least one measurement will be elevated. Two further British reviews concluded that screening for hypertension is not justified at present.

Asthma

With the increasing awareness of asthma and the apparent rise in incidence over the past few years, it has become clear that the definition of 'mild asthma' is difficult. Concordance between different ways of confirming the diagnosis is less than was previously thought, and longitudinal studies suggest that at the mild end of the spectrum bronchial hyper-reactivity may be a temporary or transient phenomenon.

Primary prevention

There is a little evidence that rigorous allergen avoidance in infants at high risk of atopy may reduce the incidence of allergic disease, at least in the short term.

Smoking by the mother in pregnancy increases the risk that the infant will develop asthma and will demonstrate increased bronchial hyper-reactivity on histamine challenge. There is controversy as to whether exposure to cigarette smoke (passive smoking) actually causes asthma. It is associated with a reduction in the size of the lungs and smaller airways, and an increased rate of hospitalization for respiratory illness.

Reduction in air pollution may also be an important primary prevention measure.

Abnormalities of the genitalia

Careful inspection of the genitalia in the neonate to detect undescended testes, hypospadias, and other anomalies is an essential part of the routine neonatal examination. The identification of hernia and hydrocoele, and concerns about medical indications for circumcision (which are often unfounded), are other common problems raised either by the parents or at a routine examination.

By far the most common problem detectable by screening examination is abnormal descent of the testicle. At birth, 6.0 per cent (60 per 1000) of males have one or both testes undescended, and the rate is some five times higher in low-birth-weight babies than in full-term infants. A high proportion of testes which are undescended at birth have descended normally by 3 months of age. The prevalence at this age is 1.6 per cent (16 per 1000). Further natural descent is unlikely after 3 months of age. Some testes apparently normally descended at 3 months may be found to be incompletely descended when re-examined between 1 and 5 years of age. The majority of these boys have had late initial descent of the testes between birth and 3 months of age, or have been judged to have incomplete initial descent at the first examination.

Infant boys thought to have incomplete descent of the testis should be referred for surgical opinion by the age of 12 months because early surgery may improve fertility and facilitate the early diagnosis of malignancy.

The screening test is a physical examination. The testis is gently manipulated into the lowest position along the pathway of normal anatomical descent without tension being applied. The most precise criterion for diagnosis of undescended testis at birth and in the first few months of life is that the centre of at least one testis should be less than 4 cm below the pubic tubercle (2.5 cm in babies weighing under 2.5 kg). Subjective classification by experienced examiners into three categories (well down, high scrotal, or suprascrotal) is as reliable as actual measurement.

Although apparently simple, the physical examination is not always straight-forward. The size of the scrotum is not a good guide to whether or not the testes are descended. The gubernaculum is sometimes mistaken for a testis.

4r   Several correspondents have reported continuing difficulties in the early identification of undescended testes, resulting in late operations. Several factors may contribute to this, including difficulties with the physical examination, or a higher incidence of reascent of an apparently descended testis than has previously been thought. There is not sufficient evidence at present to propose any revision of current policy but clinicians should be aware of the difficulty.

Recommendations

Routine reviews

+ We recommend the continuation of the neonatal and 6–8 week physical examination for every baby

+ We recommend that routine medical examinations at school entry are discontinued, except as part of research studies.

Developmental dysplasia of the hip

+ One individual should be identified to act as coordinator for training and quality monitoring.

+ The pathway of referral and the responsibility for investigation and management of suspected hip disorders in infants, and of infants with risk factors for DDH, should be agreed by specialists and primary care staff, clearly defined, and streamlined to ensure that delays do not occur. This is particularly important at the 6–8 week review, since there may be some urgency in commencing treatment for a newly discovered case at this age.

+ The child health promotion coordinator (p. 141) should ensure that each neonate is assessed for risk factors and examined once within the first 72 hours by someone who has been appropriately trained to recognize abnormalities.

+ The list of risk factors must include family history, breech presentation, foot deformity, and torticollis. Missed DDH in an infant with a positive family history is particularly distressing for parents and may result in litigation.

- A baby with a clinical examination suggestive of DDH should have an ultrasound examination and be referred to someone trained in the management of DDH. Any baby with risk factors for DDH should have an ultrasound examination irrespective of the clinical findings. This may have to be phased in, depending on resources. Ultrasound examination of those with an abnormal Barlow or Ortolani test takes precedence over those with risk factors where resources are limited.

- Every baby should have a further review of risk factors and an examination of the hips at 6–8 weeks. The indications for an ultrasound examination are the same as for the first examination.

- A child with a suspect clinical examination should not be subjected to repeated checks or reviews but should be referred promptly.

- Universal screening by ultrasound cannot be recommended except in the context of a research programme.

- Parents should be warned (e.g. by the PCHR) that no screening procedure is perfect, and informed about the physical signs of hip disorders (i.e. limited abduction, abnormal skin creases, asymmetry, and limp). They should also be told whom to contact if they have any concerns.

- Whenever a child is seen for the first time after s/he begins to walk, s/he should be observed walking to check that the gait is normal.

Monitoring the screening programme

The priority at present is the setting and monitoring of quality stand-ards for examination, recording, referral, and treatment. The training of staff is a priority, and a suitable model enables staff to learn the correct technique. (*See* HFAC4 website)

Process measures include the coverage of screening, numbers referred for specialist opinion at each age, and numbers of babies needing treatment with splints or surgery. Quality measures should also include the intervals between referral and specialist consultation, and between consultation and treatment (when needed). The presumed benefit and therefore the best outcome measure for DDH screening is reduction in hip morbidity in adult life, but radiological appearances of the joint at skeletal maturity may be an acceptable proxy measure. Monitoring of late diagnosed cases is useful as a warning of deficiencies in the system, but numbers in any one district are too small to permit generalizable conclusions.

Heart disease

+ Symptoms and signs of CHD should be routinely sought at the newborn examination and at the review at 6–8 weeks of age.

+ Parents should be aware of the significance of potentially serious symptoms, notably persistent tachypnoea, and should be encouraged to seek help if concerned. This information could be provided through the Personal Child Health Record.

+ All professionals dealing with children should be familiar with the symptoms and signs of cardiac disease in babies, and in particular with the risk of rapid deterioration in infancy once the child presents with symptoms.

+ After the 6–8 week review, the CVS should be examined in any child with relevant complaints.

+ The potential benefits of routine examination of the CVS after 8 weeks of age do not justify any more specific recommendation.

+ Children with conditions having a high risk of CHD should have a thorough assessment as soon as possible to ensure that significant heart disease is not overlooked. Babies with Down's syndrome should be managed according to the best-practice protocol.

+ Primary health care teams should be aware of the importance of early diagnosis and referral of Kawasaki disease.

Hypertension

+ We recommend that at present no attempt should be made to introduce universal screening for hypertension. Further research on the detection of secondary hypertension and the prevention of essential hypertension may eventually change this view.

+ Measurement of the blood pressure must be part of the clinical evaluation of any child presenting with a relevant medical problem.

Asthma

+ Primary prevention by reducing parental smoking should be pursued and is one of the many reasons for addressing this issue in health promotion programmes.

+ In view of the variability in symptoms of mild asthma, and the lack of sensitivity, specificity, and reproducibility of tests for bronchial hyper-reactivity, we do not think that the criteria for a good screening programme (p. 138) could be fulfilled.

Undescended testes

◆ A note should be made of testicular descent at the neonatal and 8-week examinations. The second examination is particularly important in those cases where the testis is *not* 'well down' in the scrotum.

◆ No further check need be made as a matter of routine. Parents can be shown how to check the testicular descent themselves (e.g. while the child is in the bath).

◆ If there is doubt about the descent of either or both testes after 6–8 weeks, the child should be referred for a surgical opinion to a surgeon with experience of and interest in paediatric surgery. As a few testes may descend between 8 weeks and 1 year, and most surgeons will not operate on a child before it is a year old, it may be acceptable to review the child at the age of about 1 year and refer at that stage, provided that there is not a long waiting list.

◆ Explicit guidelines are needed to ensure that the system works efficiently. These will depend on local circumstances, but we suggest that:

  • the referral should be made immediately after the 6–8 week examination or, if later, a named individual should be responsible for ensuring this indeed happens

  • the surgical clinic appointment should be sent so that the child can be seen at or before the first birthday

  • the GP should be notified of non-attenders

  • any deliberate delay in sending the parents an appointment should not be incorporated in measures of clinic waiting-list times.

◆ These checks are often neglected in children who are disabled. *All* children should be examined, though judgement is needed as to when treatment is desirable.

◆ The age of diagnosis and treatment, and the number of boys discovered to have an untreated undescended testis at the age of 5 or subsequently, may be recorded as a measure of the success of the screening programme for undescended testes.

◆ Training for primary care staff should include the indications for circumcision and the recognition and management of hernia and hydrocoele.

Chapter 8

Growth monitoring and nutrition

This chapter:
- ◆ Reviews the value of growth monitoring (GM)
- ◆ Outlines the reasons why GM may be useful
- ◆ Describes the requirements for successful GM
- ◆ Makes recommendations for GM
- ◆ Examines the value of measuring the head circumference

It is good clinical practice to measure, and plot on a suitable chart, the height, weight, and head circumference of any child where concern about growth or chronic health problems is a feature and in children requiring prolonged follow up for any reason (see also p. 350). This chapter is concerned with the more difficult question of whether, when, and how growth should be assessed, and measurements taken, in an apparently healthy child and how they should be interpreted.

Screening or monitoring?

Interpretation of growth measurements requires skill and judgement, and is easier when several measurements are taken over a period of time. It is important not to overlook children with growth disorders, but inappropriate referrals generate both parental anxiety and a substantial increase in specialist workload. With the possible exception of single height measurements (p. 182), weighing and measuring children cannot be regarded as screening and therefore we have adopted the term **growth monitoring** (GM).

Is growth monitoring useful?

Although the routine measurement of height, weight, and head circumference (HC) is strongly supported by most health professionals, there is still disagreement about the benefits, the ages when measurements should be made or recorded, and the threshold at which referral for specialist advice is desirable.

There is a substantial literature on GM in developing nations. This focuses mainly on weight monitoring and is directed at the problem of malnutrition. Not withstanding the widespread commitment to this activity, its impact on the health of children is uncertain (see box). The reasons for this observation are probably relevant in the industrialized nations as well as in the developing world. The importance of coupling GM with health promotion in developing nations is now acknowledged and the preferred term is **growth monitoring and promotion** (GMP).

Reasons for poor performance of monitoring

- Incomplete coverage—the families whose children might benefit most from GM are those with multiple social and economic problems, who have difficulty in making full use of preventive health care measures.
- Inaccurate measurement, charting, and interpretation.
- Inappropriate, rushed, or misleading counselling of parents due to inadequate staff training.
- Poverty—lack of money and/or social support enabling parents to implement the advice given.
- Cultural resistance to particular dietary recommendations.

A colloquium on growth monitoring and promotion in the developing world was held in Antwerp in November 2001 (*see* HFAC4 website)
www.itg.be.colloq2001

Requirements for growth monitoring

Effective growth monitoring depends on all of the following factors:

- availability of suitable growth charts (see box)
- correct measurement techniques
- accurate transfer of measurements to chart
- correct interpretation (requiring an understanding of normal and abnormal growth)
- time, expertise, and resources to explain the measurements to the parents and to initiate appropriate action when necessary
- access to specialist advice.

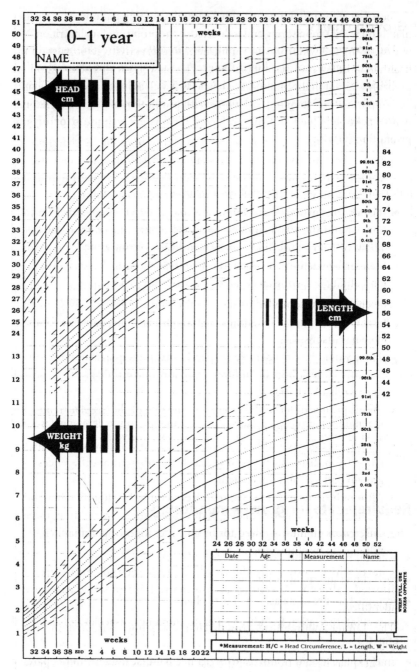

Fig. 8.1 Boys growth chart (0–1 year). © Child Growth Foundation. Available from Harlow Printing, Maxwell Street, South Shields, NE33 4PU, UK.

Growth charts

1 The nine-centile growth charts published in 1993 were recommended by an expert group of the Royal College of Paediatrics and Child Health (RCPCH) as the most suitable charts for UK children. (Fig. 8.1). They describe current growth patterns more precisely and have two additional advantages.

- ◆ Each band (the interval between each pair of lines on the chart) now represents 0.67 (two-thirds) of a standard deviation, so that crossing a complete band now has the same significance whatever the initial height of the child (T.J. Cole, *British Medical Journal*, **308**, 641–2).
- ◆ The chart now includes a minus and plus 2.67 SD line, equivalent to the 0.4 and the 99.6 centiles respectively. Only one child in 260 lies above or below these lines, whereas the figure is one in 44 for the two standard deviation line. A child below the 0.4 centile has a significant probability of having an organic cause for short stature.

2 The charts were compiled using data for white children only. Growth charts for ethnic minority groups are thought not to be desirable for the following reasons.

- ◆ There would be considerable practical difficulties in assembling a sufficiently large cohort of children from any one ethnic group to produce a reliable chart.
- ◆ Ethnic groups differ in the extent and the rate of the 'secular trend' in height and very frequent revisions would be necessary.
- ◆ Ethnic groups are not homogeneous (e.g. children whose families come from different parts of India show substantial differences in growth patterns and final height).
- ◆ Although African–Caribbean children tend to be slightly taller and Asian children slightly smaller than white Caucasian children, these differences are best allowed for by consideration of parental heights rather than by ethnic origin.

3 Charts which show only the third, fifth, or second centile are of limited value for screening, as too many false-positive cases are identified.

4 The Tanner–Whitehouse growth charts are now outdated for the following reasons

- ◆ There has been a trend over the last few decades for children to grow taller (the so-called 'secular trend').

◆ It has been noted in the last few years that weight gain in early infancy is often more rapid than is indicated on the charts and this is followed by apparent growth faltering. This is probably because of changes in feeding practices, notably a higher incidence of breastfeeding and the use of improved or 'humanized' milk formula.

Measurement techniques

Weight

Weight is easy to measure. A modern, electronic, self-zeroing scale, if properly maintained and placed on a firm surface, can weigh a nude baby to within 10–20g, a toddler in vest and pants to within 100g and children and adults in light clothing to within 150–200g. However, a baby's true weight may fluctuate by several hundred grams, depending on the contents of bowel, bladder, and stomach as well as minor fluctuations due to intercurrent illness. As far as possible, an individual baby should be weighed at the same time on each occasion and consistently before or after a feed. Weighing neonates or children in 'sacks' or on antiquated scales is not acceptable.

Length and height measurements (when indicated)

◆ *The first 12–18 months of life* In this age group, it is usual to measure supine length using a commercially available measuring device. The equipment used in specialist clinics is expensive but low-cost devices can produce measurements of acceptable accuracy. Although the error of length measurements is greater than that when measuring standing height, useful information can still be obtained because of the higher growth velocity in early infancy. (NB.: No evidence has been found to support the suggestion that extension of the hips in the neonate, in order to measure length more accurately, has any relationship with dislocation of the hips.) Length measurement requires a properly calibrated device positioned on a firm surface. Two people are needed for precise measurements. Length accurate to 1mm can be obtained with research equipment but much cheaper equipment, allowing accuracy to 0.5cm, is adequate for general use. Taking length measurements with tape is not acceptable.

◆ *As soon as the child can stand* Some 2-year-olds are upset by having their height measured and two adults may be needed to obtain a reliable measurement. Most 3-year-olds can be measured without difficulty if the examiner is patient.

◆ *Devices for measuring height* A simple 'screening' chart can be used to detect those children who are very short. It has the serious dis-advantage that for those children who 'pass' the screening test, no height measurement is recorded for future reference. Cheap measuring sticks, often mounted on weighing scales, are inaccurate. Measurement errors can be as much as 1–2 cm. For clinic or school use, good results are obtained with a Minimeter or the Leicester Height Measure. The latter has the advantage that no metre measuring stick is needed to check its accuracy. Although specialist clinics use more robust and expensive equipment, this does not necessarily increase accuracy.

Head circumference (OFC)

◆ Sewing tape should never be used and disposable paper tapes should be used only in hospital intensive care units. A re-usable plastic or fibre glass insertion tape can deliver a precise measurement if correctly used. The measurement to be taken in practice is the largest circumference since this is the only repeatable measurement.

hour). Height changes from one moment to the next and there is no exact or 'correct' height for a child.

◆ Stretching the child by applying gentle upwards pressure under the jaw does not eliminate this source of variability.

Difficulties with growth monitoring: accuracy and reproducibility

Inaccurate measurements can be due to the following

◆ Poor installation of equipment.
◆ Inadequate maintenance.
◆ Relocation of portable instruments in a slightly different position each time they are used.
◆ Loose wobbly headpieces on graduated ruler type instruments.

These errors can be avoided by checking the accuracy of the instrument with a 1m measuring stick

Poor reproducibility

◆ A correct and standardized measurement technique is important.
◆ Repeat measurements made on the same child are rarely the same, even when the same instrument is used by the same observer. This problem is not avoided by using more expensive equipment.

- Ninety per cent of the variability is in the children themselves. There is a small diurnal variation (height is greatest on first rising in the morning and decreases during the day, with the most rapid decrease during the first

Growth velocity estimations do not increase precision

- For an experienced observer measuring children under ideal conditions the SD of a single height measurement (SDshm) is around 0.25 cm. For height velocity, two measurements are needed. A child observed to have grown 4 cm between two measurements 1 year apart might in reality have grown between 3.3 cm (very low velocity) and 4.7 cm which is within the normal range (95 per cent confidence limits).

- Under field conditions these limits would be even wider since multiple observers and different conditions and instruments would be used. Differences between observers on the same occasion can be as great as 1.5 cm.

- The rate of growth (growth velocity) varies with age, sex, and initial height.

The problem of bias

- Readings of height and weight are subject to bias if the observer knows previous readings or has a preconceived idea as to whether or not the child is growing 'normally'. Ideally, measurements should be taken without knowledge of the previous figure and without prior reference to the growth chart.

Short-term variability

- Growth rates vary with the season of the year, intercurrent illnesses, and other factors. Therefore even the most precise measurements made over a short period of time (6 months or less) are likely to be misleading.

Benefits of growth monitoring

The potential advantages of GM can be listed as follows.

- *Detecting disorders* GM may facilitate the early detection of a variety of disorders (see box).

Conditions sometimes detectable by growth monitoring

- *Hypothyroidism (juvenile)*—Incidence uncertain, but uncommon. Most congenital hypothyroidism is detected by neonatal screening but a few cases are inevitably missed. Juvenile hypothyroidism is more common in girls and is usually autoimmune in nature. Only a minority of cases are short (< second centile) at the time of diagnosis.

- *Growth hormone insufficiency (GHI)*—incidence 1 in 3000–5000. GHI can occur in association with other disorders, but isolated or idiopathic GHI is the most common. Multiple pituitary hormone deficiency can present in early infancy as a short baby, sometimes accompanied by microphallus and/or hypoglycaemia and prolonged jaundice, or as short stature in early or mid-childhood. Idiopathic GHI presents with short stature and often mid-facial hypoplasia. Late-onset GHI can be difficult to differentiate from the physiological deficiency of growth hormone which may occur with delayed puberty. Because of this variable age of presentation, no single screening test could be expected to identity every case of GHI.

- *Turner's syndrome*—incidence at least 1 in 2500 females. Less than 50 per cent of cases are identified at birth, though increasing numbers are being detected antenatally. In the remainder, short stature or primary amenorrhoea are the presenting features. If tall parents have a child with Turner's syndrome, she may not necessarily be identified as short by a single measurement. At age 5, only half of all girls are below the 0.4 centile for height. The growth chart may show that the height is crossing centiles but the growth deficit becomes more obvious later in childhood.

- *Growth impairment* can be the presenting feature of many other disorders. The majority are likely to be associated with other symptoms, but short stature may occasionally be the only sign of conditions such as coeliac disease, inflammatory bowel disease, or chronic renal failure. There is no evidence that GM would make a substantial contribution to case-finding for these conditions.

- *Cranial or total body irradiation and intracranial tumours* These children should be under specialist care but occasionally they are 'missed' or lost to follow-up.

- *Syndromes* such as Russell–Silver syndrome may be identified as a result of growth impairment or short stature.

- *Some forms of bone dysplasia* can present with short stature, but without other obvious disproportion in the early stages. Diagnosis is important because genetic counselling may be required and new possibilities for treatment are being investigated.
- *Short normal children ('Idiopathic short stature')* should currently only be treated with growth hormone in the context of clinical trials. Short-term improvement in height has been shown clearly but the long-term benefits and hazards are still unknown.
- GM might also be useful as a means of detecting excessively *tall stature*—this may occur in thyrotoxicosis, congenital adrenal hyperplasia, premature sexual maturation, Marfan's syndrome, etc.
- *Psychosocial short stature* This occurs with a background of severe prolonged abuse. Hyperphagic short stature is a rare form in which there is stunting, a tendency to gorge on food, depressed mood, poor relationships, and impaired development.

- *Health promotion* GM could be used to assess and inform health promotion activity in respect of nutritional advice and overall quality of child care. For example, impaired growth may be associated with difficulties in weaning. Identification of short normal children might facilitate intervention with the psychological issues associated with short stature.
- *A focus of interest for parents* GM is valued by parents as a focus for visits to the clinic or surgery. Regular GM may be useful to reassure the parents that the child is thriving. The baby's weight gain is often used as a discussion point regarding nutrition and other aspects of child rearing. Similarly, parents take some satisfaction from recording their child's growth in height.
- *Public health aspects* Information about child growth in the whole population may be useful in several ways. First, there is a tendency for children to be taller in successive generations (the so-called 'secular trend'), though this trend is now levelling off. Second, the work of Barker and his colleagues over the past decade has heightened interest in intra-uterine and infant growth patterns, and their relationships with health in adult life, but the implications of this work for routine child health care are not yet fully worked out. Third, since there is a link between height and social circumstances, GM provides a window on the effects of poverty and changing social inequalities. Fourth, it is potentially useful to monitor the emerging epidemic of obesity.

The relationships between the size of children at any given age, their genetic background, and their social circumstances are complex. Growth patterns may to some extent reflect not only the circumstances of the present generation but also the social deprivation experienced in childhood by their parents and even their grandparents. Thus contemporary population birth-weight and height data are of limited value in assessing the *current* public health of the population, though body mass index data are relevant for monitoring the prevalence of obesity.

Data collected for public health purposes must be reliable, carefully documented, and preserved for the future. Secure long-term funding for a small number of GM projects in districts with a declared interest and track record in this field may be a more logical investment than regular GM in every district.

Weight monitoring

Parents are reassured if they know that their baby is gaining weight, although satisfactory weight gain does not rule out growth disorders and some, such as growth hormone deficiency and hypothyroidism, may be associated with normal or even increased weight gain. It is usual to plot the baby's weight on a chart before interpreting its significance, but this can be a source of considerable anxiety if staff do not understand how to use these data correctly.

Centile crossing

Few babies continue on exactly the same centile from birth onwards. About 50 per cent of babies cross at least one band on the weight chart between 6 weeks of age and 12 or 18 months and 5 per cent fall across two bands. Babies who are large at birth are more likely to show falls of this magnitude. On average, small babies catch up and large babies catch down. This is explained by the phenomenon of 'regression to the mean' (see appendix to chapter).

It is important to consider both length and weight when reviewing a possible growth problem. Staff and parents should be aware that the pattern of weight gain differs between breastfed and bottle-fed infants. There is no simple way of assessing whether a particular growth pattern is outside the limits of 'normality', although several new charts have been designed in an attempt to address the problem (box).

The pattern of weight gain differs between breastfed and formula-fed babies. Charts have been developed which show the weight gain centiles for breastfed babies, but further work is required to determine their applicability to the general population of breastfed infants.

4r   New breastfeeding charts by WHO are available. Their use in the UK is under consideration but, whatever is decided, it is important that all primary care practitioners use the same charts.

The use of charts with 'thrive lines' may make it easier for staff to assess the probability that a given rate of weight gain is abnormal. Formal assessment of these charts under field conditions is needed; their correct use and interpretation would need a good understanding of charts and of infant growth. http://www.who.int/childgrowth/standards/technical_report/en/index.html

(*see* HFAC4 website)

Undernutrition, faltering weight gain, and 'failure to thrive'

Many of the babies who gain weight slowly or whose weight graph gradually crosses centile lines downwards in the first year of life may simply be adopting a growth trajectory that is normal for them. Relative undernutrition may occur in many situations such as weaning difficulties, late weaning, minor illness, and family disturbances, and this may be associated with short periods of slow weight gain or temporary weight loss.

Deprivation and poverty increase the risk that a child will grow at a rate below genetic potential, but substantial centile shifts are seen in babies of all social classes. Some reports suggest that babies with poor weight gain may be at slightly increased risk of neglect and abuse, deficits in long-term physical growth and cognitive development, an increased incidence of cardiovascular disease in adult life, and possibly an increased risk of sudden infant death. None of these relationships have so far proved sufficiently robust to justify in themselves a formal screening programme for poor weight gain.

Concern arising when the line of weight gain crosses centile bands downwards is perhaps best described by the term 'faltering weight gain'. This is preferable to 'failure to thrive', a term that is perceived as pejorative and traditionally has been used to imply that there may be some underlying organic cause. The term 'faltering weight gain' should only be used when there is evidence that the slow weight gain is abnormal *for that baby*.

Prolonged failure to gain weight, or continuing weight loss, is more likely to have serious implications. However, it is rare that the weight chart is the only clue to a serious abnormality affecting growth in infancy. Other symptoms or signs are nearly always present as well, and in their absence hospital admission is rarely helpful since the investigation of infants whose only problem is slow weight gain seldom reveals any significant organic disease.

When psychosocial factors appear to be directly linked with, and the cause of, poor growth, the term 'non-organic failure to thrive' (NOFTT) may be used. In severe cases of suspected NOFTT, hospital admission or placement with a foster parent may result in a dramatic growth spurt, confirming the impression of insufficient food intake and an inadequate environment. However, such cases are the exception, and only a small minority of children with very slow weight gain are subsequently shown to be victims of abuse or neglect.

When is intervention indicated?

Deciding whether slow weight gain needs intervention can be difficult. Management decisions must be made on the basis of the whole clinical picture rather than from the weight chart alone, otherwise parents may be subjected to unjustified worry and unnecessary advice and intervention. This, in turn, may cause problems. Often these babies have insufficient nutritional intake, and there may be feeding difficulties which might benefit from supportive management with community-based nutritional and psychological advice. Video studies in parents' homes reveal that some parents have far greater difficulties with feeding and child care generally than would ever be suspected from the history, or from observation during a clinic visit (*see* HFAC4 website for details of training resources).

Very frequent weighing can be counterproductive as it often reveals fluctuations week by week, even though there is an upward trend. This may result in desperate attempts by the parents to increase the baby's food intake, leading in turn to further feeding difficulties.

The 'overweight' baby

Crossing centiles in an upward direction may also cause concern, primarily because it has been suggested that infant obesity might be an important, and preventable, risk factor for adult obesity. In the present state of knowledge, however, it is rarely necessary or useful to comment adversely on the fact that a baby looks chubby or fat.

Conclusion

Any baby about whom there is concern about health or growth or who has a chronic disorder should be weighed and measured, and the results must be recorded on a chart. A consensus conference proposed that a record of weight at birth, at the 6–8 week check, at other reviews (if undertaken), and at the times of immunizations would probably be sufficient to reassure parents and professionals and to identify most cases of faltering weight gain. However, there is not sufficient evidence to regard routine frequent weight monitoring as a formal screening process.

There is no reason to advise more frequent or regular weighing if the parent and primary care team are satisfied that the baby is feeding normally, is well, and has begun to gain weight. Whatever professionals may think, however, parents will continue asking for facilities for their babies to be weighed or to weigh the baby themselves. When parents or other relatives are anxious about their child's weight or food intake, plotting the child's weight on a chart may be useful as a way of reassuring them. Weighing is easy, but much anxiety is generated by uncertain or inexpert interpretation of growth charts and only staff with the appropriate expertise should advise parents on concerns arising from weighing or weight charts.

Weight in older children

Although the main focus of GM after infancy is on height gain and the detection of growth disorders, poor weight gain may also cause concern to parents and sometimes to professionals. Eating disorders are common and cause much concern to parents (*see* HFAC4 website). Any child whose health or growth is causing concern should be weighed and the height measured. Excessive thinness in a child who is otherwise well and is growing in height is rarely pathological but parental concerns must, as always, be taken seriously.

Length and height monitoring

It is usual to measure supine length until the age of 2 years and height thereafter.

Length

An accurate measurement of length in the neonate is mandatory if any abnormality is suspected. We are doubtful about the value of *routinely* measuring length in the neonate, and the logistics of ensuring that *accurate* measurements are made on all babies may become increasingly difficult with the rising number of home deliveries and very short hospital stays. Alternatively, a length measurement could be undertaken as part of the 6–8 week review.

The main benefit of length measurements in early infancy might be the identification of very short babies (length below the 0.4 centile), for example those with severe endocrine deficiency disorders, skeletal dysplasias, or Russell–Silver syndrome if these diagnoses had been 'missed' at birth.

However, critical observation ought to suggest to the examiner that such babies merit further assessment, and there are currently no data to show whether formal measurement would confer additional benefits.

It has also been suggested that a measurement of length taken at birth or at 6–8 weeks might subsequently be useful in difficult diagnostic situations. However, there is as yet no convincing evidence that records of one or more routine length measurements throughout the first year of life would simplify the differential diagnosis of 'failure to thrive' or growth disorders.

Height

It is important to monitor growth (weight *and* length/height) in cases where some abnormality is suspected or known to exist, for example in an infant who at birth was noted to be very small for dates, or who is thought to be failing to thrive, or who has a dysmorphic syndrome. Children who suffered from intra-uterine growth retardation may grow more slowly and gain weight at a lower than normal rate.

When a child presents with parental concerns about abnormal growth or unexplained long-standing health problems, the clinical assessment should routinely include measurement and plotting of height and weight. Many children with short stature are identified by parents or by paediatricians caring for the child because of other medical conditions.

Screening for abnormal stature and/or monitoring of height gain in apparently well children might be justified by the following considerations.

- It might permit the early detection of conditions which limit growth but may not be accompanied by any other symptoms or signs, for example growth hormone insufficiency, hypothyroidism and Turner's syndrome (see box on p. 175). The early identification of short stature associated with Turner's syndrome (TS) and with hormonal deficiencies is particularly important because early treatment improves the prognosis for final adult height. (The National Institute for Clinical Excellence (NICE) has accepted that TS and growth hormone deficiency are indications for growth hormone replacement therapy. *See* HFAC4 website.)
- GM might facilitate the detection of conditions causing unusually rapid growth, for example congenital adrenal hyperplasia, thyrotoxicosis, precocious puberty, etc.
- Normal short children could be identified. There is currently little evidence that this would be beneficial in terms of either treatment or psychological benefits. Short children may be more at risk of being bullied, but this is

a problem to be addressed by whole-school approaches rather than screening (p. 116).

◆ Constitutional delay in growth and puberty (CDGP) might be identified, but professional awareness of this problem and of treatment possibilities is probably more important than a formal monitoring programme.

The single measurement as a screen versus multiple measurements over time

Using the nine-centile charts, any single length or height measurement (whether opportunistic or at child health surveillance reviews) could be regarded as a screening test. Using the 0.4 centile as the cut-off for referral would identify some, but not all, children with idiopathic growth hormone deficiency or Turner's syndrome without an excessive number of false-positive cases. Raising the cut-off to the second centile would increase sensitivity but at the expense of a substantial rise in false-positive cases.

Measuring height gain over time

Acquired disorders (see box on p. 171) which affect growth can occur in any child, whatever his/her initial height. A single measurement cannot be expected to find these cases. Identification of these children by growth monitoring would therefore require sufficient measurements to demonstrate centile crossing over time.

The data in the box on p. 169 illustrate the difficulties with interpreting changes in growth patterns based on two or three measurements. Multiple measurements would improve reliability by establishing a trend and might enable the primary care team to identify children with growth disorders at an earlier stage. Considerable resources would be needed to achieve this. We have not so far seen any evidence that this would in reality improve the timeliness of diagnosis of growth disord-ers across whole populations.

Height velocity

Height velocity charts do not overcome the difficulties outlined above nor do they facilitate the detection of disordered growth. Growth data plotted on a growth velocity chart are no more informative than the same data correctly plotted on a height chart (see box on p. 169).

Correcting for prematurity

The limited evidence available suggests that growth measurements should be corrected for prematurity (i.e. born before 37 completed weeks gestation) until at least the age of 2 years (see HFAC4 website).

Parental heights

When there is concern about a child's height, it may be useful to obtain the heights of the parents and record them on the child's growth chart. However, interpretation of parental short stature as an explanation for short stature in the child needs experience and care. The height of both parents is not always available, though the height of one parent (or even a sibling) can be useful. Self-reported heights and estimated heights of partners are not very reliable. Very short parents may themselves have a growth disorder. At present, correction for parental height is too complex to be incorporated into screening.

Summary

Careful follow-up of infants at risk, responsive clinical care to parental concerns, a high awareness among all child health professionals of the importance of measuring children, and the implementation of a single screening height and weight measurement at around the age of 5 years should identify most children with abnormal growth. Facilities that allow referral from primary care for timely specialist assessment must be in place. A more intensive approach to GM, with multiple measurements, may have some benefits in terms of earlier diagnosis, but on current evidence these are likely to be very modest in relation to the extra resources required.

Obesity

The prevalence of obesity is increasing in children as well as in adults, to the extent that the term 'epidemic of obesity' is being widely used. A significant proportion (between one-third and two-thirds) of obese children will go on to be obese adults. The probability of tracking (obese child becoming obese adult) increases with the age of the child, the degree of overweight, and having obese parent(s). Obesity in children is associated with emotional and psychological distress and with an increased risk of type 2 diabetes, which is distinct from the familiar type 1 diabetes in children and the rare dominantly inherited maturity onset diabetes of the young (MODY) which begins in childhood. Obesity in adult life is associated with an increased risk of a number of disorders including coronary heart disease, hyperlipidaemia, various cancers, stroke, gall-bladder disease, type 2 diabetes, orthopaedic problems, and depression. Weight reduction is associated with a decreased risk of at least some of these disorders.

The causes of the epidemic are complex, but can be summarized as a shift in the balance between energy intake and energy expenditure. Genetic factors probably play a part but cannot explain the rapid increase in the last decade. There are several very rare single-gene disorders which cause massive obesity.

There is little doubt that reduced energy expenditure is a feature of current Western lifestyles, with more time spent in viewing television and playing and computer games, more labour-saving devices, and more use of cars as opposed to walking or cycling. There is less agreement as to whether, and how much, energy intake has increased, although changes in eating habits may be important—for example 'grazing', eating out, energy-dense snacks, fewer family meals, etc.

Identification

Identification of gross obesity is easy. Where there is concern that a child may be overweight, or frankly obese, his/her height and weight should be measured and the body mass index (BMI) calculated and plotted (see box).

Body mass index (BMI)

$BMI = (\text{weight in kg})/(\text{height in metres})^2$

BMI is the most convenient and widely used proxy for obesity. It correlates with total body fat but does not distinguish between muscle and fat. It is possible that in less fit children muscle mass is replaced by fat mass. Body proportions affect BMI. Other measures of obesity, such as waistline and skinfold, are potentially helpful but are not yet in regular use.

British BMI reference cut-offs
BMI ≥ 91st centile—overweight
BMI ≥ 98th centile—obese

The International Task Force on Obesity derived cut-off points linked to the adult cut offs of $25\,\text{kg/m}^2$ (overweight) and $30\,\text{kg/m}^2$ (obese) at age 18. These are under review.

Intervention

Children and families should be offered support to manage weight sensibly. Clinicians agree that even children who are concerned about their obesity, and wish to lose weight, have great difficulties in doing so. However, overweight children can be managed by a primary care team who have a positive attitude to weight management (*see* HFAC4 website). The child and family should want help and be willing to make lifestyle changes. They may need ongoing support to achieve small incremental changes in behaviour. A sustainable healthy lifestyle is the primary goal of management. A small number of children may need referral for specialist investigation, psychosocial help, or detailed dietetic advice.

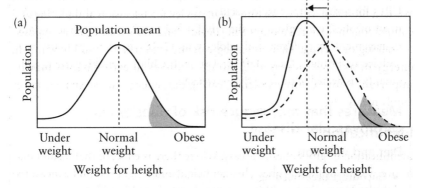

Fig. 8.2 (a) Interventions aimed at high-risk individuals who form the tail of the distribution curve. At best, only a small number of people benefit. (b) The potential benefits of shifting the whole distribution curve—small improvements in many people may improve the health of the population more than the targeted approach. Note, however, that while the concept is attractive, there is as yet no evidence either that this is achievable where obesity is concerned or that it could be done without any adverse effects. (Modified from Roberts, *What works*, Barnardos.)

Screening

The aim would be to identify the tendency to excessive weight gain early and prevent or reverse it. BMI charts are available and could be used for screening, but a consensus conference (*see* HFAC4 website) concluded that it would be inappropriate to recommend the use of BMI for population screening until there is a consensus as to what intervention programmes might be effective and a commitment to provide the necessary resources. However, population trends in BMI might be useful for monitoring the impact of public health interventions, and BMI is included in the proposed care public health dataset (see p. 347).

Prevention

A promising approach is prevention by encouraging physical activity (not only sport, but also daily activities such as walking, climbing stairs, etc.) and sensible eating, for example as part of the Healthy Schools initiatives (p. 117). This calls for a multisectoral approach and involves a wide range of measures aimed at weight control in all children, rather than targeting those who are overweight or at risk of obesity (Fig. 8.2). A programme that addresses the issue of obesity in the population as a whole will also be likely to reduce the risks of cardiovascular disease, diabetes, and cancer (box).

URLs for websites for cardiovascular disease prevention and the management of obesity are given on the HFAC4 website. An approach to weight management in children and adolescents (2–18 years) in primary care (Advice to Primary Care Staff for Use with Children Seeking Help with Obesity) is available on the HFAC4 website.

Measures that may reduce risk of obesity and cardiovascular disease

Diet and nutrition

- Encourage breastfeeding.
- Increase fruit and vegetable consumption (free fruit every school day to school children aged 4–6 years).
- Review food-related initiatives in schools (e.g. breakfast clubs, after-school clubs etc.) and involve children and young people in planning what is needed. NB Children generally *know* about healthy eating—more information is not the answer.
- Easy access to drinking water in schools to reduce consumption of sugary drinks ('Water is cool in school' campaign).

Physical activity

- Regard physical activity as a vital part of the curriculum and provide a wide range of options.
- Make school playgrounds safer and more enjoyable so that children can be more active.
- Increase access to exercise (e.g. investment in road safety schemes to promote walking and cycling, free or low-cost sports facilities).
- Promote reduced traffic speeds and introduce traffic calming or diversion so that children can play outside.
- Reduce television viewing.
- Increase accessibility and affordability of facilities for children and young people outside the home (swimming pools, skating rinks, clubs), so that going out and being active are more attractive than staying indoors to watch television or play computer games. UK provision for young people is among the worst in Europe.

Skills and self-esteem

Measures to increase self-esteem and social skills are likely to enhance children's enthusiasm for activities other than television and computer games.

Government action

Following the Government's acceptance of the National Audit Office's predicted economic loss to the economy in 2010 through overweight and obesity, the Department of Health is to lead a cross-cutting programme of measures to address the obesity epidemic.

(*See* HFAC4 website for further details)

Updates

4r

The National Screening Committee's Fetal, Maternal, and Child Health sub-group provides information on its website: www.nsc.nhs.uk/ch_screen/child_ind.htm

Growth monitoring recommendations have not changed with respect to the identification of medical disorders affecting growth. The main current issue is *obesity*. The best individual and public health approaches to tackle the obesity epidemic continue to stimulate much debate. Emerging evidence suggests that the origins of obesity can be traced back to early infancy. Changes in dietary effects are desirable and there has been much media interest in providing healthier school meals and teaching children to enjoy a wider range of foods. High energy sweet drinks are often available for purchase in schools and many authorities believe that they should be banned from school premises. Not all obese children or teenagers become obese adults and not all obese adults were obese as teenagers or children. In an environment that is conductive to obesity, diet and exercise need to be regarded as lifelong issues.

Regular weighing and measuring of school children in order to derive the BMI has been debated, partly as a result of the deliberations of the House of Commons Health Select Committee. Hall D, Cole TJ. What use is the BMI? *Arch Dis Child*, 2006; **91**: 283–286.

Current Department of Health Policy is to initiate a countrywide programme of weighing and measuring children on two occasions, so that BMI can be calculated and used for public health monitoring purposes; however, it is not intended to send that BMI measurement to the parents as there is currently no evidence that this would be beneficial and some concern that it may be confusing and even harmful. The guidance can be found at:

Measuring childhood obesity: guidance to primary care trusts: http://www.dh.gov.uk/obesity

In addition to the generic public health reports mentioned page 12, see:

Report on obesity—Royal College of Physicians of London: www.replondon.ac.uk/pubs/brochures/pub_print_SUP.htm

Australian review of obesity: *Medical Journal of Australia* 2005;**182**:130–5 www.mja.com.au/public/issues/

Jotangia D, Moody A, Stamatakis E *et al.* Obesity among children under 11. Dept of Health, 2005.www.dh.gov.uk/PublicationsAndStatistics/Publications/PublicationsStatistics

Reilly JJ, Armstrong A, Dorosty AR *et al.* for the Avon Longitudinal Study of Parents and Children Study Team. Early life risk factors for obesity in childhood: cohort study. (2005). http://bmj.bmjjournals.com

Government Response to the Health Select Committee's Report on Obesity (2004). http://www.dh.gov.uk/PublicationsAndStatistics/Publications/PublicationsPolicyAndGuidance/

Koplan JP, Liverman CT, Kraak VA eds, Committee on Prevention of Obesity. Preventing Childhood Obesity: Health in the Balance. http://www.nap/edu/catalog/11015.html

Lederman SA, Akabas SR, Moore BJ. Summary of the Presentations at the Conference on Preventing Childhood Obesity. *Pediatrics*; 2004; **114** (4); 1146.

Occipito-frontal head circumference (OFC)
Reasons for measuring the head circumference

The routine measurement of head circumference is intended to aid the detection of two groups of disorders—those characterized by a large head, and those characterized by a small head.

Conditions with enlargement of the head include hydrocephalus, subdural effusion, and haematoma, and a number of less common conditions associated with dysmorphic syndromes etc.

Hydrocephalus is characterized by a head measurement that is crossing centile lines upwards, together with the well-known features of suture separation, tense fontanelle, prominent veins, downward gaze, irritability, and sometimes developmental abnormalities. Early treatment for hydrocephalus is desirable, though there is no conclusive evidence that it improves outcome. A much more common cause of head enlargement is a familial large head, in which the growth line may cross centiles but the other symptoms are usually absent and a close relative, often the father, also has a large head circumference.

An abnormally small head is designated microcephaly. This may arise from some abnormality of brain development in the pregnancy, or may be a sign of impaired brain growth due to some peri- or postnatal brain injury. There is no specific treatment for microcephaly.

Very rarely microcephaly is associated with craniostenosis. Usually this condition results in an abnormally shaped head. A small but normally shaped head results only from total craniostensosis (i.e. affecting all the sutures of the skull), a condition which is extremely rare and is usually associated with other symptoms and signs such as irritability and vomiting. Early recognition of craniostenosis is important and should be included in teaching programmes; it is not necessarily detected by routine measurement of the head circumference.

Diagnosis of disorders affecting head circumference

These conditions cannot be diagnosed by measurement of the head circumference alone. Since 2 per cent of children have a head circumference above the 98th centile, and 2 per cent below the second centile, other evidence must be sought to determine whether a particular measurement is significant.

Head measurements well below the second centile are compatible with normal intellect. The probability of abnormality is higher if the measurement is below the −2.67 SD line (0.4 centile). Some ethnic groups tend to have smaller head measurements, and the use of growth charts not designed for them can be misleading.

There has been very little new work on head circumference measurement. The rate of head growth in the first year is often increased in children who are 4r subsequently diagnosed as autistic—this is an interesting finding on theoretical grounds but has negligible value as a diagnostic clue. *See* Courchesne E, Carper R, Akshoomoff N. Evidence of brain overgrowth in the first year of life in autism. *JAMA* 2003; **290**: 337–44.

Bigler ED, Tate DF, Neeley ES, et al. Temporal Lobe, Autism, and Macrocephaly *American Journal of Neuroradiology* 2003; **24**: 2066–76.

Screening and monitoring

A head circumference measurement in the neonatal period is potentially useful for two reasons. First, if the measurement is abnormal at this time, the problem is clearly of antenatal or intrapartum origin. Second, a baseline measurement may occasionally be useful if there is thought be rapid head growth in the early weeks of life. However, the measurement is, of little value if it is taken while there is still marked scalp oedema or moulding. A further measurement at the 6–8 week examination is usually recorded.

Continued monitoring of head growth after 8 weeks might be expected to facilitate early diagnosis of abnormalities such as hydrocephalus, but no evidence was found to suggest that there would be significant benefits from such a programme, or that they would outweigh the undoubted concerns and over-investigation that arise from over-referral of babies who are in fact normal.

Recommendations

◆ Staff training in measurement technique, the interpretation of growth charts (including the relevance of parental heights), normal growth and its variants, and the management of slow weight gain, failure to thrive, non-organic failure to thrive, and other disorders is vital.

◆ Every primary care team should have access to specialist advice for any infant or child with a possible growth disorder and the pathways for referral should be clearly established.

◆ There are opportunities to weigh the baby at each routine visit for a review or an immunization. This means that, at a minimum, babies will usually be weighed at birth, at 2, 3, and 4 months, and at 12–15 months.

◆ Accurate weighing requires that the baby is weighed nude unless there are special circumstances (e.g. a dressing or splint). In this case, the state of dress should be recorded. If the baby is weighed naked, the room must be warm.

◆ The baby may be weighed at other times if the parent or a professional considers it necessary. Facilities should be provided for the parents to weigh the baby when they wish. Professional advice should be available to help them interpret the results in private.

◆ Primary care staff must have access to suitable calibrated equipment (see p. 173) and an adequate supply of nine-centile growth charts (see p. 171) but should use the growth section of the Personal Child Health Record as the child's main growth record.

◆ Height should be measured with a Leicester Height Measure. If any other device is used, it must be calibrated regularly with a 1 metre rule.

◆ Scales should be checked and calibrated regularly.

◆ For infants born before 37 completed weeks gestation, correction for gestational age is essential up to the age of 2 years when plotting measurements on the charts.

◆ Measurements should be made in metric units (but should be converted to imperial units if parents so request), dated, recorded in figures as well as a point on the graph, and signed.

◆ Any child whose growth is causing serious concern to his or her parents should be assessed with care and considered for specialist referral.

◆ In the neonate, length should be measured and recorded in any infant who is premature, small for gestational age, or dysmorphic.

◆ At 6–8 weeks, length should be measured in any infant who was of low birth weight ($<2500\,g$), if any disorder is suspected or present, and in any infant whose health, growth, or feeding pattern is causing concern. It must be recorded on the chart.

- After 6–8 weeks, further length measurements should be taken when there are specific indications.
- Measurement of height and weight should be made at or around the time of school entry, preferably at about 5 years of age. These measurements should be stored so that BMI can be calculated and used as a public health indicator (rather than for clinical use with individual children).
- On the current evidence height monitoring after school entry can only be supported on a selective basis when there is concern about the child's health or growth or the child was not measured at school entry.
- Referral is usually indicated in any child who has a *single* length or height measurement below the 0.4 centile. Advice should be sought, though referral may not be necessary, in those with a single length or height measurement above the 99.6 centile.
- Whereas there is no dispute that single measures of height below the 0.4 centile should be taken seriously the interpretation of channel shifts over time ('slow growers') is more difficult. No firm recommendation can be made at this time but specialist advice should be requested if in doubt.
- Height velocity charts do not help to improve the accuracy of growth monitoring and are not recommended for routine use.
- Growth monitoring may be important in children with disabling conditions and dysmorphic syndromes. Growth charts are now available for children with Down's, Turner's and Noonan's syndromes and for achondroplasia, and these should be used.
- Meticulous growth data collection and storage for long-term audit and research are important and should be supported in those districts where sufficient expertise and commitment exist, but should not be regarded as a goal for every district.
- These recommendations may change in the light of further evidence about the treatment of 'normal short' children.
- Strategies to prevent obesity, such as increased physical activity and sensible eating, are to be encouraged at a community level.
- Screening of individual children for obesity is not recommended, but health professionals should offer support to children and families who want to control their weight.

Head circumference

- The head circumference should be recorded before discharge from hospital following birth. This is an important measurement and should be performed and recorded carefully. If there is excessive oedema or moulding of the scalp following birth this fact should also be recorded and if possible the measurement should be repeated a few days later.

◆ Head measurement should subsequently be undertaken at approximately 6–8 weeks of age. It should be plotted on the chart and also written in figures. If there is no concern at this time no further routine measurements are needed, but the OFC should always be measured and recorded if there is any concern about a baby's growth, health, or development.

◆ If the growth line is crossing centiles upwards and the child shows symptoms or signs compatible with hydrocephalus or other abnormality, specialist opinion is essential. If there are no accompanying symptoms or signs, two measurements over a 4-week period are acceptable. Beyond this time limit, a decision must be made either to accept the situation as normal or to refer the child for specialist examination.

◆ There is no justification for repeated measurements spread over many months, a practice which is to be deplored because it creates excessive anxiety. Modern imaging techniques make it simple to obtain a definitive diagnosis at an early stage.

◆ A head measurement above or below the ± 2.67SD line (99.6 and 0.4 centiles respectively) at any stage is an indication for more detailed assessment. A small or large head may be a reflection of genetic characteristics and the parents' head measurements should always be checked. If they are in keeping with that of the baby, and the baby appears to be developing normally, referral may not be necessary.

◆ If the growth line crosses centiles downwards but the baby is other-wise well and thriving, no special arrangements need be made. Concern should be expressed to the parents only if it becomes clear that the growth line is not only below the second centile but is also falling away from it.

◆ These apparently straightforward monitoring procedures must not be regarded as simple screening tests. Skill and judgement are required in deciding how to interpret the measurements and no single pass–fail criterion can be proposed.

Audit

The quality of measurement and charting, and the action taken when abnormality is suspected, should be reviewed. At local level, crude outcome indicators such as age of starting growth hormone treatment are not helpful because (a) numbers are small in any one district and (b) too many variables affect this indicator. The number of new cases detected by monitoring, their subsequent management, and the reasons for any delay in diagnosis are suitable topics for audit. Growth clinics should monitor their own performance in collaboration with district and tertiary services.

Research

Action research methods are needed because the speed at which the epidemic of obesity is developing suggests that we cannot afford to wait for additional data before instituting measures to tackle the problem. Specific issues include the following

♦ There are still unanswered questions regarding the definition, identification, prognosis and management of slow weight gain, failure to thrive and non-organic failure to thrive, and the role and value of 'thrive lines' in managing these problems. The relevance of regular weighing to the detection of psychosocial deprivation needs further evaluation.

♦ A study is needed to compare the recommendations set out above with a policy of height monitoring, in terms of sensitivity, specificity, and yield of new cases benefiting from treatment or intervention.

♦ There are wide variations in existing policy regarding GM in schools. In some districts, annual height measurements are still being undertaken to at least the age of 14. This 'natural experiment' should be used to ascertain the benefits of these more resource-intensive policies. It is only under these circumstances that its continuation can be supported.

♦ The optimum approach to service provision needs further study, taking account of the increase in referral rate which will inevitably accompany more determined efforts to improve early detection.

♦ BMI charts will need evaluation to determine whether and how they contribute to GM or management decisions.

♦ Assessment of measures to prevent and treat obesity are needed.

♦ Although the guidelines regarding head circumference monitoring are generally accepted in the UK, little is known about the accuracy, value, or optimal timing of regular head circumference measurement or the relative merits of different referral criteria.

Appendix: Regression to the mean*

Charts of weight attained, also known as weight distance charts, are derived from cross-sectional data, and they allow weight to be expressed as a centile

* Reproduced with permission of the BMJ Publishing Group from T.J. Cole, (1995). Conditional reference charts to assess weight gain in British infants. Archives of Disease in Childhood, 73, 8–16.

relative to the reference population, adjusted for age and sex. Such charts are also used to monitor weight velocity, on the grounds that a normally growing infant stays close to his or her chosen weight centile. This means that weight faltering is often inferred from the infant's weight falling across centiles. However, weight distance centiles should not be used in this way, as they are derived from cross-sectional data and cannot quantify changes in weight.

Over a period of time, infant weight tends to drift (or regress) towards the median—the tendency is to become less extreme with passing time. Thus an infant on the second weight centile is likely to show catch-up growth, whereas 98th-centile infants tend on average to catch down. A weight velocity reference that compensates for regression to the mean is called a conditional reference. It answers the question: 'Knowing the infant's previous weight, what is her likely weight now?'

The concept of regression to the mean is a statistical phenomenon. It states that if individuals or groups of individuals are weighed once, and later weighed again, their weight centile on the second occasion tends, on average, to be nearer the median than on the first occasion. This may seem counter-intuitive—surely an infant on, say, the second weight centile ought on average to stay there rather than move to a higher centile?

This phenomenon is about averages—it does not say that *every* infant on the second centile will catch up, only that a majority will. To see why, consider a randomly selected child at, say, 12 months of age. Knowing nothing about her we expect her to be average for her age, with an expected weight on the population median. Now imagine that we are given the information that her weight at 9 months was on the second centile. How should this extra knowledge alter our expectation of her weight at 12 months? The fact that she was below the median 3 months earlier obviously means that she ought still to be below the median, but by how much?

There is a range of possibilities. At one extreme, if weight tracks perfectly between 9 and 12 months, then we should expect her to remain on the second centile. Conversely, if there is no tracking at all between the two ages, our initial expectation will be unaltered, and we should still expect her to be on the median at 12 months. Thus the alternatives range from the second to the 50th centile, depending on how strongly weight tracks between 9 and 12 months. (Her *actual* centile at 12 months may well be below the second centile, but her average or expected centile will be above it.)

In this context tracking is synonymous with correlation, and perfect tracking requires perfect correlation. This is impossible, and so the extreme case of expecting her to remain on the second centile is ruled out. Her predicted weight centile at 12 months has to be above the second centile—less extreme than her weight centile at 9 month—and so her weight appears to regress towards the median. The same argument, in the reverse direction, applies to infants with weight centiles above the median.

The amount of regression to the mean depends on how highly correlated weights are at the two ages, and so the way to adjust for regression to the mean is to quantify this correlation.

Chapter 9

Laboratory and radiological screening tests

> This chapter covers:
> - Phenylketonuria and hypothyroidism
> - Other metabolic disorders
> - Cystic fibrosis
> - Duchenne muscular dystrophy
> - Urine analysis and urine infections, reflux
> - Haemoglobinopathies
> - Liver disease in infancy
> - Hypercholesterolaemia
> - Lead poisoning
> - Neuroblastoma and coeliac disease

In general, screening procedures requiring laboratory or radiological tests have been subjected to more critical evaluation than clinical examinations, presumably because of the obvious costs involved and the requirements for careful organization. Parents should be fully informed about each test and informed consent sought before it is performed.

4r   The National Screening Committee's Fetal, Maternal, and Child Health sub-group Electronic Library for Health provides information on screening at http://libraries.nelh.nhs.uk/uk/screening/

Neonatal blood-spot-based programmes

Neonatal phenylketonuria and congenital hypothyroidism screening

Screening programmes for phenylketonuria (PKU) and congenital hypothyroidism (CH) are well established. Their value is now accepted, and although they are expensive they are thought to be cost effective. The results of the PKU programme are good if care is coordinated by expert clinicians and dieticians. Age at the start of treatment and quality of phenylalanine control in the first few years of life are important determinants of psychological outcome. Therefore rapid referral of infants with positive screening tests to a specialist unit is mandatory.

The benefits of CH screening are worthwhile but are less impressive than in the case of PKU. The level of thyroid-stimulating hormone at the time of diagnosis, which is an indicator of the severity of hypothyroidism, is an important prognostic marker, suggesting that in severe cases the impairment of neurological development is not fully reversible.

Importance of audit, monitoring, and feedback

Streetley and Corbett co-ordinated a national audit of the programme in England and Wales from 1994 to 1997 (*see* HFAC4 website). A group of standards were developed and then the programme was audited. At that time few of the standards were met. A number of recommendations were made, including several that were to be undertaken on a national basis.

A Programme Centre has been set up under the National Screening Committee to undertake these functions for the PKU and CH screening programmes. In due course, it will take on this role for any other programmes that may be introduced for other inborn errors of metabolism. Audit and monitoring of the neonatal sickle cell screening programme (see p. 194) will also probably fall within its remit eventually.

It is vital to ensure continuing laboratory quality control, very high coverage, and prompt follow-up of positive screening tests. Litigation costs for 'missed' cases are already considerable and will rise inexorably. Audit reveals that there are several reasons why coverage may fall short of 100 per cent including long stays in neonatal intensive care units, homelessness, travelling families, etc.

Careful monitoring and clear accountability are essential if disasters are to be avoided, since the programme involves many different staff and procedures: blood sampling by midwives, testing by laboratories, processing of results by community child health departments, repeat tests done by health visitors, and referrals arranged through GPs.

Parents must be informed about the tests; this may involve both written information (nationally prepared leaflets and the Birth to Five book) and verbal explanation. They should be given the results—it is not safe for parents or professionals to assume that the result is normal unless they hear otherwise.

It may never be possible to screen 100 per cent of the population and no laboratory test can ever be totally reliable. The diagnoses of PKU and

CH should always be considered in appropriate clinical circumstances and there should be no hesitation in repeating the investigations whenever there is doubt. This is particularly important in the case of CH since, for a variety of reasons, the screening procedure misses a few cases.

Other inherited metabolic disorders

Screening for many other disorders is possible and is undertaken in some parts of the UK and in several other countries. Examples of conditions whose early detection may be both useful and cost-effective include galactosaemia, maple syrup urine disease, homocystinuria, medium-chain acylCoA dehydrogenase deficiency (MCADD), and biotinidase deficiency. A study of a screening programme for MCADD is under way. A decision whether to roll this out nationally is expected this year (2006). There are a number of issues that need to be resolved when introducing such a programme, as described in Dezateux C (2003). Newborn screening for medium chain acyl-CoA dehydrogenase deficiency: evaluating the effects on outcome. *European Journal of Pediatrics* **162(suppl 1)**: S25–S28. *see* link to article at www.springerlink.com

As predicted, the need for infrastructure to manage positive screening results and cases is proving quite a challenge. A useful parent information sheet can be found by following the link to 'Blood spot screening for MCADD' at www.bch.org.uk/departments/clinicalchemistry/neonatalscreeningservices.htm

Haemoglobinopathies

The two most important haemoglobinopathies are sickle cell disease (SCD) and the thalassaemias, although there are a number of other less common abnormal haemoglobins.

Approximately 3.3 per cent of the total UK population belongs to a racial group with a significant risk of having an abnormal haemoglobin. One person in 80 of West African origin and 1 in 200 of Jamaican origin has SCD. There are said to be over 9000 people with SCD in the London alone, and it is estimated that between 75 and 300 babies are born with the condition each year.

There is a significant morbidity and mortality from SCD particularly in the first 3 years of life. SCD is associated with impaired immunity and fulminating pneumococcal infection. This can be prevented by penicillin prophylaxis which needs to be started by 3 months of age. Pneumococcal vaccine may also be useful. Parents can be taught to recognize splenic sequestration crises.

In the UK there are an estimated 600 people with homozygous thalassaemia, mostly of beta type, and about 60 children are born each year with the condition. Children with thalassaemia usually present with anaemia and failure to thrive. These features should lead to early diagnosis, followed by treatment with blood transfusion and iron chelation therapy.

Screening programmes aim to reduce the morbidity and mortality rates of infants born with haemoglobinopathies. Antenatal screening followed by fetal diagnosis allows parental choice as to whether to continue with a pregnancy. The National Screening Committee has recommended that screening programmes for haemoglobinopathies should be introduced antenatally and neonatally. The precise details have yet to be finalized. In the neonatal period screening will be for haemoglobiopathies, making use of the blood already collected to screen for hypothyroidism and PKU. In the antenatal period thalassaemia and haemoglobinopathies will be screened for.

People with SCD often feel that their condition is poorly understood and that they do not receive the help they need when acutely ill. Screening for haemoglobinopathies should be undertaken in parallel with other improvements in the programme of care offered to individuals with these conditions. It is a complex undertaking, involving health education together with obstetric, haematological, genetic, and paediatric services. People with SCD may need practical help to improve quality of life, for example better housing to avoid cold damp conditions which may precipitate crises.

All children with SCD or thalassaemia should have access to a specialist team.

Progress in newborn biochemical screening   4r

◆ For an overview and regular updates, and information for parents, (including cystic fibrosis) *see*: www.newbornscreening-bloodspot.org.uk. Neonatal haemoglobinopathy screening is also under way *see* www.kclphs.org.uk/haemscreening/.

Cystic fibrosis

Screening for cystic fibrosis in the neonatal period is carried out in a number of places worldwide and parts of the UK. Irrespective of screening, the prognosis in this condition has improved considerably, and at least one country (Canada) has achieved improvement without screening that is equal to that attained in countries where screening has been implemented. Evidence from the largest controlled trial of screening suggests some improvement in growth and pulmonary function, but this is not conclusive. In view of the balance of the evidence and the fact that a significant part of the country already screens for the condition, it has been decided that neonatal screening should be universal in the UK. A screening algorithm has been agreed and implementation of this is underway.

4r

Muscular dystrophy

It is technically possible to screen all boys for Duchenne muscular dystrophy at birth, and some authorities have advocated this. The advantage of early diagnosis would be that the birth of further affected boys could be avoided. The main argument against this procedure has been that the total number of births thus prevented would be very small, so that the procedure might not justify its cost. A programme along these lines has been running in Wales for over 10 years. The Child Health sub-group of the NSC reviewed the evidence in 2004 and concluded that newborn screening could not be recommended at present

4r

An alternative approach is to screen all boys who first walk later than 18 months (the third centile), since 50 per cent of cases are late walkers (conversely, it can be calculated that between 0.5 and 1.0 per cent of late-walking boys have Duchenne muscular dystrophy). This proposal has not been widely adopted as formal screening policy and where implemented has not proved successful. However, a high index of suspicion should be maintained in this situation.

Liver disease in infancy: extrahepatic biliary atresia

The incidence of clinically significant liver disease in infancy is at least 1 in 3000 births. Of these, about one in five have extrahepatic biliary atresia (EHBA). Early referral of babies with this condition is important because surgery (the Kasai operation) is probably more effective if carried out at a major centre, preferably by 6 weeks of age. Other liver diseases (hepatitis, alpha-1 antitrypsin deficiency, galactosaemia, etc.) would also benefit from early diagnosis. In addition, the problem of bleeding due to vitamin K deficiency could be avoided.

There is currently no simple screening procedure for liver disease or EHBA. The clinical features of these conditions include prolonged jaundice with yellow sclerae, a high conjugated ('direct') bilirubin, and, in some cases, hypoglycaemia. Pale stools (white or chalky coloured) are an important feature of liver disease but are rare in healthy babies. When combined with jaundice, they are an indication for immediate referral.

From a screening perspective the difficulty is that benign prolonged jaundice (so-called 'breastmilk jaundice') is very common in breastfed babies, affecting around one baby in 10. Jaundice may persist to 6 weeks of age and sometimes considerably longer than this. Therefore, in breastfed babies, prolonged jaundice alone lacks specificity as a 'screening' test.

Any baby with prolonged jaundice combined with pale stools, any signs of illness, or any other abnormal feature should be referred immediately. In exclusively formula-fed babies, prolonged jaundice (beyond 3 weeks) is very uncommon and is in itself sufficient indication for referral.

Familial hypercholesterolaemia

This is a dominantly inherited disorder with an incidence of 0.1–0.2 per cent (1 in 500 to 1 in 1000). It carries a higher risk of early heart disease than does polygenic hypercholesterolaemia. It is not feasible at present to screen all children for this condition or for the other hyperlipidaemias. Screening and management of the relatives, including children, of any person suffering coronary heart disease at a young age (i.e. below 50 years for a male and below 60 for a female) remains controversial.

Subclinical lead poisoning

There is a robust association between elevated lead levels in the blood and teeth and reduction in intellectual functioning. It is not clear whether the association is causal. The magnitude of the effect is small and there is little evidence that intervention in children with no other clinical evidence of lead intoxication is likely to be beneficial or cost-effective. The American Academy of Paediatrics has proposed a screening programme for subclinical lead intoxication but there has been little support for this in the UK.

Miscellaneous
Screening in specific syndromes and disorders

In some conditions there are specific disorders that ought to be tested for at intervals. The management of any uncommon disorder should include a review of the recognized features and complications, and a plan should be made to ensure that relevant problems can be identified promptly. A familiar example is the high risk of hypothyroidism and hearing problems in Down's syndrome. Recommendations for screening in Down's syndrome can be found at the website of the Down's Syndrome Medical Interest Group (*see* HFAC4 website).

Urine infections

Urine examination as a screening test

Screening for proteinuria and for asymptomatic bacteriuria has been advocated in the past on the grounds that chronic pyelonephritis resulting in chronic renal failure might be a preventable condition. We could find no convincing evidence that this is a worthwhile procedure.

Management of urine infections

Primary care staff should be aware that urinary tract infection (UTI) is common in infants. UTI should be considered in any infant with an unexplained pyrexia of 38.5 °C or above and, if possible, a urine specimen should be obtained. Infants with a first UTI should be referred for investigation.

Vesico-ureteric reflux has an important association with urinary infections and there is a familial predisposition. It has been suggested that the siblings or children of any individual with this condition should undergo a micturating cystogram to ensure early identification.

The issues raised by antenatal ultrasound screening for urinary tract anomalies are outside the scope of this report.

Other screening programmes

There have been proposals that screening should be undertaken for neuroblastoma and for coeliac disease. The evidence to date does not support the introduction of either programme.

Recommendations

PKU, hypothyroidism, cystic fibrosis, and sickle cell disease

- ◆ Commissioners should identify one individual to take an overview of these screening programmes and ensure that referral, investigation, and management are well coordinated.
- ◆ Parents should know the reasons for doing these tests and should receive the results, whether positive or negative, in a timely fashion.

Other inherited metabolic disorders, and Duchenne muscular dystrophy

At the present time we recommend only that a high level of awareness is maintained regarding the presenting features of these conditions. Suspect cases should be referred for the appropriate diagnostic tests without hesitation. Purchasers should be aware that DNA technology may greatly extend the feasibility of and demand for screening in the next few years. This will bring with it new issues such as that of carrier detection. These must be addressed for each condition before screening can be introduced.

Urine analysis as a screening test

+ This is not recommended, but there should be a local policy regarding the referral and investigation of infants with urinary infections.

Further research is needed in this subject. There are practical difficulties in ensuring that all UTIs in infants are accurately diagnosed and appropriately investigated. The optimal approach to investigation of infants with a family history of reflux also needs further study. In July 2007, The National Institute for Health and Clinical Excellence (NICE) will be publishing guidelines on the diagnosis and management of urinary tract infections in infants and children. Screening for asymptomatic infection will not be covered.

Liver disease in infancy

+ Primary care staff should be aware of the possible significance of prolonged jaundice and should not readily dismiss it on the assumption that it is caused by breastmilk. The finding of pale stools and/ or yellow urine (provided that the baby is not dehydrated) should heighten suspicion and is an indication for immediate specialist opinion.

+ Some of the reported late diagnoses are due to delays in referral to specialist units. Paediatricians in turn should ensure that such babies are investigated promptly and, if conjugated hyperbilirubinaemia is found, consider referral to a specialist centre.

+ Until further evidence is available, no formal screening programme can be recommended.

Familial hypercholesterolaemia

+ Screening should be confined to the families of known sufferers from this condition.

Subclinical lead intoxication

◆ Screening for elevated blood lead levels is not recommended.

Neuroblastoma and coeliac disease

◆ Screening for these conditions is not recommended. (*See* HFAC4 website)

Chapter 10

Iron deficiency

This chapter:
- ◆ Defines iron deficiency
- ◆ Describes its effects
- ◆ Discusses screening and primary prevention
- ◆ Outlines recommendations

Definition

Iron deficiency anaemia (IDA) is defined in early childhood by a haemoglobin (Hb) level of less than 11 g/dl, together with other evidence of iron deficiency and a response to iron administration. Iron deficiency is not necessarily accompanied by anaemia. It can be defined by a transferrin saturation of less than 16 per cent, a serum iron of less than 14 μmol/l, a total iron-binding capacity of more than 40, or a serum ferritin of less than 10 mcg/l. Zinc proto-porphyrin (ZPP) levels have also been used to define iron deficiency. ZPP increases when erythropoiesis is ineffective, as in iron deficiency states, and a ZPP level of greater than 50 is suggestive of iron deficiency (although this may also occur in other disorders). Transferrin receptor concentration is also increasingly being used.

The predisposing factors and causes of iron deficiency include inadequate dietary intake of iron, often in association with drinking unmodified cow's milk ('doorstep' milk), prematurity and low birth weight, and the use of food stuffs and beverages (notably tea) which reduce the availability of iron for absorption. Unmodified cow's milk increases intestinal blood loss, although the significance of this is uncertain.

Effects

IDA is associated with deficits in a variety of developmental and behavioural measures, typically of between 10 and 15 points on standard tests such as the

Bayley test. These deficits are probably due to a direct effect on the brain rather than being a result of anaemia. The behavioural and intellectual deficits are reversible with iron therapy and, in view of the lower prevalence of IDA in older children, are assumed to recover spontaneously in many cases as the child's diet becomes more varied.

Long-term follow-up of children who have recovered from IDA shows some small persisting intellectual deficits, but these may reflect the adverse environment which caused the iron deficiency and should not be interpreted as evidence of irreversible impairment of brain development. The research evidence is currently unclear, especially as many studies have been performed in non-industrialized countries where there is significant comorbidity. Nevertheless, it seems undesirable for young children to suffer easily treatable nutritional deficits which might affect their developmental progress.

4r   The jury is still out on the importance of iron deficiency as a public health problem in the toddler age group; however, a recent systematic review found little evidence of motor or mental impairment in this age group: Sachdev, HPS, Tarun G, Nestel P (2005). Effect of iron supplementation on mental and motor development in children: systematic review of randomised controlled trials. *Public Health Nutrition* **8**, (2) 117–132. *see* www.ingentaconnect.com

Prevalence

IDA is a common disorder in pre-school children (Table 10.1). Various studies suggest a prevalence in the UK of between 5 and 40 per cent. It is thought to be more common in the underprivileged and in ethnic minorities, but in the population as a whole the correlation with socio-economic status is weak and it is by no means rare in the better-off. Less information is available for schoolage children, but the prevalence appears to vary between 3 and 10 per cent.

Table 10.1   Iron deficiency and anaemia*

Measurement	Prevalence (%)		
	$1^{1}/_{2}$–$2^{1}/_{2}$ years	$2^{1}/_{2}$–$3^{1}/_{2}$ years	$3^{1}/_{2}$–$4^{1}/_{2}$ years
Hb < 11 g/dl (all)	12	6	12
Hb < 10 g/dl	2	1	0
Ferritin < 10 mcg/l (all)	28	18	30
Ferritin < 5 mcg/l	9	3	7

* Based on a representative sample of 2101 children.
Source: Gregory, J.R., Collins, D.L., Davies, P.S.W., Hughes, J.M., and Clarke, P.C. (1995). *National diet and nutrition survey*, Vol. 1. HMSO, London.

Screening

A strong case has been made for the introduction of screening programmes for IDA, particularly in areas of poverty. Screening is acceptable to and popular with parents, the screening test appears to be simple and cheap, and an effective treatment is available.

Nevertheless, there are some arguments against screening.

1 The test requires a blood sample which some parents might see as an unnecessary intrusion.

2 Although haemoglobinometers are simple to use, meticulous technique in collecting the sample and using the instrument is essential, particularly when the diagnosis of IDA is based solely on the Hb level. The instruments available to primary care teams have a higher measurement error than those used in laboratories, and little is known about the sensitivity, specificity, and positive predictive value of Hb measurements carried out in the primary care setting. Severe IDA would probably be identified without difficulty, but detection of the mild cases who would form the bulk of the screen-positive children might be less reliable.

3 The timing of the screening test presents problems. Iron intake probably falls to a level below daily requirement in the second half of the first year in many at-risk children, but the child does not necessarily show biochemical evidence of iron deficiency or develop anaemia until considerably later. Thus many children who would pass the screening test at the age of 12 or 18 months become iron deficient in the third year. Conversely, some children who are iron deficient in the second year undoubtedly recover as they eat a more varied diet in the third and fourth years of life. The ALSPAC study found that a level of Hb below 9.5 g/dl at 8 months old is associated with a lowered locomotor score on the Griffiths Scales of Mental Development, measured at 18 months (*see* HFAC4 website). There was no such association at 12 and 18 months. This finding highlights the difficulty of deciding on an optimum age for screening.

4 The identification of children who are iron deficient but who have not yet developed anaemia could be facilitated by the use of other tests in addition to Hb, but this would complicate the procedure and increase costs. Some of the recommended tests would require a venepuncture rather than a capillary specimen. However, the evidence that iron deficiency without anaemia is harmful is still not convincing.

5 Iron deficiency is potentially preventable and resources should be devoted to primary prevention rather than screening (which is secondary prevention).

Primary prevention

In theory, this could be achieved by the following measures.

1 Provision of iron supplements for premature and low-birth-weight infants; this is now standard practice.

2 Not using unmodified cow's milk ('doorstep' milk) in the first year of life as the child's main milk drink (it is not necessary to eliminate it altogether). Note that although breastmilk has a low iron concentration, the bio-availability is very high.

3 Not giving young children tea.

4 Continued use of infant formula or follow-on milks in the second half of the first year of life.

5 Weaning onto mixed feeding at about 6 months of age.

6 Providing a source of vitamin C (fruit juice or ACD drops)—this increases iron availability.

7 As far as possible, use haem iron (i.e. from meat) as this is more bio-available.

8 Iron supplementation for *all* infants has been suggested and is the usual practice in some countries, but in the UK is only used to treat diagnosed IDA.

In some circumstances nutrition education may reduce the incidence of IDA but the impact appears to be variable and in some situations minimal. It must depend on a complex interaction between biological, cultural, and social factors.

All infant formula sold in the UK is iron fortified (5–8 mg/l). 'Follow-on' milks have no advantage over standard infant formula in the prevention of IDA and are not available under the Welfare Food Scheme. The use of infant formula or follow-on milks reduces the incidence of IDA, although the higher cost compared with doorstep milk is a problem for some parents. We are not aware of any direct comparison of standard and follow-on formula in the UK. A Canadian trial showed that follow-on formula was superior in preventing iron deficiency, but the level of iron in the standard 'comparison' formula was much lower than is usual in Europe.

The universal prescription of iron supplementation is routine in some countries and reduces the incidence of IDA substantially but has some disadvantages.

1 Some infants are reluctant to take iron medicine and this may cause feeding conflicts with the parent.

2 Iron in overdose is dangerous, and it is undesirable to keep hazardous medicines in homes with young children unless absolutely necessary.

3 It has been suggested (although the evidence is not persuasive) that iron treatment may increase the risk of infection and also may affect growth adversely.

4 Iron treatment could in theory increase iron overload in a child with undiagnosed thalassaemia. However, most cases of thalassaemia have presented before the age at which IDA becomes a common concern.

Recommendations

◆ Avoid early cord clamping at delivery.

◆ Encourage breast feeding with the introduction of a varied weaning diet after about 6 months of age.

◆ All parents should be informed about the advantages of infant formula feeding over doorstep milk and the use of doorstep milk as the main drink should be discouraged, at least until the first birthday.

◆ The use of ACD vitamin drops (available free under the Welfare Food Scheme) should be encouraged.

◆ All members of the primary health care team should be aware of the high incidence of IDA.

◆ In districts or localities where there is severe socio-economic deprivation and a substantial proportion of ethnic minority families, existing screening programmes should be continued provided that they are adequately monitored, are shown to be reaching those members of the community most at risk, and are accompanied by continuing efforts at primary prevention.

◆ We do not think that the evidence supports the extension of whole-population screening programmes at present, *except* as a means of measuring the effectiveness of intensified efforts at primary prevention in a carefully planned project.

◆ Efforts at primary prevention should be intensified. However, advice on good nutrition for young children should not be given in isolation but should be part of a wider programme of support, particularly for vulnerable families who need extra support (p. 30).

◆ The advice of a dietician familiar with the dietary customs of other ethnic groups and cultures should be available to the primary health care team.

+ Iron supplementation for premature and low-birth-weight (small for gestational age) infants should be given.

+ Universal iron supplements are not recommended. A 4–6 week course of iron therapy should be given to any infant whose Hb is below 11 g/dl, unless there is any other obvious explanation, and the Hb should then be re-checked.

+ The Hb should be checked in any infant whose diet is causing concern. This can best be achieved by ensuring easy access to a haemoglobinometer in the primary care setting, but those who use it must be familiar with the technique and interpretation.

+ Any infant whose Hb is below 7.5 should also have a full blood count and an assessment of iron status. If thought to be indicated by the laboratory, thalassaemia and sickle cell disease should be excluded. The laboratory should advise the primary health care team on the interpretation of the results. (NB: It can be difficult to exclude thalassaemia trait in children with iron deficiency, but it is doubtful whether this is necessary if the Hb level responds to iron, since the diagnosis is of no relevance in infancy or childhood.)

Research needs

It is still not clear why some infants become iron deficient while others do not. Dietary variables do not seem to be the complete explanation. Differences in weaning practices, temperamental differences in the readiness of infants to eat new foods, variations in iron stores earlier in infancy, and individual differences in the absorptive capacity for iron may all play a part.

The apparent lack of effectiveness of health education measures in changing feeding practices needs further study.

Although the short-term impact of IDA on development seems to be beyond question in early infancy and in toddlers, less is known about these effects in older children or teenagers.

Chapter 11

Screening for hearing defects

> This chapter:
> - describes and defines hearing loss
> - summarizes the epidemiology
> - describes the impact of hearing loss on development
> - lists and discusses the various approaches to screening
> - makes recommendations for practice, monitoring, and research

Hearing impairment is of two main types.

- **Sensorineural hearing loss (SNHL)** is caused by a lesion in the cochlea or the auditory nerve and its central connections. It may be unilateral or bilateral. Important causes and risk factors are summarized in Table 11.1.

- Conductive hearing loss is related to abnormalities of the ear canal or middle ear.

Permanent childhood hearing impairment (PCHI)

This term includes SNHL and the small percentage of children with permanent conductive hearing losses who require the same intervention as SNHL cases with equivalent degrees of hearing impairment (e.g. bilateral atresia, branchial arch syndromes affecting the ossicles, etc).

Impact of PCHI

In the absence of early and appropriate intervention, children with PCHI suffer substantial impairment of language acquisition. Educational difficulties follow and lead in turn to social isolation, an increased risk of mental

Table 11.1 Epidemiology, risk factors, and causes of hearing loss

- The estimated birth prevalence of congenital sensorineural or mixed hearing impairment ($40 dBHL in the better ear averaged over the frequencies 0.5,1,2, and 4 kHz) is 1.16 per 1000.

- 1.3 per 1000 children have this degree of hearing loss and require a hearing aid; the difference is accounted for by acquired and conductive hearing loss.

- Meningitis is the most important cause of acquired hearing loss and accounts for up to one-fifth of profound hearing loss although this figure has fallen since the introduction of Hib and meningococcal vaccines and the consequent fall in the incidence of the respective forms of meningitis.

- Ascertainment of less severe hearing loss in pre-school children is incomplete, but at least 0.3 per 1000 have a hearing loss which, although less than 40 dB, is clinically significant and requires a hearing aid.

- The incidence of SNHL is at least 10 times higher in babies admitted to neonatal intensive care units (NICUs) than in the 'normal' population. There are a number of risk factors including low birth weight, gestational age below 32 weeks, prolonged ventilation, prolonged jaundice, ototoxic drugs, hypoxic ischaemic encephalopathy, neonatal meningitis, etc., but in practice a simple guideline, such as a NICU stay of more than 48 hours, may define the at-risk population more simply. A substantial proportion (over half in some series) of these babies have other disabilities as well.

- Other factors which increase the risk of hearing loss include congenital infections (rubella, cytomegalovirus), dysmorphic syndromes, particularly those affecting the head and neck, family history of a close relative who needed a hearing aid before the age of 5 years, acute bacterial or tuberculous meningitis, and mumps (usually unilateral).

- If all high-risk factors are considered, between 40% and 70% of all cases could be identified by testing between 5% and 10% of all babies. This yield can only be obtained by a systematic and well-organised approach to the identification and testing of at-risk babies. Universal neonatal screening is a much better option.

- Conductive hearing loss is extremely common. At least half of pre-school children have one or more episodes of OME. A much smaller number of children (perhaps around 7%) have OME for at least half of the time between 2 and 4 years (see Fig. 11.1).

health problems, and reduced prospects for independence in adult life. Intervention through quality early years support including auditory habilitation, educational input, and social input will help the child acquire a means of communication by speech, signing, or both.

Acquired conductive hearing loss

Acquired conductive hearing loss is associated with middle-ear pathology. In developed countries this is usually due to secretory otitis media, now more commonly known as otitis media with effusion (OME). Chronic suppurative

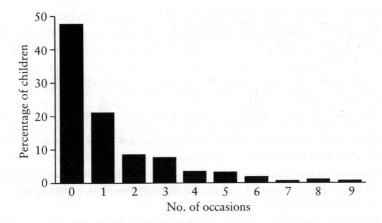

Fig. 11.1 Persistence diagram of OME. The definition of OME was bilateral flat tympanograms, indicating fluid in both ears. Over 1000 children were tested on nine occasions at 3-month intervals. In 69 per cent of cases, OME either did not occur or was transient. In 7.3 per cent of cases, OME was present for at least half the study period. There is as yet no way of identifying the group with prolonged OME except by serial testing of all children (at least four times), and therefore no feasible screening programme which could select this high-risk group. The solution is (a) to find markers which will indicate persistence of OME without the need to test every child serially or (b) to focus on the disability caused by OME (clinically evident hearing impairment, language delay, or unexplained behavioural problems). Solution (a) is preferable as it would offer the possibility of primary prevention; solution (b) is the only option available at present.

Based on Nijmegen cohort, data reworked by Stephenson et al., presented and discussed by Haggard. Acknowledgments to authors and Nuffield Hospitals Trust.

otitis media with discharge and perforation is much less common, although the prevalence may be higher in poorer communities. SNHL and middle-ear disease may coexist.

The list of known risk factors for OME reflects the three major influences: ear infection, nature of the mucosal immune response, and anatomical maturity for clearing secretions from the Eustachian tube. Parental smoking is also important. Breastfeeding may be protective. The role of allergy is uncertain but is probably relevant only to a few. Some children are at particular risk of developing persistent OME, including those with Down's syndrome, cleft palate, Turner's syndrome, and facial malformation syndromes.

The nature and extent of the disability caused by OME is still controversial. It is likely that in those children with occasional self-limiting episodes, OME probably has a minimal influence on speech and language development, but severe persistent OME may result in significant delay in language acquisition, behaviour disturbance, and in some cases temporary impairment of balance. However, few research studies have differentiated between those children with transient OME and minor hearing impairment, in whom the effects are likely to be transient, and those with persistent disease and more marked hearing loss which may have more impact. In addition, it is highly likely that hearing loss interacts with other factors, such as environmental deprivation, temperament, and genetic influences, on the rate of language acquisition. Unilateral or asymmetric hearing loss may cause short-term deficits in the ability to localize sound and to distinguish important sounds such as speech from back ground noise.

Treatment

Conservative management is advocated for the majority of children who are not severely affected. Decongestants are not effective. Antibiotic and steroid therapy have limited benefits and significant side-effects.

Surgery to ventilate the middle ear is effective while the inserted grommets remain patent. The persistence of the condition, and hence the ability to benefit from treatment, will be short-lived for many children but nevertheless these benefits may be important for the young child during the phase of rapid language acquisition, the long-term benefits of surgery are uncertain but are enhanced by adenoidectomy, particularly in those children who are prone to repeated ear infection. Adenoidectomy is of less value in those whose problem is persistent OME.

The provision of a hearing aid can help the most severely and persistently affected children, who often face repeat operations. Continued audiological and educational supervision is essential.

Simply explaining the nature of the problem to parents or teachers is often helpful. Once they understand that the child has a hearing loss, they can communicate more effectively. Written information such as leaflets on glue ear (see HFAC4 website) and access to other sources about OME should be available. A copy of the child's test results or audiogram, with appropriate explanation, is reassuring.

Unilateral hearing loss

Unilateral hearing loss is generally assumed to be primarily a social disadvantage in school, but it has been suggested that there may be subtle yet significant effects on cognitive development. When identified early, there may be benefits to both child and parents in terms of earlier aetiological diagnosis. Unilateral hearing impairment will be detected as part of the universal programme. Further research is needed on this issue.

Early diagnosis and intervention for PCHI

There are several reasons for the current professional commitment to early diagnosis of PCHI.

♦ There is growing confidence that early diagnosis and intervention do improve the outcome in terms of speech and language quality, communicative skill, and emotional development. A definitive demonstration of this presents considerable research problems, since the age of diagnosis and of commencing intervention depend on many factors, including the family's social and communicative skills and attitudes which are in turn an important determinant of outcome. Furthermore, the potential benefits of early intervention are unlikely to be realized unless families receive good quality support (from health, education, and social care services) and counselling, as well as guidance on amplification and communication.

♦ Animal studies suggest that there is a sensitive or critical period for learning. Brain plasticity is greatest early in life, and meaningful sound input may be necessary to facilitate the development of neural connections. Current experience with cochlear implantation in children suggests that the first 6 months of life may be of particular importance, although good results have been obtained in some children up to the age of 10 years.

♦ It is easier to achieve high coverage for screening and early detection services for babies in the first year of life than at any time subsequently until school entry.

♦ Most parents welcome early diagnosis of disabling conditions and have a low opinion of services which fail to identify serious long-term problems in their children.

♦ It is easier to establish the cause of PCHI if it is diagnosed early. In particular, intra-uterine infections become increasingly difficult or impossible to diagnose after the first few months of life.

Views of the Deaf community

Deaf children of deaf parents are a special case. The aim of early diagnosis is to improve oral communication, but the strong views of some members of the Deaf community on signing should be remembered and respected. It should not be assumed that every hearing-impaired parent will unreservedly welcome early screening for their infant.

Arguments in favour of screening

Parents sometimes recognize severe hearing loss themselves, but hearing loss of moderate degree, or predominantly affecting high frequencies, is easily missed, sometimes for several years. Therefore a good case can be made for screening.

Since most cases of significant SNHL are congenital and the process of language acquisition begins at birth, the obvious time to screen is in the neonatal period. However, even universal neonatal screening would not detect all children with hearing loss for the following reasons.

• SNHL due to congenital rubella and cytomegalovirus may deteriorate during the first 2 years of life, even though not readily detectable in the neonatal period.

• Some types of genetically determined SNHL are progressive and may present at any time in childhood. Until recently it has been thought that this applied only to a very small proportion of cases, but follow-up of large cohorts who had been shown to have normal hearing in the neonatal period suggests that hearing loss with an onset in the first year of life may be rather more common, perhaps at least 10 to 15 per cent.

Are there any disadvantages to screening? In studies on universal neonatal screening, a small percentage of parents refuse the offer of a screening test. Some parents observe their baby respond to sound and decide that screening is superfluous. A few parents may suspect that their baby has a hearing loss but would prefer to put off the moment of diagnosis. The psychological reasons for these behaviours are probably complex and need further study. They might represent protection of self or partner against intolerable stress in the face of other life problems. It is clear that sensitivity to parental feelings is important. A screening test which seems routine to staff might be a major life event for the parent if the child turns out to have a hearing loss. Better information before and with the test may overcome some of these problems.

Approaches to screening

There are many possible strategies for screening for hearing loss.

Neonatal screening

Universal neonatal screening

This is now regarded as the ideal approach since it allows early diagnosis and intervention. It offers access to a 'captive population', making it possible to achieve high coverage rates, although the rapid turnover and early discharge policy in most maternity units makes this more difficult than might first appear.

All areas in the UK now have universal neonatal screening, either in hospital, or in the community. The primary screening test is automated otoacoustic emissions (AOAE), followed, for those who fail, by automated auditory brainstem responses (AABR)—see below for more details. Most areas aim to screen babies before they leave the maternity unit, while a few only screen babies after they have gone home. Systems are in place to test those babies 'missed' by hospital screening programmes, because they go home too early. Clinical management of babies found to have a unilateral hearing loss, as a byproduct of the screening protocol, will also be considered.

The main cost of universal neonatal screening is in personnel. The tasks of providing training for screeners, ensuring that all infants are tested (including those discharged from hospital early, born at weekends or holidays, or at home), and maintaining standards present challenges which should not be under-estimated.

Selective neonatal screening of high-risk groups (Table 11.1)

Case-finding may be achieved via antenatal departments, neonatal intensive care units, postnatal wards, and the primary care team. The programme can be brought to parents' attention at antenatal classes and by devoting a page to hearing and risk factors in the Personal Child Health Record. This is a second-best approach as only about 40 per cent of cases of congenital SNHL will normally be detected in this way; the rest are in the low-risk population.

Methods used for neonatal screening

The auditory response cradle (ARC) is an automated behavioural method which detects changes in the infant's head turns and bodily movements in response to a sound stimulus. This device was not designed, and is not suitable, for premature babies. Its sensitivity for the less severe degrees of SNHL is relatively low and it is unlikely to detect all cases with losses of 50 dB or greater, which is usually regarded as the desirable criterion for neonatal screening. It is not currently recommended.

Automated otoacoustic emissions (AOAE) are acoustic responses produced in the inner ear by the outer hair cells of the cochlea and detected with a sensitive microphone placed in the ear canal. AOAE screens the auditory pathways as far as the cochlea. It is a very sensitive test and detects hearing losses as low as 30 dBHL. In the Rhode Island study, for example, AOAE screening resulted in identification of six cases per 1000 births (including unilateral). In the New York State demonstration project 154 children out of 43 081 had a hearing loss, but only 42 had bilateral SNHL that was moderate, severe or profound. The test is easier and quicker than AABR (see below) and has been used in several centres for universal screening. Unfortunately, there is a high rate of inconclusive responses in the first 2 days of life; around

60 per cent pass at or before 6 hours of age, 80 per cent pass between 6 and 12 hours, and over 95 per cent pass thereafter. Half the inconclusive responses are unilateral and half are bilateral. Ambient noise and technical difficulties may be partly responsible but can be overcome. Fluid in the middle ear and maturational delays are thought to be the main reasons for the high rate of inconclusive responses.

Automated auditory brainstem response (AABR) audiometry is an 'objective' method involving the computer analysis of EEG signals evoked in response to a series of clicks. AABR screens the auditory pathways as far as the brainstem. A full auditory brainstem response study is a skilled undertaking, but automated screening devices can be operated by unqualified staff after appropriate training and have been used for neonatal screening of high risk babies. AABR is generally thought to be too time consuming as the primary test for universal screening but may be appropriate in high-risk populations such as premature babies where prevalence of PCHI is greater. Even in skilled hands, diagnostic ABR testing may produce results which are difficult to interpret, particularly in NICU infants, and in some cases hearing loss has been incorrectly diagnosed. For this reason, audiologists are careful to confirm the diagnosis of PCHI before fitting hearing aids.

The recommended procedure

Current recommendation is that all babies should have an AOAE. Those who have a normal response are regarded as passing the screen, although it is possible for an infant to have a 'normal' emission with a limited frequency range of normal hearing. Those with an unsatisfactory or inconclusive response undergo a second AOAE screening. All babies who do not pass the second AOAE screen should then undergo an AABR. Parents are told that the child has, or has not, shown a clear response to the newborn hearing test, rather than using the terms 'pass' or 'fail'.

Making use of parental observations

These can be enhanced by the use of a check list in the Personal Child Health Record, which alerts parents to the existence of hearing loss in babies and tells them what to look for. Parents are more likely to identify severe and profound hearing loss and may easily overlook less severe or high-frequency impairments.

Behavioural testing during the first year of life

The technique, which is known as the **distraction test**, was the mainstay of screening in the UK for some decades. It required two people working in collaboration and depends on the infant's ability to turn and localize a sound source. A developmental maturity level of around 7 months is optimum for this test. Before this age, sitting balance, head control, and sound-localization ability are imperfect. Beyond 10 months of age, the development of object permanence and increasing sociability make the test more difficult.

Pre-requisites
Quiet conditions, adequate sound-level monitoring, and careful technique are essential. Good results can be obtained if initial and regular refresher training courses are provided to ensure that technique is meticulous and standard guidelines are observed. Adequate testing conditions, proper equipment, and protected time are essential.

Hazards and problems of the distraction test
Many staff are still very committed to the distraction test and believe that it is valuable. It is possible that there is a publication bias and that districts whose results are satisfactory do not publish them. However, the published studies on the performance of this screening procedure under field conditions are not encouraging. This is partly because few districts fulfil all the conditions set out above. Problems include the following.

◆ The main limitation of the test is that it cannot pick up children until they are at least 6–7 months old, and so an opportunity has been missed to institute management earlier.

◆ Uptake is often unsatisfactory and the incidence of hearing loss is higher in non-attenders.

◆ The sensitivity of the test in practice is often low and many cases are missed.

◆ Poor test technique generates a large number of false positives.

◆ The procedure, if properly performed, identifies many genuine but transient cases of hearing loss due to middle-ear disease. These rarely require treatment, but increase waiting times for definitive diagnosis for those children with more serious problems.

◆ Parents' concerns and important risk factors are often ignored and inappropriate reassurance is given on the basis of inadequate testing—in these circumstances the screening test is not merely valueless but can be positively harmful, because the child's apparent responses to sound may persuade parents that their own worries about the child's hearing were unfounded. This can lead to delays in identification.

◆ The test has also been used, inappropriately in our view, to 'screen' babies with high-risk factors such as a positive family history or a long stay in

NICU. For several reasons such babies may be particularly difficult to test and should be referred for definitive diagnosis if this was not done in the neonatal period.

Dual pathology

Children can have both CSNHL and middle-ear disease. Sometimes the hearing impairment is attributed only to the middle-ear disease and the child may be referred for ear, nose, and throat (ENT) management. Unless the hearing is re-checked at intervals, the sensorineural component of the hearing loss can easily be overlooked for many months.

Improving the distraction test

Costs can be reduced if the test is done by one health visitor and one assistant. This can be done without any fall in standards. It has also been suggested that the hearing level at which the baby 'passes' might be raised, since this would reduce the number of false-positive results while missing very few significant cases of SNHL.

Economic aspects

With increasing public awareness of hearing problems and high-risk factors, many children (including most of those with risk factors) are diagnosed before the age at which the test is normally performed. If 40 to 50 per cent of all cases are found by a high-risk screening programme and parents identify a further proportion themselves, it is unlikely that the distraction test will detect more than one-third of the total number of cases and a quarter or a fifth may be more realistic. Thus, the 'incremental yield' (p. 138) will be relatively small and the cost per case detected correspondingly high.

The cost per case detected is greatly reduced if cases of OME discovered by screening are included. However, this is not generally regarded as the function of the distraction test, for reasons set out previously.

Testing between the ages of 18 and 42 months

In this age group it becomes possible to test hearing by methods involving cooperation.

Speech discrimination tasks, such as the McCormick Toy Test, require the child to respond by pointing to a series of objects named by the examiner in a very quiet voice. An automated version of the Toy Test is now available. These tests are enjoyed by children, and are easily learnt and applied accurately. Most children can perform these successfully by 39 months of age. At or beyond this age, inability to cooperate with the Toy Test is suggestive either of a hearing difficulty or some more general developmental problem.

The child may be required to give some behavioural response to measured sound, produced either by voice or by a warbler or audiometer. These 'performance tests' are capable of giving accurate results if the tester is adequately trained and are particularly useful when testing children whose first language is not English and no staff are available who speak the child's own language.

The more mature and cooperative child can be tested with headphones (pure-tone audiometry).

The 'intermediate' screen

We considered whether any further pre-school screening test of hearing should be undertaken after the age of 7 months. This has been called the 'intermediate' screen. The argument in favour is that a few children with acquired or progressive SNHL and those with severe OME may otherwise elude diagnosis until they start school, with possibly serious consequences for their learning and education.

The disadvantages of such a policy are as follows.

+ The low yield of important new cases.

+ The high incidence of transient OME.

+ The difficulty of determining which cases of OME are transient and which are persistent (see Fig. 11.1). The ability to predict which cases would suffer some disability from their OME would be a useful advance, but as yet no such method is available.

Children with problems which might be associated with hearing impairment (delayed language development, behavioural disturbance, etc.) need a hearing assessment (see Chapter 13).

The school entry 'sweep' test of hearing

This test consists of a modified pure-tone audiogram performed at fixed intensity level. Criteria for referral on this test vary from 20 dB, through 25 dB, to 30 dB at one or more frequencies and after one or two tests. Many variables affect the results of this procedure, including ambient noise, the skill of the screener, and the maturity of the child.

A questionnaire to parents has been developed on a large sample. This has not yet been evaluated in a further field trial. It may not be effective in deprived areas or ethnic minorities but the cost is low and it may complement case-finding by teachers.

The school entrant 'sweep' test is used in most districts in the UK. Following the introduction of universal neonatal hearing screening in Wessex, the number of children with significant bilateral SNHL diagnosed after 6 months old has fallen from 69% to 34% (Kennedy C, McCann D, Campbell MJ, Kimm L, Thornton R.Universal newborn screening for permanent childhood hearing impairment: an 8-year follow up of a controlled trial. *Lancet* 2005; **366**: 660–2). In addition to this group, at school entry, there will be some children who are newly moved into the UK or have an acquived or progressive loss. A significant number of milder cases are detected, and unilateral losses are usually identified for the first time. OME is very commonly detected at this stage, and may have educational implications even though few children require active treatment. Since the referral criteria and management of OME remain controversial and treatment resources are overstretched, each district and health board should define precisely its own policy and referral pathways, and monitor the results.

Further screening tests of hearing after school entry appear to have a very small yield and we do not think that they can be justified. However, hearing should be assessed in any child experiencing learning, behavioural, or speech and language difficulties.

Impedance measurement

Impedance measurement is a technique for assessing middle-ear function and therefore for detecting fluid in the middle ear. It does not give a direct measure of hearing levels. It is a very sensitive test which detects even minor degrees of middle-ear dysfunction and is best reserved for use as a diagnostic procedure in specialist clinics. It should not be used as a primary screening procedure for pre-school children. Although it has been suggested that school entrant screening might be improved by addition or substitution of impedance screening, this proposal on its own would introduce too many non-specific referrals to be practicable.

Acquired hearing loss—meningitis

Early diagnosis reduces the incidence of most complications of acute bacterial meningitis. *All* young children who have had this condition should have an audiological assessment before or soon after discharge. Profound hearing loss following meningitis in a young child is an educational emergency, since the benefits to the child of having had previous experience of sound will be squandered if amplification and teaching are not provided promptly. An early assessment for cochlear implantation is also mandatory as this may become technically difficult or impossible if delayed too long.

4r Updates

Audiology services for children have been reviewed and proposals made for further work: www.rcpch.ac.uk

Newborn hearing screening is now established throughout the country. For a progress overview in implementing newborn hearing screening: http://www.nhsp.info/.

See also two useful reports on screening in Victoria, Australia:

Hearing impairment: a population study of age at diagnosis, severity, and language outcomes at 7–8 years. Wake M, Poulakis Z, Hughes EK, *et al.* (2005). *Archives of Disease in Childhood* **90**(3):238–44. http://adc.bmjjournals.com/cgi/content/full/90/3/238

Russ SA, Poulakis Z, Wake M, *et al.* (2005). The distraction test: the last word? *Journal of Paediatric and Child Health* **41**:197–200.

Hearing screening policy offers a good example of how research should be put into practice. Early results suggest that neonatal screening not only works as a screening programme but results in better outcomes for children. *See* C Kennedy and D McCann (2004). Universal neonatal hearing screening—moving from evidence to practice. *Archives of Disease in childhood: Fetal and Neonatal Edition* **89**;378–383. http://fn.bmjjournals.com/cgi/content/full/89/5/F378

Recommendations

Need for a well-organized audiology service

The first step in considering the following recommendations for screening must be to examine the whole paediatric audiological service and to review present and future staffing needs. There is no point in creating an excellent screening network if the facilities for behavioural testing, definitive AABR studies, ENT assessment, diagnosis, or education and rehabilitation are inadequate. All parents with hearing-impaired children should have access to a centre with such facilities, and the need for paediatric, educational, social care, psychological, and genetic advice must be met. The term 'family-friendly hearing service' has been proposed to capture these demanding requirements.

Working together is essential for a well-organized service and an **audiology working group** (children's hearing services group) should be created as defined by the National Deaf Children's Society with a named co-ordinator to act as a contact and reference point (*see* HFAC4 website) This group must include parental representation.

A systematic approach to increasing parental awareness about hearing loss, such as the use of a check list (*see* HFAC4 website for examples), should be adopted in all districts, irrespective of any other measures to ascertain children with hearing loss. The full potential of this approach has yet to be adequately explored and evaluated but there is sufficient professional support for us to recommend it as a matter of policy.

Parental suspicions about possible hearing loss must be taken seriously and a rapid efficient referral route to an audiological centre must be available in *every* part of the country. No parent who expresses concern about a child's hearing should be denied prompt referral to the audiological service.

Neonatal screening

Following a recommendation from the National Screening Committee, universal neonatal hearing screening has been set up throughout the UK. The primary screening test is automated otoacoustic emissions (AOAE), followed, for those referred, by automated auditory brainstem responses (AABR). Those units that aim to test babies before they leave hospital must have systems in place to test those babies discharged before being tested. A few areas aim to test babies after they leave hospital. Babies with a unilateral hearing loss should be followed up.

The distraction test

♦ Once universal neonatal screening has been in place for more than 8 months, universal distraction testing should be abandoned

♦ Distraction testing should only be undertaken by those properly trained, with regular updates

♦ Parental awareness, perhaps via PCHR (Chapter 17), and staff receptiveness need to be maintained and in some areas improved

'Intermediate' screening

Intermediate screening (screening between the first year and school entry) is not recommended. However, it should be routine to ask the parents of pre-school children whether they have any concerns about the child's hearing. An audiological assessment should be arranged for any child who has:

♦ significantly impaired language development

♦ a history of chronic or repeated middle-ear disease or upper-airway obstruction

♦ developmental or behavioural problems.

Quality standards for services have recently been published (*see* HFAC4 website).

We emphasize that, even when universal neonatal screening has been implemented, substantial numbers of children will need assessment in the 'intermediate' years. Most of these will have OME. A well-run clinical service can ensure that those few children who need a surgical opinion or intervention are selected for referral to an ENT surgeon without creating long waiting lists.

Children with conditions which put them at high risk of middle-ear disease should be assessed at regular intervals in a clinic with full diagnostic facilities including impedance equipment.

The **school entry sweep test of hearing** should be continued while further evidence on its value is collected. The diagnostic and referral pathway must be evaluated as well as the sweep test itself. After this, no further routine screening test of hearing is recommended.

Impedance tests should not be regarded as a screening procedure.

Acquired hearing loss

Audiological assessment and follow-up should be arranged for any young child who has had bacterial meningitis, prolonged treatment with ototoxic drugs, or severe head injury, either before or soon after discharge from hospital.

Organization and equipment

It is important that health authorities provide adequate conditions for hearing testing and that the staff involved have their own hearing tested every 2 years.

All staff involved with screening tests of hearing should have access to the necessary equipment (sound-level meters, warble-tone generators, etc.) and proper training in their use. Equipment should be checked and calibrated regularly.

Coordinator

Arrangements should be made in each PCO, district, or health board for co-ordinating the local paediatric audiology programme, including screening, monitoring, training, and refresher courses. Information should be collected on the uptake of screening programmes, the number of referrals, delays experienced between referral and diagnosis and between diagnosis and treatment, and the age at which each child with SNHL is diagnosed. Liaison with other disciplines and agencies is vital to ensure that nationally agreed standards of service are achieved and that the requirements of relevant legislation and guidance are fulfilled.

Research

Research is needed on many aspects of screening for hearing loss, including techniques, organization, and yield.

- The optimum management and follow-up of unilateral hearing loss needs further study (see above).
- Continuing surveillance of babies who 'pass' the newborn screen seems desirable but there are no data on the most cost-effective approaches to this task.

- Although there is good evidence that early intervention improves outcome, further work is needed to confirm that and to address the question of whether there might be any adverse effects of early intervention.
- Can we predict which children will suffer persistent OME? If we could, would treatment improve their quality of life and behavioural outcomes sufficiently to justify screening and, if so, which children would benefit most?
- Comparison of AOAE-based programmes with AABR-based programmes.

Monitoring and outcomes

Single measures such as age of detection or age at fitting of first hearing aid in children with SNHL must be treated with caution for the following reasons.

- It can be difficult to define these points precisely.
- Ascertainment is often uncertain, particularly in areas of high population mobility. For example, 'missed' cases may eventually be detected in other parts of the country.
- Ascertainment is never complete until around 5 or even 6 years of age even in districts with a good service. Therefore mean ages of diagnosis or aiding are always several years out of date and respond slowly to changes in service delivery.

There is no substitute for comprehensive audit and quality monitoring of the performance of the audiological programme. It is important to keep under review not only ages of diagnosis, but false-positive referral rates, waiting times at each point in the network of services (including ENT), and the differences between age of diagnosis for high-risk and low-risk cases. Standardization of records would facilitate comparisons between districts.

Evaluation of screening programmes for hearing loss in childhood

It is difficult to evaluate the sensitivity of screening programmes for hearing loss because 'missed' cases may not be diagnosed for several years, by which time they may have moved to another district. The follow-up of very large cohorts of children to detect missed cases is difficult and prohibitively expensive.

Creation of a **national register** of children with hearing impairment would (if well designed and adequately funded) help to overcome this problem in addition to providing other research opportunities. Such a register could allow long-term outcomes such as educational achievements and employment status in early adulthood to be monitored.

Chapter 12

Screening for vision defects

This chapter:

♦ Describes defects likely to cause disabling impairment of vision

♦ Defines the terms used to describe the common disorders such as squint, refractive error, and amblyopia

♦ Reviews the tests and procedures used for assessing vision in pre-school and school-age children

♦ Sets out the arguments for screening

♦ Gives a brief account of colour vision defects and vision problems associated with 'dyslexia'

♦ Makes recommendations for screening and early detection

Disorders of vision can be subdivided into the following categories:

♦ serious defects likely to cause a disabling impairment of vision ranging from partial sight to complete blindness

♦ the common and usually less incapacitating defects including refractive errors, squints, amblyopia, and defects of colour discrimination.

Conditions causing a disabling vision impairment as the primary problem

These are individually and collectively uncommon, with a combined prevalence of visual impairment (acuity less than 6/18 in the better eye) about 1 per 1000. This may underestimate the true prevalence of visual impairment in the community, as it is likely that there is under-recognition and/or under-reporting of visual loss in children with multiple other impairments.

Early detection

Early detection of serious visual impairment is important for four reasons:

1 Ophthalmic symptoms or signs such as squint or progressive visual failure can be the presenting feature of serious systemic disease.

2 Some conditions are sight- or life-threatening and are treatable—for example, cataract, glaucoma, and retinoblastoma. This also applies to some acquired eye diseases, notably retinopathy of prematurity, uveitis in association with juvenile chronic arthritis, and diabetes.

3 Many visual disorders have widespread and/or genetic implications. Over half of children with visual impairment have multisystem disorders. Impaired visual function may be associated with, and occasionally be the presenting feature of, severe learning disability.

4 Developmental guidance and early educational advice by specialist teachers is much appreciated by parents and may reduce the incidence of secondary disabilities such as behaviour problems. Multidisciplinary support may be needed for children with additional impairments.

How early detection is achieved

Many cases are detected by parents or other family members. A significant number are found at the neonatal examination by simple inspection of the eyes. Some are found by specialist examination of known high-risk groups, including low-birth-weight infants at risk of retinopathy of prematurity and babies with a first-degree relative known to have a potentially heritable eye disorder.

Screening for common non-incapacitating vision defects
Definitions

The terms used in this section are defined in the box. The most important of these is amblyopia, and the prevention, identification, and referral of this condition should be the main aims of a pre-school vision screening programme.

Amblyopia

Untreated amblyopia results in permanent vision impairment, and affects *at least 2 per cent* of children in the UK. Although it usually (although not invariably) occurs in only one eye, it may be a bar to certain careers and may leave the individual effectively partially sighted if the other eye is lost through disease or trauma. It has been estimated that this happens to at least 150 people per year in the UK (*see* HFAC4 website).

Amblyopia may be suspected in infants who present with other eye problems such as squint, but unless refraction is performed it is difficult to diagnose with confidence in the clinical situation before the child can cooperate with visual acuity testing. Prompt referral of infants with squint or other obvious

Definitions of terms used in the text

Visual acuity is a measure of how well a person is able to separate adjacent visual stimuli such as the features of a letter.

Refractive state: the optical system of the eye is designed to produce a focused image on the retina. The eye that does this perfectly without refractive correction is known as *emmetropic*. Few eyes have a perfect optical system, and so most people have some refractive error—*ametropia*.

The common refractive errors are:

Myopia (short sight) in which distance vision is blurred. This is uncommon in early childhood, but is increasingly common in the teens.

Hypermetropia (long sight), which, if significant, blurs both distance and near vision.

Astigmatism, in which the degree of refractive error is different between the two axes of the eye.

Anisometropia in which the refraction is significantly different between the two eyes.

The refractive state of the eye changes throughout life, concomitant with eye growth, but particularly in infancy and childhood. Accordingly, hypermetropia is frequent and physiological until at least the age of around 2 years.

In children referred following screening, it is important to accurately measure refraction and to carry out a fundus examination. This will be facilitated, in many cases, by instilling cycloplegic eye drops which paralyse accomodation and dilate the pupils.

The *correction of impaired visual acuity* related to refractive error usually involves the prescription of spectacles. Severely impaired visual acuity may affect school work and sporting prowess, but minor impairments caused by slight refractive errors seem to have little impact on education or performance. Children may be reluctant to wear spectacles prescribed for these minor errors.

A *manifest squint (strabismus)* is a deviation of the eyes which is apparent at the time of examination. It is demonstrated by use of the cover–uncover test. The prevalence of squint in infancy is around 1% and in early childhood it is between 3% and 7%.

A *latent squint* is detected only when the two eyes are dissociated by testing, using the cover test. It may become manifest under conditions of stress, fatigue, or illness.

> **Amblyopia** is a condition of reduced vision in which the eye itself is healthy, but, because of a refractive error, a difference in refraction between the two eyes (anisometropia), a squint, or opacities in the refractive media, the brain has either suppressed or failed to develop the ability to perceive a detailed image from that eye. It is usually unilateral but may be bilateral in some circumstances (e.g. extreme hypermetropia).

vision problems may help to avoid the development of amblyopia or reduce its severity. In many cases, however, amblyopia presents for the first time after the age of 3 years, without any other obvious signs of eye problems.

Treatment

There are two phases in the management of amblyopia. First, any obstacle to clear vision (e.g. cataract) is removed and the eye is presented with a focused image by the correction of any refractive error, usually by spectacles. This is followed by occlusion with patching or penalization of the better eye. Although gains in visual acuity are usually achieved, they are not always maintained, nor can the development of binocular vision be guaranteed.

Patching is easier, and is said to be more effective, in younger children but is thought to be of doubtful benefit beyond the age of 7 or 8 years.

Determining the effectiveness of treatment is clearly important and a randomized trial of treatment of amblyopia is needed to settle the issue. The first trial comparing conventional treatment with no treatment of children aged 3–5 years with anisometropic amblyopia has been completed—see page 232.

Prevention

There has been some interest in the prevention of amblyopia by detection and treatment in infancy of the more common antecedent causes, which include refractive error and strabismus (squint), although the natural history of amblyopia and its relationship with these potentially amblyogenic factors is unclear. Currently, neither amblyopia nor strabismus can be reliably predicted or prevented (see box).

Criterion of success

At present, the immediate criterion by which the success of a pre-school vision screening programme should be judged is its ability to *detect* amblyopia as early as possible rather than *prevent* it. The long-term aim is to reduce the number of children with permanent vision deficits; the achievement of this goal

---

Limited scope for preventing amblyopia by screening in infancy

- Studies have been conducted to determine the effectiveness of retinoscopy or photo-refraction in detecting defects in the first year of life.

- It has been suggested that provision of spectacles for babies with hypermetropia may reduce the incidence of squint and amblyopia, but the evidence for this is not conclusive.

- The overall impact on the number of cases of these conditions would be small.

- Refraction is changing rapidly in infancy, and so close supervision and frequent skilled monitoring would be needed for a successful early intervention programme.

---

depends not only on screening but also on the effectiveness of, and compliance with, treatment.

Assessing vision in young children

The measurement of visual acuity in children under the age of 3 years

There is currently no satisfactory way of assessing visual acuity suitable for the universal screening of children who are too young to perform standard acuity tests.

Various tests have been used to demonstrate that the child has reached a developmental stage at which visual fixation and concentration on tiny objects is possible. These provide only a *qualitative indication* of overall visual behaviour but cannot offer any quantitative measurement of visual acuity or any direct or indirect indication of refractive error. Examples include Sheridan's graded balls and matching toys tests, and the use of tiny sweets known as hundreds and thousands (1 mm diameter). While these tests do indicate the presence of vision, they can very seriously underestimate the severity of a vision defect.

Direct measurement of visual acuity in infancy requires special tests, such as forced-choice preferential looking methods. However, some inferences can be drawn about the likelihood of significantly impaired vision in either or both eyes from the assessment of fixation. The examination requires considerable skill, and non-specialist staff need thorough training to achieve competence.

Available evidence suggests that formal visual screening of every infant during the first year of life has a very small yield and is probably not justified.

The pre-school child: 3–5 years

Although it is important to use the best possible test for children, the limiting factor with pre-school screening is the difficulty in obtaining reliable responses when testing visual acuity in the less mature or mildly delayed child, resulting in unacceptably high recall or false-positive rates. It is possible to test the vision of some children between the ages of 2 and 3 years; around 80 per cent of children can perform visual acuity tests at 3 years of age but the figure rises to 90 in the cohort aged 4 to 5 years. Several studies suggest that there is a substantial difference in yield, sensitivity and specificity of vision screening carried out by orthoptists as compared with non-specialist health professionals. In practice, however, the greatest difficulty is in maintaining high uptake rates, with few screening studies reporting rates above 60–75 per cent.

Although it is usual to test distance vision in adults at 6 m, distance testing of children with the appropriate tests at 3 or 4 m gives acceptable results. It is often easier to maintain rapport and attention control at the shorter distance when testing young children, and many clinic rooms are too small for testing at 6 m.

School-age children

Children aged 4 and 5 years can perform visual acuity tests more easily than 3-year-olds. By the age of 5 years, when UK children start compulsory schooling, linear charts are usually satisfactory, although single letters may be needed for a few very anxious or developmentally immature children.

Tests of visual acuity The visual acuity for distance vision can be assessed using picture tests, single letters, or charts with lines of letters (such as the Snellen chart). Any of these can be used with a letter-matching card or with plastic letters, so that the child does not have to be able to name the letters. A linear chart is preferable to single letters because the latter may seriously underestimate amblyopia (the so-called 'crowding phenomenon') or even miss the diagnosis altogether. It is essential to occlude each eye in turn, otherwise the result indicates only the vision in the better eye.

The principle is to use the most difficult test the child can do because this will give the most robust result.

1 The gold standard is now the linear logMAR tests because the Snellen chart, although still the most widely used visual acuity test, has several defects. The progression of letter sizes on the chart is irregular, the number of lines on the chart increases with each step, so that the task becomes relatively easier with larger letters, and the scale is too coarse for precise measurement of small changes. These problems have been overcome by

the use of the logMAR charts. The 3 metre logMAR cards were designed to combine the advantages of existing tests with those of the logMAR design.

2 The Snellen chart. (NB All Snellen charts are effectively single-letter charts towards the top.)

3 Single-letter charts: the 3 metre logMAR cards are the best because they are logMAR based.

4 Picture cards and other similar tests.

Near vision   The routine testing of near vision adds very little to the detection of significant visual defects. Children with hypermetropia do not necessarily have a significant reduction of near-visual acuity. Near-vision testing can safely be omitted from the vision screening of children, although it does of course have a place in the assessment of the child with a suspected visual problem.

Referral criteria   If the child does not achieve 0.2 in either eye (roughly equivalent to 6/9 on a Snellen-based linear chart), despite good cooperation, referral is indicated.

Pre-school screening for vision defects

Although the disability caused by vision defects in early childhood is not known, several arguments have been offered in support of pre-school vision screening.

◆ The experience of older children and adults suggests that correction of a visual acuity of 6/12 or worse is likely to improve quality of life. Neither the disability and economic loss caused by squint and amblyopia, nor the benefits or adverse effects of treatments such as patching, have been established. It is, therefore, difficult to know how much weight to place on this argument.

◆ Treatment for amblyopia can be initiated and sometimes completed before the child starts school.

◆ The results of intervention for amblyopia might be better if started before the age of 5 years. This is an important and difficult issue. If the treatment of amblyopia is more successful at 3 than 5 years, early diagnosis would be important. Evidence to date suggests that age of starting treatment for amblyopia makes little difference to outcome within this age range. However, amblyopia diagnosed at 3 years is often associated with squint whereas when diagnosed at 5 years it is more likely to be associated with straight-eyed anisometropia, so that the cases are not strictly comparable. Thus the question is not yet finally resolved (see page 232).

Detection of strabismus (squint)

The majority of manifest squints are first *recognized by parents or relatives*. The parents should always be asked whether they have noticed any squint, laziness, or turning of one eye. Some parents are incorrectly informed that squint is normal under the age of 6 months. This serious misconception can lead to delay in diagnosis of serious eye disease. There is a high incidence of strabismus in children born preterm and those with neurodevelopmental problems. A family history of high refractive error or squint in a first-degree relative may be significant. Any such history may justify referral for more detailed examination. The detection of squint is summarized in the box.

Detection of squint

A careful inspection of the eyes should be made to identify any squint (strabismus) which has been overlooked or ignored by the child's parents.

Some squints are not instantly apparent to simple inspection. In order to demonstrate these, the following tests may be used:

- the corneal reflections test
- the cover test
- a prism test
- examination of the eye movements by moving a small target of visual interest through the horizontal, vertical, and oblique planes
- tests of stereopsosis may be used—a normal result is said to imply that both eyes are healthy and functioning as a pair.

Some or all of these procedures are widely used for screening, but the skill required for their proper performance and interpretation is not generally appreciated.

Pseudosquint A common difficulty is the distinction between squint and pseudosquint (i.e. the appearance of squint caused by epicanthic folds). Squint and prominent epicanthic folds may coexist. Pseudosquint is very common.

Screening for latent squint involves the use of the cover test. It is doubtful whether the detection of a presymptomatic latent squint is of any significant benefit to the child.

Community screening—evidence and options

Universal screening of all infants in the first year of life (after the 6–8 week contact) would result in detection of some vision defects that otherwise would be missed. The yield would be very small and would not justify this use of professional expertise.

Universal vision screening of all pre-school children is carried out in many areas by doctors or health visitors, but it has a significantly lower yield and less satisfactory sensitivity and specificity than a programme involving orthoptists. Testing before the age of 4 years appears to produce too many unreliable results for a satisfactory screening programme. Waiting until all children are in school at age 5 years may result in a less satisfactory outcome for the treatment of amblyopia. Therefore, on the evidence available, the Working Party believes that the gold standard would be an examination of all children between 4 and 5 years of age. This programme would remove the need for a further test at formal school entry at age 5 years. However, universal coverage may still be a problem in the pre-school years and it is as yet uncertain whether orthoptists will be in a position to deliver such a programme.

Secondary screening by a community-based orthoptist involves examining children referred by parents or by other professional staff, whenever a concern is expressed, and selecting those who require a more detailed assessment. This results in a substantial reduction in the number of referrals to ophthalmologists and considerable financial savings. It may also help to reduce inequity by improving ease of access to eye care, as social class plays a significant part in determining age of presentation for children with amblyopia.

An *assessment of visual acuity at school entry* is routine in most districts. This is usually done by school nurses. The detection of vision defects in school is easier and therefore cheaper than in the pre-school years because school children are a 'captive population' and high coverage can be achieved easily. The importance of the best available test materials, satisfactory distance and lighting conditions, and high standards of testing is emphasized. If a school entry programme is adopted in preference to the pre-school screen, we suggest that it should be supervised and quality monitored by the eye care team.

New cases of myopia and other vision defects continue to present throughout the school years, raising the question of whether any further universal screening is needed **after school entry**. Some children recognize for themselves that their vision is not as good as that of their peers, but often impaired visual acuity is only discovered by formal testing. There is evidence that those adults who are socially disadvantaged are less likely to have their eyes tested and more likely to have undiagnosed treatable eye diseases, including refractive errors. If this is also true for children, a further universal vision test may be needed to offer more equitable care.

The role of vision screening after school entry remains controversial—the disability caused by uncorrected refractive error, the need for further screens, the number of occasions, and the optimal ages have not been established.

4r Updates

The questions posed in 2003 have to some extent been answered by a randomised trial of screening and patching in preschool children. The findings were as follows: Nearly half the children identified as cases by repeated community screening do not have unilateral acuity loss; combined treatment with patching and glasses has useful effect for acuity = or <6/18, but none for = or <6/12; patching causes moderate distress to children, but probably has no lasting emotional impact; treatment is as effective at age 5 as at age 4.

Clarke MP, Wright CM, Hrisos S, Anderson JD, Henderson J, Richardson SR (2003). A randomised controlled trial of treatment of unilateral visual impairment detected at pre-school vision screening, *British Medical Journal*. **327**:1251–4.

Richardson S, Wright CM, Hrisos S, Buck D, Clark MP (2004). Stereoacuity in unilateral visual impairment detected at pre school screening: outcomes from a randomised controlled trial. *Investigative Ophthalmology & Visual Science* **46**: 150–4.

Hrisos S, Clarke MP, Wright CM (2004). The emotional impact of amblyopia treatment in pre-school children: randomised controlled trial. *Ophthalmology* **11**:1550–56.

In another study, by Williams et al, an intensive screening programme with several examinations between eight and 37 months resulted in a lower incidence of amblyopia in the screened group, suggesting that very early detection and treatment do make a difference; however, such a programme would be difficult to generalise and would be very expensive in relation to the magnitude of the benefits.

Williams C, Northstone K, Harrad RA, Sparrow JM, Harvey I, and the ALSPAC Study Team (2003). Amblyopia treatment outcomes after preschool screening v school entry screening: observational data from a prospective cohort study. *British Journal of Ophthalmology*; **87**:988–993.

Williams C, Northstone K, Harrad R A, Sparrow J M, Harvey I, ALSPAC Study Team (2002). Amblyopia treatment outcomes after screening before or at age 3 years: follow up from randomised trial *BMJ* **324**:1549–1551.

Screening by orthoptists has been introduced in more districts but it is too early to determine how much this has resulted in improvements in service or outcomes. Screening in school after the age of school entry is still a contentious issue but current recommendations are unchanged.

Colour vision defects

Congenital (mainly X-linked) deficiencies in colour vision, primarily affecting the perception of reds and greens, occur in 8 per cent of boys and about 0.5 per cent of girls. Blue deficiencies and total colour blindness are extremely rare. The Ishihara test is widely used, although it is very sensitive and detects even very minor defects which might be of trivial significance in some careers. The City University test is preferable as a detailed diagnostic test, but not as a screening tool. Two reasons are advanced for the early detection of colour vision defects.

1 It has been suggested that they might cause learning difficulties, particularly with regard to colour-coded materials used in the teaching of reading and mathematics. In fact there is little evidence that colour vision defects do cause learning difficulties and most affected children can distinguish different coloured materials despite reduced colour discrimination.

2 Some defects preclude people from entering certain careers and it is helpful for a person to know that they have this deficiency at an early stage in career planning. Screening at the beginning of secondary schooling might be useful, by providing information that would be important in career planning. A case can be made for including only boys in view of the much higher incidence.

Little is known about whether adolescents benefit from or value this screening process. It might be equally effective to provide health education. For example, those whose career planning might be affected by a colour vision impairment could be advised to visit an optometrist for assessment.

Colour vision update

4r

Recent evidence supports the contention that colour vision has little importance in educational attainment and occupational choice. Screening for colour vision defects cannot be justified:

Cumberland P, Rahi JS, Peckham CS (2004). Impact of congenital colour vision deficiency on education and unintentional injuries: findings from the 1958 British birth cohort. *British Medical Journal* 329:1074–1075.

Cumberland P, Rahi J, Peckham CS (2005). Impact of congenital colour vision defects on occupation. *Archives of Disease in Childhood.* May 24; (ADC Online First, published on May 24, 2005 as 10.1136/adc.2004.062067).

Vision and 'dyslexia'

There has been much interest in recent years in the relationship between visual deficits, such as eye-movement disorders and delay in establishment of dominance, and dyslexia or reading problems. A disorder known as 'scotopic sensitivity syndrome' has also been described.

The evidence on these conditions is still equivocal and further research is needed. There is no dispute that any child with reading or other learning problems needs a vision assessment, but we do not think that this need routinely include tests or treatment for the conditions mentioned above except in the context of a special development or research programme.

Recommendations

Referral pathways

Each district will need to ensure that children can access an ophthalmic team comprising those professions most closely involved with vision assessment, ophthalmic examination, correction of refractive error, and the management of ophthalmic conditions, i.e. ophthalmologists, orthoptists, and optometrists. Guidance on how hospital and community services may be provided is contained in the report Children's Eye Health Working Party of the Royal College of Ophthalmologists, the British Orthoptic Society and the College of Optometrists (*see* HFAC4 website).

Every parent with concerns about their child's vision should be able to enter a planned referral pathway from first suspicion to diagnosis and management. In the case of concerns about possible serious visual impairment, the referral process should bypass routine waiting lists. Since many causes of visual impairment are part of a multi-system disorder, the referral and assessment process is likely to involve a developmental paediatric clinic working with an ophthalmologist and the eye care team. Management should take account of good practice guidance, for example the RNIB report 'Taking the time: telling parents their child is blind or partially sighted' (*see* HFAC4 website).

Parents should be aware that their child is entitled to free NHS eye examinations up to the age of 16 (19 if in full-time education) by community optometrists, who are trained and equipped to provide the support they need.

Detection of severe visual impairment

- A careful inspection of the eyes and examination for the red reflex is an essential part of the neonatal examination. Fundoscopy is not essential but the ophthalmoscope may be used, focused on infinity from a distance of 20–30 cm (8–12 inches), to detect cataract as a silhouette against the red reflex. The inspection and the examination should be repeated at 6–8 weeks. Urgent referral is mandatory if there is any suspicion of abnormality. Photographs of the baby which show an absent or disturbed red eye reflex are also useful (parents reporting this phenomenon should be referred *promptly* to an ophthalmologist).

- The parents should be asked if there is a family history of visual disorders. Children at risk of having a genetically determined disabling visual disorder should be examined with extra care, preferably by an ophthalmologist. This is important, even if the usual age of presentation is much later.

- Parents should be asked soon after the birth and at each sub-sequent contact whether they have any anxieties about the baby's vision. An age-related check list in the Personal Child Health Record can be used. For example, they can be asked if the baby looks at the parents, follows moving objects with the eyes, and fixates on small objects.

- Primary health care team staff should be familiar with the visual development of the normal baby, and should be alert to the various symptoms and signs which first warn parents that there may be a visual defect (e.g. abnormal appearance of the eyes, wandering eye movements, poor fixation and visual following, photophobia, etc.).

- All children with dysmorphic syndromes or neurodevelopmental problems should undergo a specialist eye examination as some may have serious defects of vision.

- Forty per cent of children with sensorineural hearing impairments have eye problems, some very severe. All children with sensorineural hearing problems should undergo a specialist eye examination.

- Babies with a birth weight of less than 1500 g, or born at 31 weeks gestational age or less, should be screened for retinopathy of prematurity, according to current recommendations. The increased risk of other eye problems including myopia, squint, and cortical visual impairment should also be remembered.

- It should be remembered that poor visual fixation in the first year of life is sometimes the presenting feature of learning disability, but a vision defect should always be excluded.

Screening for non-disabling visual defects

◆ Screening for non-disabling visual defects in children under 2 years of age should be confined to history and observation.

◆ Children of any age with suspected vision defects, a significant family history, or any neurological or disabling condition should be referred routinely for visual assessment.

◆ A visual assessment by an orthoptist should be carried out on all children between the ages of 4 and 5 years. Some districts already have the staff to do this and need only to restructure their community programme, but in others it may take a few years to introduce.

◆ Until a programme of screening by orthoptist can be established, we recommend that screening of pre-school children should not be offered. Children should be screened at school entry. If this cannot be done by an orthoptist, the programme and the quality of testing should be supervised by an orthoptist or optometrist.

◆ Screening of vision at school entry and during primary school years should cease in areas where a satisfactory pre-school (4–5 years old) orthoptist screening programme has been established.

◆ The evidence available is insufficient to allow a firm decision about screening in secondary school. The working party recommends that, if already in place, screening on a single occasion should continue, but any more than this should cease. No new screening should be introduced.

◆ Any child undergoing assessment for educational under-achievement or other school problems should have a visual acuity check.

◆ It is important to ensure that vision screening is undertaken in schools for children with hearing impairment because (a) good vision is particularly vital for a person with impaired hearing, and (b) conditions such as Usher's syndrome, which have important genetic and educational implications, may present with insidious loss of vision.

◆ One person in each district should take responsibility for monitoring the results of vision screening. This person should have links with the hospital children's eye service to set up links, agree protocols, etc., and may also be involved in developing children's eye services on a community basis.

◆ The relevance of more subtle eye problems to reading difficulties and 'dyslexia' is controversial. Screening programmes for such problems could not currently be justified but ophthalmology and paediatric services must decide how to respond to parents who are worried about this possibility.

Colour vision defects

◆ No attempt should be made to screen for colour vision defects in primary school.

◆ The value and timing of screening for colour vision defects in older children is uncertain. We recommend that where screening is already in place it should continue, but if not in place it should not be introduced. If screening is not in place, all pupils and carers should be made aware of any occupations that may be barred to someone with abnormal colour vision.

◆ Children found to have a colour vision defect should be told that they have a difficulty in discriminating colours which *may* be important with regard to certain career choices. In cases where such a defect could have important career implications, expert advice should be obtained from an optometrist, an ophthalmologist, a special clinic, or a careers adviser.

Research

◆ The nature and degree of disability caused by impaired visual acuity and amblyopia in later life need further evaluation.

◆ Research is continuing on the natural history of amblyopia and the development and evaluation of vision in infancy, with the eventual aim of *preventing* amblyopia.

◆ An improved visual acuity test for young children based on the logMAR design has been developed and initial trial results have been reported.

Sonsken P and Salt A: Newsletter of the British Academy of Childhood Disability. http://www.bacdis.org.uk/publications/newsletters/2005_autumn.pdf   4r

The value of testing all secondary school children for visual acuity defects has been questioned. It is said that adolescents are unlikely to wear spectacles unless they themselves recognize a visual difficulty. The alternative approach might be self-referral, encouraged by the inclusion of eye care as a topic in health education curricula. It is not known whether children value and make use of the discovery of a colour vision defect. An alternative approach has been suggested—to include eye care and colour vision defects in a health education lesson. Children who felt that they might have a vision problem, or a defect that might be relevant to their career plans, would be offered an eye examination. However, there has been no research in these areas and these approaches need to be evaluated.

Chapter 13

Identifying children with developmental and behavioural problems

This chapter deals with:

- ◆ The definition of disablement and the epidemiology of disabling conditions
- ◆ The importance of identifying, detecting, and caring for children with disabling conditions
- ◆ The distinction (for convenience only) between two categories of disabling condition—low-prevalence high-severity disorders, and high-prevalence low-severity problems
- ◆ The ways in which disabling conditions are identified
- ◆ Screening for autism
- ◆ The place of developmental screening
- ◆ The early identification of speech and language impairments and how they may be managed
- ◆ Motor disorders and specific learning disabilities
- ◆ Psychological, behavioural, and emotional disorders and service provision for them
- ◆ The vital importance of collaboration between health, social services, and education in the planning of early identification activities

In Chapters 2 and 3 we considered the primary prevention of developmental and behavioural problems and the promotion of parenting skills. The aims of pre-school health care include the timely identification of disabilities and disorders that may be relevant to education and the provision of whatever intervention may be appropriate, including suitable arrangements for the child's education. However, it will never be possible to identify all children in advance of starting school, since some problems only emerge when the child has to conform to the expectations of the teacher and the discipline of the classroom.

We suggested (p. 130) that many problems in children's health and development are found by means other than screening. The services and systems needed to achieve comprehensive early identification of disabilities and disorders are summarized in the box. In this chapter, we review the definition and epidemiology of disability, and then examine the detection and initial management of conditions affecting development, such as cerebral palsy, learning difficulty, disorders of speech and language, and autism, with a particular focus on early identification and screening. This is followed by a review of behavioural and emotional problems, where many of the same issues apply. Some of these conditions cause long-term disability, while others resolve partially or completely. Service provision for children with special educational needs is outlined in Chapter 14.

Services and systems required for early identification of disabilities and disorders

- Competent, thorough neonatal examination.
- Planned follow-up of newborns judged to be at high risk.
- Follow-up of infants and children suffering any form of neurological insult.
- A core programme of professional reviews and contacts at agreed ages, with inclusion of both open and structured questions to parents about the child's progress.
- Recognition that parents are often right when concerned about their child's development, coupled with easy access to specialist assessment when needed.
- A holistic approach to assessment that recognizes how the impact of several minor problems can be cumulative and cause significant disability.
- Training and support of child care staff to identify possible problems and act appropriately when concerned.
- Network of health, social, and educational services that can provide a prompt coordinated response to referrals.

4r **National service frameworks**

The relevant NSF standards are:

Standard 1 (Core standards): 'Promoting Health and Well-being, Identifying Needs and Intervening Early'.
Standard 9: 'The Mental Health and Psychological Well-being of Children and Young People'.
www.dh.gov.uk/policyandguidance/healthandsocialcaretopics/childrenservices

Child and adolescent mental health is still an under-served area, with serious inequalities of access to services due partly to lack of funding and partly to recruitment difficulties. Following publication of the NSF, an important Executive Letter (March 2005) reminds chief executives of their duty regarding CAMHS — 'Delivering A Comprehensive Child And Adolescent Mental Health Service By 2006'. This sets targets in three areas:

♦ 24 hours, 7 days a week cover

♦ Services for children and young people with learning disabilities

♦ Services for 16 and 17 year olds

Follow link from:

www.dh.gov.uk/PublicationsAndStatistics/LettersAndCirculars/DearColleagueLetters/

Definition of disablement

The definition of disability is hotly disputed and our understanding is still evolving. Most recent national research is based on the World Health Organization scheme entitled the **International Classification of Impairment Disability and Handicap (ICIDH)**. This was criticized as being too medical and focused on the individual, and allowing no account to be taken of environmental factors. In November 2001, WHO replaced it with a new publication called the **International Classification of Functioning, Disability and Health (ICF)** (Table 13.1 and box); this is the framework for the future. However, our present knowledge of the prevalence and severity of disability must be quoted using the concepts and language of the past.

4r   This topic has been reviewed recently:

Colver A. A. shared framework and language for childhood disability. *Dev Med Child Neurol* 2005; **47**: 780–84.

Epidemiology

The largest British survey of disability was undertaken by the Office of Population Censuses and Surveys (OPCS) in 1986. The 11 areas of disability

Table 13.1 An overview of the ICF*

Part 1: Functioning and disability			Part 2: Contextual factors	
Components	Body functions Body structures	Activities Participation	Environmental factors	Personal factors
Domains	Body functions Body structures	Life areas (tasks, action)	External influences on functioning and disability	Internal influences on functioning and disability
Constructs	Change in body function (physiological)	Capacity: Executing tasks in a standard environment	Facilitating or hindering impact of features of the physical, social, and attitudinal world	Impact of attributes of the person
	Change in body structure (anatomical)	Performance: Executing tasks in current environment		
Positive aspects	Functional and structural integrity	Activities Participation	Facilitators	NA
		Functioning		
Negative aspects	Impairment	Activity limitation Participation restriction	Barriers Hindrances	NA
		Disability		

NA, not applicable.

* See HFAC4 website.

and the prevalence found are shown in Table 13.2. In reality these disabilities do not usually occur singly. Most children have combinations of disabilities. Clusters have been identified by a re-analysis of the OPCS data (*see* HFAC4 website). Eleven distinct clusters, which formed a natural hierarchy of severity, were found (Table 13.3).

The challenge—identification of developmental disorders and disabilities

Table 13.2 shows that disability in childhood is an important problem. In summary, there are 360 000 disabled children in the UK (32 per thousand or 3 per cent of the child population), and 189 000 of these have severe disabilities;

Table 13.2 Areas of disability and their prevalence

Type of disability	Rate per thousand childhood population
Locomotion	9
Reaching and stretching	2
Dexterity	3
Seeing	2
Hearing	6
Personal care	7
Continence	9
Communication	11
Behaviour	21
Intellectual function	9
Consciousness	5

Definitions

- The concept of impairment remains. **Impairment** is a loss or abnormality of body structure or of a physiological or psychological function.

- The concept of disability has been replaced by measures of activities. An **activity** is the nature and extent of functioning at the level of the person. Activities may be limited in nature, duration, and quality.

- The concept of handicap has been replaced by measures of participation. **Participation** is the nature and extent of the person's involvement in life situations in relation to impairments, activities, health conditions and contextual factors. Participation may be restricted in nature, duration, and quality.

- The term disability had been dropped while the term disablement has been adopted as an umbrella over the concepts above.

5500 live in residential care and 16 000 attend residential schools; 1.8 per cent of all children attend special schools. Disabled children are eight times more likely to be looked after by the local authority than non-disabled children and constitute 28 per cent of all children looked after. There are increasing numbers of children with disability who attend mainstream schools and many need considerable support.

Table 13.3 Clusters of children aged 5–15 years and their disabilities

Cluster	Description	Total in Great Britain (% of disabled population)
1	**Mild disabilities**: 85% have just one (e.g. locomotion 28%, or continence 28%)	40 000 (14)
2	**Behavioural disabilities**, but 47% have other mild disabilities	74 000 (25)
3	**Continence disabilities**, but 36% have behaviour disability	22 000 (8)
4	**Consciousness disabilities**: fits, often with another disability such as behaviour (33%)	12 000 (4)
5	**Hearing disabilities**, but 51% have communication disability	21 000 (7)
6	**Communication and behaviour disabilities**: 38% have learning difficulty and 21% have locomotion disabilities	42 000 (14)
7	**Personal care disabilities** with a wide range of other disabilities: 52% have disabilities of locomotion	15 000 (5)
8	**Hearing and behaviour disabilities**: 58% have communication disabilities	21 000 (7)
9	**Multiple disabilities**: 80% have four or more disabilities. All have personal care disability and 62% have learning disability	22 000 (8)
10	**Multiple and severe disabilities**: on average, 6.6 disabilities	15 000 (5)
11	**Multiple and very severe disabilities**: on average 9 disabilities	8000 (3)

Disability may involve motor, intellectual, language, or emotional development. It may be trivial or profound, transient or permanent. It is useful to distinguish two groups of problems.

- Low-prevalence high-severity conditions: this group includes conditions for which a pathological basis has been demonstrated or can be presumed. Examples include cerebral palsy, aphasia, and severe learning disabilities (mental handicap).

- High-prevalence low-severity conditions: this group includes delayed speech acquisition, clumsiness, and minor psychological pathology. In these children, a pathological basis for the child's difficulties is rarely found. They

are best understood as an interaction of genetic predisposition, environmental factors, and ill health of various kinds. For example, a child may
have a family history of slow language acquisition, live in a poor family, and
suffer repeated episodes of respiratory infection associated with conductive
hearing impairment.

The distinction is made solely for convenience and has no rigorous scientific
basis. Some children in the second group may be more disabled than some of
those in the first. However, there are some differences between these two
groups in the approach to prevention, detection, and management.

4r Normal child development

Sure Start commissioned a review of the literature and some educational
material about child development. The result may be useful for those working
with infants and pre-school children.

Review of the literature to support 'Birth to three matters': A framework to
support children in their earliest years. Tricia David, Kathy Goouch, Sacha
Powell and Lesley Abbott. http://www.dfes.gov.uk/research/

Developmental disorders and disabilities—identification and management

In the following sections we consider in more detail the question of how these
conditions can be detected.

Low-prevalence high-severity conditions

These conditions, although rare, have serious effects on the individual child
and collectively form a significant health care burden for society. The list
includes cerebral palsy, muscle disease, learning disability, hearing and visual
impairment, autism, epilepsy, osteogenesis imperfecta, and many others.
Details of the most common are shown in Table 13.4.

Primary prevention

There is currently little scope for primary prevention of these conditions
within child health services. The early recognition of genetically determined
conditions such as Duchenne muscular dystrophy may avoid the birth of a
second affected child within the same family (see p. 196). Prevention of
acquired brain injury involves reducing risks of head injury by accident prevention programmes, prevention and prompt treatment of infections of the
central nervous system, etc. (Chapter 4).

Table 13.4 Conditions causing disability in childhood

◆ Cerebral palsy: 0.15%–0.3% (1.5–3 per 1000)

◆ Duchenne muscular dystrophy: 0.03% of males (3 per 10 000 male births)

◆ Severe learning disabilities (previously mental handicap): 0.37% (3.7 per 1000)

◆ Speech and language impairments, including developmental and acquired dysphasia, pseudobulbar palsy, and unknown causes: incidence depends on the definition, but for persisting severe cases it is at least 2 per 1000

◆ Classic autism: 0.03%–0.04% (3–4 cases per 10 000 births) Autism spectrum disorder: 1–2 per 1000

◆ Many other disorders may lead to disability, such as osteogenesis imperfecta, head injury, and juvenile arthritis

Periconceptional and antenatal health surveillance and health promotion

The health of the fetus and of the parents during pregnancy has long-term effects on morbidity and mortality. The Working Party has not attempted to review this subject, but this is not to deny its importance. Preparation for parenthood, access to genetic services, family spacing, measures to reduce identifiable risks (such as rubella vaccination and folic acid supplementation), screening programmes, and advice on alcohol, smoking, drug abuse, diet, and safe eating may all play a part in improving pregnancy outcomes and therefore the health of the child. The mental health of the parents, and in particular of unsupported mothers, is equally important.

Detection

Serious impairments can be detected in a number of ways.

Screening Formal screening for hearing and vision defects is discussed in Chapters 11 and 12 respectively. Formal screening for learning disabilities, developmental delay, and cerebral palsy are not currently recommended. We argued in previous editions of this book that routine developmental screening makes little contribution to the detection of serious impairments. Although routine developmental examinations are capable of detecting extreme deviations from normal development, most are found by other means.

Autism, autism spectrum disorder, and related conditions are uncommon, but there is currently much interest in their early diagnosis and in the possibilities for early intervention (see box). Children with these global impairments of communication skills are less common than those with 'simple' language delay but have a worse prognosis and often make enormous demands on services. For American and Australian perspectives, with reviews of screening policy, *see* HFAC4 website.

Autism, autism spectrum disorder, and pervasive developmental disorder

◆ This is a group of specific developmental disorders in which there are qualitative impairments in social interaction and communication combined with a restricted repertoire of interests, activities, and behaviours, with onset in early childhood. The prevalence is between 1 and 2 per 1000, although two recent studies suggest up to 4.6 per 1000. Boys outnumber girls. The incidence of reported cases is increasing but it is uncertain whether this is a true rise or is due to changing diagnostic criteria and increased awareness.

◆ In many cases symptoms are present and recognized by parents before the age of 2 years. Long delays in diagnosis are commonplace. In 15–30 per cent there is regression and frank loss of skills, usually during the second year of life but sometimes earlier or later.

◆ Early diagnosis is important because (a) early intervention may be beneficial, although this is still uncertain, (b) parents are very dissatisfied and lose confidence in professionals when delays occur in diagnosis, and (c) genetic advice is needed so that parents can make choices about further children—the risk of recurrence of autism in another child is 5 per cent and is several times higher than that for related disorders of communication.

◆ Several screening tests for autism have been proposed. The one that would be most suited to UK screening and the best researched is the Checklist for Autism in Toddlers (CHAT). This must be administered at 18 months (±2 months). CHAT is a five-item test aimed at behaviours that are typical of autism—impairment of joint attention and of pretend play. CHAT has good specificity but low sensitivity. The authors do not currently recommend its formal introduction for screening; however, learning how to use CHAT is an excellent way of improving health professionals' awareness of autism and this may facilitate earlier diagnosis.

◆ Each district needs access to a multidisciplinary team for assessment and management of suspected autism.

- There is *no* support for the proposition that the MMR vaccine causes or precipitates autism: see for example
  - Incidence of autism spectrum disorders: Changes over time and their meaning. Rutter M. Acta Paediatrica **94**: 2–15, 2005.
  - Sengupta N, Bedford H, Elliman D, Booy R. Measles: prevention. Clinical Evidence. BMJ 2005. (http://www.clinicalevidence.com)
  - MRC Review of Autism Research. Epidemiology and causes. 2001. (http://www.mrc.ac.uk/pdf-autism-report.pdf)
- A national plan for autism has been published: http://www.nas.org.uk/nas/jsp/polopoly/

See HFAC4 website

High-risk follow-up The early recognition of many children with cerebral palsy is facilitated by a high-risk follow-up clinic for infants who have been in neonatal intensive care. Between 8 and 20 per cent of cases of cerebral palsy are related to neonatal encephalopathy and a further substantial proportion to the problems of prematurity and low birth weight. A combination of information regarding clinical progress and imaging data allows the neonatologist to offer increasingly reliable predictions about the probability of permanent impairment. Identification of dysmorphic syndromes and of the underlying genetic abnormality is also becoming more accurate, and there are more data on which to predict long-term outcomes.

Diagnosis of hearing and vision defects, and of moderate and severe motor impairments, can usually be achieved within the first year of life, although the interpretation of motor or developmental deficits is complicated by the need to correct for prematurity (see box). The more subtle cognitive and behavioural problems commonly associated with very low birth weight may not be easily identifiable until school entry or even later.

Similarly, follow-up of children who have experienced postnatal insults to the nervous system, such as trauma or infection, should identify a further significant proportion of children who are or become disabled.

Listening to parents If asked carefully chosen well-structured questions, most parents can provide detailed reliable information about their child. Inappropriate reassurance of parents by professionals continues to be a common cause of delay in diagnosis of disabilities. Staff should be familiar with the normal 'milestones' of development and their variability and with the various presentations of severe learning disabilities, muscular dystrophy, autism

> ## Correction for prematurity
>
> ◆ In 1947, Gesell and Amatruda recommended that full correction for prematurity should be made when assessing the development of preterm infants. This seemed logical and is the usual practice.
>
> ◆ Normative data for available developmental tests were obtained on populations of mainly full-term or slightly pre-term infants. The relevance of these data to very pre-term infants is uncertain.
>
> ◆ If full correction is made for prematurity in the very pre-term infant, some infants with unequivocal motor abnormalities will have developmental quotients within the normal range. In other words, if developmental assessment is considered asa 'screening test' for cerebral palsy, the sensitivity is greater if no correction is made; specificity is greater if full correction is made.
>
> ◆ In the first year of life, for infants with no identifiable neurological deficit, prediction of IQ at age 5 is slightly better if scores corrected for prematurity are used; thereafter, prediction is better if uncorrected age is used.
>
> ◆ From the primary care team's perspective, there are two practical points. First, interpretation of developmental assessment in very pre-term infants is difficult and usually needs specialist help. Second, concerns about development in general and motor development in particular in these infants should not be dismissed as being due solely to prematurity.

spectrum disorder, etc., and they should remember that in a significant number of these children (including those with cerebral palsy) no high risk factors can be identified.

'Evolutionary' diagnoses   The period of uncertainty while a diagnostic problem evolves often leads to delay in commencing a formal intervention programme for children with cerebral palsy or severe learning disability. There is no evidence that this delay has any adverse effect on functional outcome, but the early involvement of therapy and educational disciplines is perceived by parents as highly beneficial and supportive, and this is particularly true in situations where the diagnosis is uncertain.

Management
Above all else, parents value the quality of communication between themselves and the professionals. Badly handled news breaking (see HFAC4 website) is

still one of the most common concerns voiced by parents of disabled children. This issue is important not only in cases where the child has a serious disorder but also when the problem is perceived by the professional to be relatively minor—it may not be minor to the parents.

The conditions described above are rarely amenable to treatment in the medical sense, but much can be done to improve quality of life. The prevention, identification, and management of disability involves many other disciplines and agencies in addition to those professionals directly concerned with child health. Parents and voluntary organizations have made it very clear that they expect a high standard of care, and there is a strong professional commitment to provide this, bringing together the perspectives of social services, education authorities, and voluntary agencies.

The multiple nature of childhood disability has profound implications for planning. For example, the services that are needed by a child with cerebral palsy do not depend on the diagnosis but on the pattern of disabilities and family circumstances. Services set up to deal with only one disability will run into difficulties. A comprehensive multidisciplinary service, usually although not invariably based in a child development centre, is essential for the assessment and ongoing care of children with major disabilities (see Chapter 14 for further discussion).

There is a strong link between disability and both social class and income. Lower-income families have more children with disabilities, while having a disabled child costs money and limits the earning power of families. Current benefits are from 20 to 50 per cent too low to meet the minimum essential costs of disabled children and their families. The 1991 UK Census confirmed the correlation between poverty and enumeration districts with high levels of limiting long-term illness.

High-prevalence low-severity conditions

Some developmental problems give rise to much concern in early childhood and are likely to affect educational progress, but are not sufficiently severe to prevent the attainment of independence in adult life. Many of these tend to improve as the child matures and some resolve completely. The most important of these, delay in speech and language acquisition, will be considered in some detail, because the identification of these children has been a contentious issue in preventive child health care and has important implications for social services and education authorities.

Other examples of developmental impairments include mild global learning disabilities, clumsiness, minor or mild psychological problems, and specific learning disabilities such as 'dyslexia'.

Developmental screening

This can be defined as 'systematic repeated measurements of the developmental progress of apparently normal children, at specified key ages in infancy and early childhood, in order to detect children whose development is suspect in one or more areas, or to confirm normality'. The term should be restricted to procedures whose philosophical aim is to meet the classic criteria for screening tests (p. 133).

In previous editions, we did not recommend formal screening tests to identify children with severe disorders because they are not needed, and we questioned the value of developmental screening programmes for mild and moderate developmental disorders. This was not because the problems are unimportant—they obviously are—but because there are more constructive ways of approaching the issue. We argued that developmental screening programmes perform poorly when tested against the classic screening criteria and that this is because of fundamental difficulties with applying the concept of screening to child development (see box), rather than to shortcomings of available tests.

Reasons for shifting the emphasis from developmental screening to primary prevention and opportunistic intervention

- *Many disabling disorders are identified in the neonatal period, or by parents, relatives, and friends, or by playgroup leaders, child care staff, etc.* The additional contribution of screening would be modest. Its main benefits might be in detecting mild developmental problems.

- *Defining who should be regarded as a 'patient' or 'case'* There is no absolute distinction between, for example, normal and abnormal speech, or between excessive clumsiness and acceptable motor competence; nor is there any precise age at which failure to achieve a certain milestone can be said to be abnormal.

- *The definition of 'caseness' is compounded by parents' perceptions* which depend on educational background, social status, expectations for their children, professional views, and the opinions of voluntary organizations.

- Referral for learning problems in school-age children is often governed more by the *availability and ease of access to diagnostic and remedial services* than by any other factor.

- *Poor sensitivity and specificity of screening tests.*

- *Development is a continuum* Children who 'fail' a screen but then 'pass' a definitive assessment show a higher rate of subsequent problems than those who 'passed' the screen.

- *Inverse care law* Children and parents who are most in need of help are least likely to access it. Poverty is an important predictor of developmental delay and educational failure—in fact, on a population basis it may be as good a predictor of poor educational outcomes as results of screening tests.

- *Lack of evidence* that formal developmental screening programmes have either short- or long-term benefits.

- *Positive evidence* that outcomes can be improved by intervention programmes aimed at communities or populations.

Tests for use by non-specialists

- The *Macarthur Communicative Development Inventory (MCDI)* is a parent-report instrument designed for use by non-specialists. It provides a useful review of a child's speech and language progress up to the middle of the third year. It (and the PEDS—see below) is being used in Sure Start evaluations (see box on p. 55).

- The 10-item *Parents' Evaluations of Developmental Status (PEDS)* was devised by Dr Frances Page Glascoe in Nashville, Tennessee. It taps into parents' knowledge of their child. Referral decisions depend on the pattern of parental responses. Data are available comparing it with a range of more formal tests.

- *First words and first sentences test* (*see* HFAC4 website)

- The *Denver Developmental Screening Test (DDST)*, devised by Frankenburg, is a popular developmental screening test in North America and extensive data are available regarding its psychometric characteristics and its performance as a screening test.

- The *Schedule of Growing Skills* is a widely available UK developmental scale based on the work of Dr Mary Sheridan. Data are available comparing it with the Griffiths scale.

For further literature and availability of these tests, and the *Framework for assessment* pack of assessment methods, *see* HFAC4 website.

Professionals sometimes need to use a developmental test for reasons other than screening. For example, they may wish to check on their suspicions, demonstrate problems to a parent, or teach trainees. Currently popular methods are listed in the box. Of these, the Denver scale is the best known and is easy to apply. The Schedule of Growing Skills takes longer to administer but allows a more considered appraisal of the child's skills. PEDS is designed to elicit parental concerns in a systematic way (see HFAC4 website). It has been used in Australia to help not only health professionals but also a range of other staff to ask structured questions to parents about their child's development (box). This is important because many problems come to light through community child care and early years networks.

Platforms—the Australian approach

Platforms is an evidence-based approach to the early detection of problems and major risk factors in the community. It is based on the fact that young children and their families make contact on numerous occasions with a number of different professionals—community nurses, child care centres, preschools, schools, GPs, and paediatricians. Platforms attempts to reconceptualize these encounters as 'platforms' from which professionals engage in conversations with parents about their child and themselves, systematically elicit and respond to their concerns, make informed referrals for further assessment or intervention, and work closely with other professionals in the community.

Platforms has three components.

1 Improved coordination of services at a community level—setting up a steering group of professionals and consumers, mapping existing resources for children and families, establishing data collection systems, etc.

2 Detecting problems and those major risk factors which have been shown to have a deleterious effect on child outcomes, and where an effective intervention exists. This uses the Parents' Evaluation of Developmental Status (PEDS), a 10-item parent-completed questionnaire covering the age range birth to 8 years, plus additional questions designed to detect risk factors.

3 A series of age-relevant activities and interventions which have been shown to improve child outcomes, such as breastfeeding, immunization, appropriate nutrition, secondary prevention of obesity, reading to young children, etc.

See HFAC4 website

For assessment of other aspects of the child's progress, in the context of the family, the guidance in *Framework for assessment* should be consulted (page 21).

'Delay' in speech and language acquisition

It is said that 20 per cent of parents are concerned about their child's speech development and 70 per cent of the UK's speech and language therapy budget is spent on children. Yet there is still little reliable information on which to base service planning.

Delays in the acquisition of speech and language require special consideration for the following reasons.

- They are common.
- They are probably the most common single cause of parental concern about development.
- They can be the presenting feature of other serious disorders (secondary language impairment)—deafness, severe learning disability, cerebral palsy, rare disorders such as congenital pseudobulbar palsy, auditory agnosia (children who show no response to sound but have normal peripheral hearing), and autism.
- Severely impaired children may need special educational facilities.
- Intervention at an early stage might avoid irreversible impairment of language acquisition.
- Early developmental problems, psychosocial and behavioural problems, and environmental adversity may interact to create a series of negative experiences for the child and parent, which seriously affect subsequent health and progress. Early intervention might break this downward spiral of disadvantage.

Causes of delayed language development   The causes of language delay, although widely debated, are still uncertain. Language difficulties do run in families, and both genetic and environmental factors contribute to this finding. This observation is of practical importance because the use of written materials as a means of 'screening' for or identifying language delay in children may present particular difficulties to these parents.

Normal variation   There are wide variations among normal children in the rate of language acquisition (Fig. 13.1) and in the way children acquire language. Genetic influences play a substantial role in determining the rate of language development among the slowest 5–10 per cent of children. Fast developers are more likely to be found in professional families and slow developers are more likely to have parents who are poor and unskilled or semi-skilled, but these are generalizations.

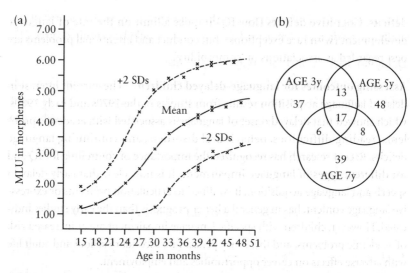

Fig. 13.1 (a) The mean length of utterance (MLU) (a standard measure of language production which is roughly equivalent to the number of syllables per sentence) plotted against age. The variability between children is such that one-sixth of children aged 4 years have an MLU equal to the 50th centile for a 3-year-old; in other words, one child in six can be said to be one year behind in expressive language development. (Reproduced with permission from Wells, G. (1985). *Language development in the pre-school years.* Cambridge University Press.) (b) The language development of 857 children was assessed at 3, 5, and 7 years. Many children were 'delayed' at one assessment, but only 17 were considered delayed at all three. (Reproduced with permission from Silva, P.A. (1987). Epidemiology, longitudinal course and some associated factors, an update. *Clinics in Developmental Medicine*, Vols 101/102, p. 6. Blackwell Scientific, Oxford. In *Language Development and Disorders* (ed. W. Yule and M. Rutter).)

Specific language impairment   Many authors have drawn a distinction between 'simple delay in language development' and 'language disorder', although there are no absolute differences between these categories and the value of distinguishing them is still uncertain. The term 'specific language impairment' (SLI) is now preferred to 'language disorder' since the former makes no assumptions about the nature of the problem. Operational definitions of this term vary between authors, but most accept that a child can have difficulties with one or more aspects of the use of language which are out of keeping, or out of step, with other intellectual functions and are not explained by hearing loss, deprivation, or overt neurological disorder.

Comorbidity   Delayed language development may be an isolated phenomenon but it is commonly accompanied by other problems such as generalized cognitive impairment, behaviour and conduct disorders, and attention deficits. Cognitive deficits (low IQ) impose a limit on the rate of language development (with rare exceptions), but conduct and attentional problems are best regarded as associations or 'comorbidity'.

Assessing outcomes for language-delayed children   The current interest in delayed language acquisition results from studies in the 1970s and early 1980s, which showed that delayed onset of language is associated with academic problems, reading difficulties, behavioural disorders, and continuing language deficits. Recent research has recognized the importance of controlling for IQ and for different types of language impairment. It is now clear that early delay in speech and language acquisition, if confined to articulation problems or expressive language content, has in general a better prognosis than the early studies indicated. However, children with specific language impairment are at increased risk of academic problems, and these may persist into secondary school and adult life with adverse effects on career opportunities and employment.

Identification   Parents are often surprisingly lacking in knowledge about normal language development, and even highly educated parents may benefit from guidance and information. There is a natural tendency to focus on the quantity and clarity of speech, and professionals need to appreciate and explain the importance of *comprehension* and *social communication*.

Educating parents about *hearing behaviour* is also important, and the need to assess hearing in any child with language delay, especially if comprehension is suspect, should be stressed (Chapter 11).

Formal screening is not needed to identify the majority of children whose speech and language development is obviously normal or the very small number who, equally obviously, have gross delay or abnormal development. In the latter case, the child's difficulties may be highlighted by a health professional, early years leader, or a friend or relative. Parents may need guidance in defining the nature of the problem and in accepting that there is something wrong, but they are often aware that the child is 'different' (*see* HFAC4 website).

Screening to identify children with less severe delays in speech and language development is a much more difficult issue. The development of new tests is unlikely to be helpful because, although screening tests tend to have rather low sensitivity, the main problem does not lie primarily in the tests themselves. It is the disappointing overall performance of the whole process which raises serious doubts as to whether a screening model is appropriate.

What is the current best policy?   A systematic review did not find evidence in support of formal population screening for speech and language delay (*see* HFAC4 website). Chapter 3 explained why the evidence favours a primary

prevention approach. Universal access to health professional advice is important to ensure that the aims of this approach are achieved—to facilitate key
learning skills including language development, to inform parents about normal and abnormal language acquisition, and to explain how this links with the
first steps to literacy.

Nevertheless it is still important to identify children with specific language
impairment and with 'secondary' language delays. Professionals can do this by
drawing on parental concerns, using structured questions that tap into parents' knowledge of their child, supported by the insights of relatives, child care
staff, play group leaders, etc. If there is doubt as to whether language is developing normally, the child can either be referred immediately (if the problem
seems to be severe or the parents are very concerned) or a test can be used to
help decide on further action.

The identification of children with comprehension deficits can be difficult
even for experienced professionals. A formal checklist or test can help parents
and professionals to decide whether to refer a child for formal assessment by
specialists or simply observe progress; it could also be useful in monitoring the
progress of large numbers of children on a community-wide basis, for instance
in monitoring progress of projects like Sure Start.

Few tests fulfill the criteria of being quick and easy for non-specialists to
use, standardized for the kind of use envisaged here, and reasonably cheap for
community services to purchase. The Sure Start programme plans to adopt
MCDI and PEDS (p. 251), applied at ages 2 and 4 years. A recent review (*see*
HFAC4 website) suggested that in the UK the test best meeting the criteria for
use by health visitors is the First Words, First Sentences test, although the data
on this are still scanty.

Intervention   For the child with difficulties in speech and language development, gains can be demonstrated from intervention programmes. The best
evidence is for children in the 3–4 year age group. The benefits are less clear
for younger and older children, and some disorders, notably pragmatic skills,
are more resistant to intervention. Children with secondary delays due to
hearing loss, cognitive deficits, or autism spectrum disorder, for example, need
a different approach. Those who have severe disorders such as the various
forms of aphasia usually need to learn ways of coping with their disability as
this is likely to be permanent.

Parents, teachers, and other non-specialists who spend time with the child
can learn relevant skills from the speech and language therapist. Early identification allows time for progress to be assessed and for appropriate liaison
with the education authority. It is important that joint planning for the child's

educational placement and programme be undertaken between health (in particular the speech and language therapist) and education, as conflicts can easily arise in this area.

Managing referrals—a service for children with speech and language problems Since speech and language delays are so common, a high referral rate is inevitable. Managing referrals to the speech and language therapy service is important to avoid services being overwhelmed, resulting in long waiting lists and consequently high non-attendance rates. Unless this is done, children recognized as having a potentially serious problem have to take their place in the queue and may wait months to be seen. One approach is to ensure that initial assessments ('triage') are done by an experienced therapist with the confidence to make decisions. An explicit process of prioritization and regular periodic caseload review facilitates caseload management. The system needs to be integrated with an audiological service so that hearing can be assessed promptly in any child where this is in doubt.

The findings of intervention research are summarized in the box.

Interventions for speech and language problems

◆ Research in intervention is difficult because the range of severity is wide, the rate of spontaneous improvement is variable, there are many differing profiles of language delay, each with a different prognosis, controls for non-verbal IQ and socio-economic status are essential, and apparent short-term gains with intervention may 'wash out' over time so that longer follow-up may reveal a diminishing advantage for the intervention group against controls; conversely, there may be 'sleeper' effects and there may be no apparent benefit in early childhood but the advantages of early intervention might be seen in the teens or adult life. Single case studies can contribute useful information but it must be shown that the findings generalize to other children.

◆ Specific speech and language teaching procedures can accelerate the child's acquisition of vocabulary, phonological skills, and grammatical structures, but there is little evidence that these changes confer any long-term benefit to the child. This may be because of continuing spontaneous improvements in many untreated children, but the necessary long-term studies have not been done. Little is known about the length of treatment needed for maximum benefit or the extent to which treatment generalizes to other areas of language.

- Parents can carry out intervention programmes under the guidance of speech and language therapists; the results are probably as good as those obtained with one-to-one professional therapy, although not all parents are able or willing to do this.

- Most children are treated on the assumption that they will acquire language in the same way as 'normal' children, but this may not be true for those with severe SLI. Different approaches may be needed for these, perhaps requiring a more individualized programme.

- Because of the association between language problems and other behavioural and attentional difficulties, intervention often needs a substantial behaviour management component.

- In cases of environmental deprivation, language delay may be the most visible of the child's deficits but rarely occurs in isolation. Effective intervention programmes should probably address the child's development and family situation rather than focusing solely on language.

- Verbal interaction between staff and children in an early years setting is often less than is needed (in both quality and quantity) to bring about improvements, and early years placement should not on its own be regarded as a 'treatment' for language delay of predominantly environmental origin (although it may have many other benefits for parent and child). More structured educational programmes are likely to be more beneficial.

- Communication groups in early years settings may result in significant gains not only in communication skills but in other aspects of cognitive development, attention control, and behaviour.

- Intervention is needed for other forms of speech and language problems, for example, early recognition and treatment of speech impairments associated with cleft palate, palatal dysfunction, and hypo- and hypernasality, and explanation and counselling for parents of preschool children with problems of fluency, as this may reduce the incidence of true stammering in adult life.

Borderline or mild learning disabilities (so-called 'developmental delay')

Causes   This may be due to specific conditions, non-specific genetic factors, environmental 'deprivation', or, most commonly, to an association and interaction of such influences. 'Subcultural deprivation' as a cause of learning difficulties in the mild to moderate range is an important problem, particularly in poor inner-city areas and is, at least in theory, amenable to intervention (p. 54).

Detection and intervention   These children are likely to be identified by parents, relatives, or child care staff such as play group leaders. In some families, however, particularly those living in poverty, slow development may not be recognized or parents may not have the resources to seek and use help for the child.

In cases where biological rather than environmental factors are the basis for the child's problems, early intervention will be requested and expected by parents. Programmes such as Portage appear to have little effect on the overall pace of learning or the eventual IQ, but are a great help to parents in understanding and meeting their child's needs. Early liaison between health, education, and social services is the necessary prelude for long-term planning for the child's future.

Motor delay and 'clumsiness'

Leaving aside those children already diagnosed with a motor disorder in early infancy, delay in walking is most commonly a normal variant and is often associated with bottom shuffling. The majority of late walkers who have neurological reasons for the delay have been identified before 18 months of age, although 50 per cent of boys with Duchenne muscular dystrophy (DMD) walk later than 18 months. We do not recommend formal screening for DMD (p. 199). Smith *et al.* (*see* HFAC4 website) examined the effect of screening all boys who were identified as not walking at 18 months as part of the routine developmental screening programme. The yield was small and they concluded that a population screening programme was not justified, but it was worthwhile testing non-walking boys at 18 months on an opportunistic basis.

We are not aware of any formal studies on this issue; however, we suggest that any late-walking boy who does not have a family history of bottom shuffling, or who has evidence of language delay (common in DMD), or who shows evidence of clumsiness or weakness, or difficulty with running or stairs should have a creatine phosphokinase estimation to exclude DMD. An evaluation of this clinical policy would be helpful.

Developmental coordination disorder   'Clumsiness' is the colloquial term used to describe children who have poor coordination, sometimes but not always in association with other developmental difficulties. The term 'dyspraxia' is widely used, but the preferred description (DSM-IVR) is 'developmental coordination disorder' (DCD). The more obvious motor difficulties tend to resolve over time, but in many children subtle problems persist and are accompanied by a variety of social and relationship difficulties in school. It is unclear whether these are intrinsic to DCD or are simply common comorbidities. Various treatment regimens have been described, although the value of these in the longer term remains uncertain and the availability of the necessary expertise is limited.

Although screening has been proposed, such a programme would not currently meet the criteria for screening (p. 133). Case definition is elusive and the performance of the available screening tests in routine use is uncertain. This does not mean that parental concerns should be ignored. However, evaluation of motor problems is difficult in primary care settings and needs the resources of a multidisciplinary team, and so children with motor problems should be referred for assessment.

Specific learning disabilities

These are defined as unexplained difficulties in mastering individual skills such as reading. These conditions are only rarely recognized in the pre-school years, but are occasionally suspected when alert parents or nursery teachers recognize potential difficulties; this may be more likely to happen when there is a positive family history of disorders such as 'dyslexia'.

There are links between delayed language development and reading problems, and also some associations with anomalous patterns of eye movement. Some promising results have been reported with respect to the predictive value of rhyming skills.

Several approaches to screening for dyslexia have been proposed and are attracting some interest in educational research, but at present there is no screening procedure designed for use by health professionals. Schemes for the general promotion of reading skills and the early identification of reading problems in school look more promising. Regrettably, it is difficult for primary health care staff to know where they should refer children whose parents are worried about specific learning disabilities. Each district needs to set out guidance and details of what it can offer within both health and education sectors.

Developmental disorders are often defined in terms of discrepancy between one sphere of ability and the child's overall profile, but Dyck *et al.* question the validity of this approach: a study in Wales showed the difficulty in defining coordination disorder with sufficient precision for efficient referral guidelines to be developed.

4r *Recent publications on child development and screening* O'Connor TG (2002). The 'effects' of parenting reconsidered: findings, challenges, and applications. *Journal of Child Psychology and Psychiatry* **43**:555–572.

Rutter M (2003). Nature-nurture interplay in emotional disorders. *Journal of Child Psychology and Psychiatry* **44**:934–944.

Dyck MJ, Hay D, Anderson M *et al.* (2004). Is the discrepancy criterion for defining development disorders valid? *Journal of Child Psychology and Psychiatry* **45**:979–975.

Dunford C, Street E, O'Connell H *et al.* (2004). Are referrals to occupational therapy for developmental coordination disorder appropriate? *Archives of Disease in Childhood* **89**:143–147.

Language development is influenced both by genes and by environment, with genetic factors playing a bigger role in the slowest 5–10% of children: *See* Bishop DV (2001). Genetic influences on language impairment and literacy problems in children: same or different? *Journal of Child Psychology and Psychiatry* **42**:189–198.

Glascoe FP, Oberklaid F (1999). A method for deciding how to respond to parents' concerns about development and behaviour. *Ambulatory Child Health* **5**:197–208.

An ingenious study design used twins who often have mildly delayed language to tease out the role of exposure to language in facilitating language development. *See* Thorpe K, Rutter M, Greenwood R (2003). Twins as a natural experiment to study the causes of mild language delay: II: Family interaction risk factors. *Journal of Child Psychology and Psychiatry* **44**:342–355.

Parents views on speech and language monitoring and therapy were considered in a useful qualitative study; parents were generally grateful when real problems were identified and assessed but there were also a number of negative responses and worries about medicalisation of development, stigma etc:

Glogowsk M, Campbell R (2004). Parental Views of Surveillance for Early Speech and Language Difficulties. *Children & Society* **18**:266–277.

The team who devised the CHAT (a checklist for screening for autism in toddlers) has reviewed the outcomes at age 7 of children identified at age 2 and found significant changes in the pattern of impairment compared to what was expected at 2. Prediction at age 3 was more reliable: *see*

Charman T, Taylor E, Drew A (2005). Outcome at 7 years of children diagnosed with autism at age 2. *Journal of Child Psychology and Psychiatry* **46(5):** 500–513.

Nutbrown C, Hannon P, Margon A. Early literacy work with families. London, Sage Publications, 2005.

Psychological, emotional, and behavioural problems

In Chapter 3 we considered the prevention of emotional and behavioural disorders. Here we examine the identification of, and intervention for, a range of common problems affecting behaviour and emotional, moral, and psychological development*. Although in the majority of cases these problems are 'mild' or 'moderate' and are not the same as psychiatric disorder, they are clinically significant and represent a health care need. They include behaviours or distressed emotions which are common or normal in children at some stage of development, but become abnormal by virtue of their frequency or severity, or their inappropriateness for a particular child's age compared with the majority of ordinary children. Therefore they are more than the annoying behaviours displayed by most children at some time. Prevalence rates are summarized in the box.

Prevalence rates for psychopathology in childhood and adolescence

◆ The point prevalence rate for problematic psychological conditions in childhood and adolescence is approximately 20 per cent. The prevalence is much higher in deprived districts—in one survey, 68.6 per cent of pre-school children had at least one psychological problem and 29.1 per cent had three or more problems.

◆ About 10 per cent exhibit 'considerable distress and substantial interference with personal functions' and are sufficiently severe for assessment by a psychiatric service. Another 10 per cent have mild or moderate psychopathology—emotional, behavioural, relationship, or psychological abnormalities which are clinically significant but are not sufficiently severe, pervasive, distressing, or handicapping to be regarded as psychiatric disorders. This includes subjective mental distress which is complained of by the child or adolescent but often goes unnoticed by parents or teachers.

In pre-school children (under 5 years of age)

◆ Waking and crying at night: 15 per cent
◆ Over-activity*: 13 per cent
◆ Difficulty settling at night: 12 per cent
◆ Refusing food: 12 per cent

---

* Some of this material has been used previously in D. Hall and P. Hill, Community child health services. In *Health care needs assessment* (ed. A. Stevens and J. Raftery) (2nd edn). Radcliffe Medical Press, Oxford, 2002. Acknowledgements to Professor Peter Hill.

♦ For polymorphous pre-school behavioural problems involving a combination of high activity levels, disobedience, tantrums, and aggressive outbursts, associated with tearfulness and clinging, a point prevalence figure of about 10 per cent can be estimated among 3-year-olds.

In middle childhood (age 6–12 years)

♦ Persistent tearful unhappy mood: 12 per cent

♦ Bedtime behavioural rituals: 8 per cent

♦ Night terrors/other disturbances of sleep: 6 per cent

♦ Bedwetting: 5 per cent

♦ Inattentive over-activity*: 5 per cent

♦ Fecal soiling: 1 per cent

♦ Between 12 and 25 per cent of children in this age group have psychological disorder, with 7–14 per cent having overt handicapping psychiatric disorder and 5–11 per cent having 'mild' emotional and behavioural problems with various combinations of anxious unhappiness, difficult or antisocial behaviour, and poor relationships with other children.

In adolescence (age 13–18)

♦ Appreciable misery: 45 per cent

♦ Social sensitivity: 30 per cent

♦ Evident anxiety: 25 per cent

♦ Suicidal ideas: 7 per cent

♦ About 10 per cent of the general adolescent population suffers from more complex depressive moods ('marked internal feelings of misery and self-depreciation'). This is in addition to those diagnosed as having psychiatric disorder (including major depression, with a point prevalence rate of 2–3 per cent).

* Prevalence depends on the definition used—for definitions of hyperkinesis and attention deficit hyperactivity disorder (ADHD), and for further details of diagnosis and management, see HFAC4 website.

Characteristics of minor psychological problems

♦ They are a source of considerable misery. Although often described as 'mild' or 'minor' they reflect a poor quality of existence for many children and parents in the community. They are clinically significant because they are commonly associated with evident distress in the child or parents.

◆ They are relatively persistent. It is commonly assumed that children will grow out of such problems (presumably because they are similar in form to ordinary difficult behaviour which often is transitory), yet they are remarkably persistent over years. In young children some such problems can develop into or predispose to psychiatric disorder later in childhood, yet they are, to a certain extent, susceptible to prevention and treatment.

◆ They tend to be polymorphous. They present with varying combinations of difficult behaviour, angry outbursts, restlessness, moodiness, irritability or nervousness, eating and sleeping difficulties, poor relations with other children, aggressive behaviour, unusual fads or habits, continence problems, and social sensitivities.

◆ There are also more discrete patterns or problems existing as single entities: enuresis, encopresis, feeding disorder of infancy or childhood, pica, sleep disorders, conduct and oppositional disorders within the family, separation anxiety disorder, sibling rivalry disorder, and transient tic disorder.

◆ Psychological problems interact with physical ill health, and in many cases the distinction between organic illness and psychological disorder is far from clear.

Predisposing factors   The risk factors include:

◆ poor parenting
◆ inner cities
◆ socially deprived families (see Fig. 13.2)
◆ boys rather than girls
◆ children with learning difficulties and, in young children, delayed language development
◆ children with other problems of health or development
◆ adolescence rather than earlier childhood
◆ being 'looked after'.

Associated family relationship problems are common although not universal. They include:

◆ marital discord/altercations/divorce
◆ mental health problems in other family members
◆ parental coldness or irritability towards the child
◆ low degree of parental supervision of the child.

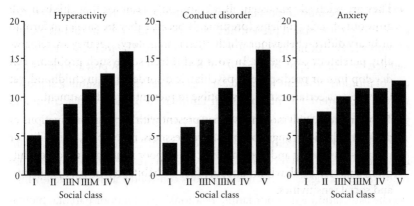

Fig. 13.2 Behavioural problems at age 10 years by social class, Great Britain 1980. (From Spencer 2000, based on Woodruffe *et al.* 1993)

Persistence   Minor psychological problems are relatively persistent, particularly when linked with continuing abnormalities in family relationships. This is true even for young children. Nearly half the psychiatric disorder in 14–15-year-olds is constituted by conditions which have persisted since childhood.

Identification   Currently, we do not recommend embarking on a formal behaviour screening exercise. The problems are the same as those described for developmental screening (p. 255). In the present state of knowledge it is more sensible for advice and help to be offered when parents seek help or when a professional identifies serious difficulties in child rearing and has concerns about the parent's ability to cope with the child's behaviour. Prevention is discussed in Chapters 2 and 3.

This recommendation, like those related to language and developmental problems, is *not* based on a lack of satisfactory screening instruments. There are many behavioural checklists (*see* HFAC4 website) whose psychometric properties have been established.

Intervention   The key issues in deciding whether treatment is necessary are the child's age, the number of psychological (emotional, behavioural, or developmental) abnormalities present, and the severity of their expression.

A single psychological abnormality does not necessarily indicate psychiatric disorder, although it can do in a minority of instances. Like indigestion or headache, a psychological abnormality can be a problem in its own right in some children but a symptom of underlying disease in others. The prognosis for untreated single problems is considerably better than for polymorphous problems.

Therefore the most important distinction in planning treatment is between a psychological problem presenting in isolation and a polymorphous picture of multiple emotional and behavioural problems. The former can often be handled by a direct approach to the presenting problem. A polymorphous picture of multiple problems will need a more complex time-consuming approach which takes parental mental health or family relationships into account and may exceed the capabilities of many primary care teams.

The inverse care law again   The families who might benefit the most from help with psychological problems in their children are often unable to make use of the strategies suggested, because of various constraints such as the following.

- The association with poor family relationships and poor parental mental health. This directly impairs the quality of parenting required to contain difficult behaviour and anxious insecurity in young children or encourage discussion of emotional difficulties in older children and teenagers.
- Associations with social deprivation and poverty. For instance, cramped housing conditions and shared bedrooms do not allow for the mainstream treatments applied to sleep problems, enuresis, or defiant behaviour.

Intervention is effective in some circumstances   There is evidence for the effectiveness of specific interventions in enuresis, fecal soiling, oppositional, defiant, or antisocial behaviour, and sleep settling/ waking difficulties. Medication can be effective in attention-deficit hyperactivity disorder and in a number of other psychiatric disorders (see HFAC4 website).

How to provide the services needed

There are serious shortages of expertise in the field of child mental health (*see* HFAC4 website). The potential volume of referrals for minor psychological pathology could quickly overwhelm the specialist child psychiatry and psychology services. Therefore the effective use of available services is particularly important. Primary care staff need to be aware of normal development and the variations that commonly occur, the conditions and factors which must be considered when deciding on the most appropriate referral, and the availability of expertise within the district.

Health visitors and school nurses with appropriate training can work effectively with cooperative families where the child presents with the common isolated problems listed above. Difficulties with sleeping, eating, temper tantrums, toileting, enuresis and encopresis, and separation anxiety are the topics most frequently cited in reports of successful interventions by health visitors.

Services are generally inadequate for children whose problems do not respond quickly to simple intervention or who have multiple difficulties, yet are not considered to require formal psychiatric help. There are wide and unacceptable discrepancies in service provision between districts, with some spending six times as much as others on child mental health.

Many of the problems affecting older children and young people are closely related to their circumstances, and their management requires multi-agency collaboration. Self-harm and breakdown of placements with foster parents or in residential units often precipitate a crisis, but currently paediatric departments, mental health teams, and social services are not well equipped to deal with these.

Most current service models are based on a four-tier structure (see box). Some services deal with a range of conditions, whereas others offer help for specific problems such as sleep disturbances or enuresis. Service provision may involve community-based teams (involving, for example, a paediatrician, psychologist, and nurse), outreach child psychiatry programmes, community psychiatric nurses, and school nurses or health visitors with special training in behavioural management.

The tiered structure of child and adolescent mental health services

Services promoting the mental health of children are provided by several different agencies, of which health is one; linkage between agencies is national policy. A tiered model for dealing with child and adolescent mental health problems is described in *Together we stand* (*see* HFAC4 website).

Within the NHS:

+ Tier 1 is primary health care.
+ Tier 2 consists of child and adolescent mental health professionals working solo. (The 'child mental health worker' typically operates at the interface between tiers 1 and 2. Some have been employed to work in close association with general practice, and others from a clinic base.)
+ Tier 3 is multidisciplinary teams, most obvious in child and adolescent psychiatric (child guidance, child and family consultation) clinics.
+ Tier 4 comprises highly specialized provision such as child or adolescent psychiatric in-patient units or tertiary clinics for rare problems.

Across the UK there is only a very weak relationship between the volume of local relevant services and local need.

Links with educational and social services are increasingly important in developing behaviour support plans and in developing new models of care, such as the Southampton Behaviour Resource Service (*see* HFAC4 website). Intensive programmes like Multi-Systemic Therapy, which aim to empower parents to cope with difficult young people, look promising.

Recommendations

1 The duty placed on social services to establish a register will encourage each PCO to identify the children with significant impairments in their district.

2 All health professionals should be aware of the main routes by which children with significant impairments are usually identified and there should be explicit pathways of care for parents with concerns about their children's development.

3 Formal universal screening for developmental delay and disorder, speech and language delay, autism, and coordination disorder are not currently recommended.

4 Child health professionals should have the skills to elicit and interpret an account of a child's development.

5 Availability of a formal test to support the initial assessment of a child whose development is in doubt is desirable, but this should be done as part of a network of child development services.

6 A child assessment and development programme and team should be available for children, wherever in the UK they may live. Parents with concerns should be able to access competent advice and help easily.

7 Children with speech and language delay need a rapid assessment service, often combined with a hearing test; a 'seamless' way of providing these services is needed.

8 The high prevalence of emotional and behavioural disorder suggests that community-based care is needed for both prevention and treatment. The demands are too great to be met solely by specialized child and adolescent psychiatry teams, which should provide leadership for community-based services and provide clinical care for the more complex and difficult problems.

Chapter 14

Children with disabilities and special educational needs

This chapter reviews:

- The legislative framework for children with disabilities and special educational needs
- Statutory duties and underlying principles
- Joint agency working
- Service planning
- Service provision for individuals
- Standards for services for disabled children and for child development centres
- Disability registers
- Special educational needs
- Role of the designated doctor for liaison with the education authority

In the previous chapter we considered how to prevent and identify conditions affecting children's intellectual, physical, and emotional development. Here we examine the provision of services for children with disability and children with special educational needs (SEN) in more detail. There is some overlap between the topics but not all disabled children have special needs, neither are all special needs due to disability.

National service framework

The relevant NSF standard is Standard 8: 'Disabled Children and Young People and Those with Complex Health Needs'. www.dh.gov.uk/policyandguidance/healthandsocialcaretopics/childrenservices

Report by Audit Commission—Services for Disabled Children and their Families. 2003. A hard hitting report: refers to the lottery of provision but also notes examples of good practice: www.audit-commission.gov.uk/disabledchildren/

Children with disability

Legislation, statutory duties, and principles

Legislation and statutory duties

The relevant legislation and statutory duties are summarized in the box.

Legislation

- The Children Act 1989 puts a duty upon local authorities to provide services designed to:

  Minimize the effect on disabled children in the area of their disabilities

  Give such children the chance to lead lives which are as normal as possible.

- The need for '*well established and close liaison between the SSD*, the health authority and relevant NHS Trusts and the Local Education Authority*', is emphasized.

- UN convention: *Article 2.3 states that disabled children must be helped to be as independent as possible and be able to take a full and active part in everyday life.*

- **Statutory duties of health authorities**
  The health service has a duty to work with local authorities to **identify children in need** (including those with disability), to contribute to the assessment and to **provide advice to Local Education Authorities** about children with special educational needs (SEN) when requested. Advice for SEN may have resource implications for health services, e.g. funding for special placements or services may be needed. It is important that consistent and accurate advice is given. This work is usually carried out or coordinated by consultant community paediatricians who may also be designated doctors for education, named doctors for child protection, and service managers.

- Removing barriers for disabled children: the service values and principles described in *Removing barriers for disabled children*, section 3.1 and

---

Appendix B, are appropriate for health services as well as social services (see Appendix 2 and Appendix 3). The same document describes standards of service regarding equality of opportunity in service provision (Standard 2) and service delivery to a disabled child and his/her family (Standard 3).

- *Disabled children: directions for their future care.*
- *Framework for the assessment of children in need and their families*: Practice Guidance, Appendix 4.
- Education Act 1996
- The Human Rights Act is important when considering the provision of services. For example, services must be provided in a way which is not discriminatory or degrading and with respect for the child's and his/her family's privacy and family life.
- * Social services department

Principles of service provision

The aim is that, wherever possible, disabled children are to be included in mainstream schooling, leisure activities, and services. The health service should support this inclusion and the provision of equal opportunities for disabled children, although this may be more difficult and more expensive than providing services for children in special schools or segregated in other ways. Furthermore, health and safety regulations and child protection concerns (accusations against care and teaching staff) have affected the way that mainstream schools cater for disabled children. Services also need to be aware of cultural differences with respect to disabled children and their care (p. 35).

Joint agency working

Social services, education services, and health services should work cooperatively to provide the following.

1 **Joint plans** to ensure the appropriate provision for all children, including those with complex or high level of need.

2 **Joint agency reviews** of children with complex needs to ensure that all agencies continue to work efficiently with each other and have a holistic picture of the needs of the child and his/her family.

3 **Joint assessments** Wherever practicable, professionals from different agencies or disciplines should undertake joint assessments in order to minimize

the number of assessments of the child and family, and to improve joint
4r working. The introduction of the 'Common Assessment Framework' will
aid communication between all professionals involved with a child and promote early identification of problems
(http://www.everychildmatters.gov.uk)

4 **Single assessments** Coordination of health assessments is needed to reduce
the number of clinic visits. For example, a single paediatric assessment
could meet the need for the annual health assessment of a 'looked after'
child and the annual review of his/her special educational needs.

5 **Support for children cared for at home and their families** The boundaries of
health care and social care are not clear. Parents and trained carers can often
manage children at home who would previously have been cared for in hospital and by nurses. The statutory agencies must have clear guidance for parents
and professionals about how this type of care can be provided and funded.

6 **Respite** Assessment of need and provision of respite is usually the responsibility of social services. However, services for children with complex health
care needs may be jointly provided or provided by the health
service. Health and social services must cooperate to avoid delays in
providing for individual children.

7 **Care packages** Efficient processes should be in place for obtaining agreement about and funding for unusual or expensive packages of care, placements, or equipment. Local **continuing care** criteria and processes need to
be agreed between social services and health services, with clear routes to
joint commissioning (including education).

8 **Transition to adult services** Community child health services should work
with social services and education departments to identify young people
who will need to transfer to adult services and plan for smooth transfer
when these young people leave school. Problems can be exacerbated by
lack of appropriate adult health services to provide for complex needs (e.g.
combined physical and learning disabilities).

9 **Sharing of information** Health professionals should share information
about an individual child to allow other services to fulfil their duties and to
facilitate smooth inter-agency working, for example for special educational
needs, 'looked after' children, child protection investigations, and children
with complex needs. Parents should receive copies of all reports and
correspondence. Parents' permission (and where appropriate the child's permission) should be obtained, but this is not essential if the child is thought to
be at risk of significant harm. The child's welfare is paramount.

Early support is a DfES programme to improve services for parents with a young disabled child. It is currently undergoing an extensive evaluation. www.earlysupport.org.uk/pilot2/index.html

4r

Service planning

Children's Service Plans

Services for disabled children should be addressed within the children's services plans of Local Authorities and should involve health, education, and voluntary agencies. User and carer involvement in service planning is now expected. Mechanisms for ensuring that user's and carer's views and ideas are considered are essential. Primary care organizations (PCOs) and other NHS trusts should also consider the needs of disabled children and incorporate plans within the local health improvement plans where appropriate. Examples of good practice are given in *Disabled children: directions for their future care*, pp. 27–32.

'Of all the children who may use social care services, children with a disability are the most visible. . . . And yet they remain poorly served. They frequently find it harder to gain access to services, wait longer for assessment, and receive poorer quality services—often from staff lacking specific knowledge and skills.'

Getting the Best from Children's Services: Findings from Joint Reviews of Social Services, 1998/99.

See HFAC4 website

Service provision for the individual child

Meeting normal needs and access to generic health services   Families with a disabled child want easy access to a wide range of therapeutic and support services without multiple assessments. Health services should develop and apply the following standards:

1 Primary care services (e.g. the child health promotion programme, health education, contraception, counselling, etc.) provided for all children must be accessible and appropriate for disabled children and young people.

2 Staff are aware that disabled children are at increased risk of abuse and neglect, which are more likely to remain unrecognized than in other children. The same thresholds for action are applied for all children.

3 Community services are needed to minimize the effects of disability and enable the child to lead as full a life as possible.

4 Relevant health care (e.g. therapy to prevent deformity and improve function) should be available.

5 Information about treatment, services, and benefits is provided to carers and, as appropriate, to children and young people.

6 There is prompt transfer of information and care when a child moves or professionals involved change. This is particularly important for children who are 'looked after' or are part of a travelling family. Efficient transfer of community child health records (immunization details, special educational needs, and medical history), primary care records, and specialist services information is needed, as well as referral to appropriate specialists. Personal Child Health Records and copies of professional letters and reports assist rapid information transfer and encourage full involvement of parents in their child's care.

7 Specialist health services (community or hospital based) are accessible. Multidisciplinary teams and joint clinics can reduce clinic visits and ensure good coordination of care.

Standards for child development services   Facilities for children with disabilities are best provided on a local basis by a child development service. Detailed standards and a 'charter' for this service are published and are summarized in the box.

- A child development service includes specialist services for assessment and management of children with disabilities including physical, learning, hearing, vision, speech, and language problems. This is a multidisciplinary team process functioning in the child development centre, in special and mainstream schools and nurseries, in community clinics, and in the child's home.
- Access to services via a 'single front door' is the ideal. There should be a single information base to support such a team whose work will be made most efficient within a unified management structure.
- Assessment of a child must involve parents fully and result in a written report and sharing information with parents and professionals. The assessment should lead to an action plan which is agreed with parents and a process for coordinating treatment.

- The management of disclosure of distressing or sensitive information should be carefully planned; there are now comprehensive guidelines for giving news.
- One professional should take on the role of key worker in order to provide a single point of contact and coordination for the family's care package.
- A complete assessment should look at the needs of the family as a whole as well as the child as an individual. Therefore it is best done by health, social services, and where appropriate education departments in collaboration.
- These teams have traditionally worked mainly with children under 5 years old. Their service should be strengthened to include children of school age and particularly those undergoing transition to adult services.
- Relationships with primary care and also with hospital and tertiary services are important and should be actively managed to achieve efficiency and good communication.
- Children and families should receive flexible provision according to their requirements. Families should be fully involved in assessment and later treatment according to management plans they have been part of creating.
- The therapy needs of children should be planned following recommended staffing levels. Clinical psychology, child psychiatry, and social work should be part of the team.
- A team base in a child development centre is not essential but is an efficient and effective way to support team working. There should be adequate secretarial and administrative support. Suitable waiting and play areas are needed, with rooms for assessment, treatment, and equipment storage. Parent facilities, information libraries, and Internet access should be available.
- Parent support groups are an essential component of the service. There should be special support for ethnic and cultural minorities.
- The transfer to identified adult services should be carefully planned in agreement with the young person and his/her family. There is a lack of suitable adult services in many areas (e.g. for children with multiple and complex physical, learning and emotional difficulties).
- For recommended staffing levels and supporting services, *see* HFAC4 website.

Disability registers

Primary care trusts will need to continue the development of locality-based information systems for disabled children in collaboration with their coterminous social services and education departments. Within the health service, registers are lists of people kept for four main purposes.

1 **Service planning:** for example, determining the numbers and ages of children with severe communication disability who need health and education resources in a particular locality.

2 **Epidemiology and research:** for example, the evaluation of perinatal care by looking at the level of disability in children who have been born prematurely.

3 **Clinical audit:** for example, using the register to identify a group of children, such as those with disabilities of continence or challenging behaviour, for whom standards of care can be evaluated.

4 **Individual care of patients:** for example, the coordination of multidisciplinary or inter-agency case reviews or planning meetings.

NHS registers

In England and Wales there is a legal duty enshrined in the Education Act 1996 to inform education authorities of children who may need special educational help.* This has led to the development of registers where the attribute that determined inclusion was not a diagnosis but a disability for which children needed special help. Health authority registers were usually set up without explicit family consent, being seen as little more than extensions of medical records. Electronic registers are now held by 60 per cent of the 166 health districts in the UK (as of 2000).

Disability registers within social service departments

In England and Wales, the Children Act 1989 required social service departments to keep a register of children in need (of local authority services) because of disability. The Quality Protects initiative aims to raise standards of care for *all* children in need, including those with disabilities. It requires the registration of children with disabilities for planning purposes.

----

* The relevant legislation in Scotland is (a) the Education Act (Scotland) 1980 and (b) the Standards in Scotland Schools etc. Act 2000. The legislation is currently under review in Scotland.

Problems with registers

The Children Act 1989 legislation did not define disability in a way that was practical for the use of registers. Methods of implementation and the degree of collaboration with other agencies have been very variable. Information is often collected but is stored by different agencies in different forms. Considerations of consent and confidentiality may preclude transfer of identifiable individual patient data between agencies or even within agencies. The Children Act guidance on registration stated that specific parental consent must be sought to hold information. Within the health service, transfer of information should be subject to the principles outlined in the Caldicott Report (*see* HFAC4 website).

Special educational needs

One child in six has learning difficulties at some time in his/her school career and one child in 60 has severe and persistent needs. The legal basis is summarized in the box. SEN is a *relativistic* concept, depending not only upon the child's intrinsic difficulties, whose impact will change over time, but also on the provision. This varies between local education authorities and from school to school. It is needs rather than diagnosis driven, so that there is no direct relationship between a medical diagnosis (e.g. autism, Down's syndrome) and the type of provision necessary, or even whether there should be special provision.

Legal basis

- Special educational needs (SEN) are defined as follows by the Education Act 1996, Section 312: 'A child has special educational needs if they have a learning difficulty which calls for special educational provision to be made for them'.

- **Section 322** of the Education Act 1996 requires health authorities to comply with requests for help from a local health authority in connection with children with special educational needs.

- **Section 332** requires health authorities and NHS trusts to inform the parents and the appropriate local education authority when they form the opinion that a child under the age of 5 may have special educational needs.

Definition

A *learning difficulty* is defined in three ways. A child has a learning difficulty if he/she:

(a) has a significantly greater difficulty in learning than the majority of children of the same age;

(b) has a disability which prevents or hinders the child from making use of educational facilities of a kind generally provided for children of the same age in schools within the area of the local education authority;

(c) is under 5 and falls within the definition of (a) or (b) above or would do so if special educational provision was not made for the child.

Children with SEN may include those with sensory, physical, and emotional and behavioural difficulties.

Special educational provision means:

(a) for a child of two or over, educational provision which is additional to, or otherwise different from, the educational provision made generally for children of the child's age in maintained schools, other than special schools in the area.

(b) for a child under two, educational provision of any kind.

Code of Practice

The Code of Practice on the Identification and Assessment of Pupils with Special Educational Needs offers guidance to schools, other professionals, and parents on the interpretation of the legislation and good practice. While non-statutory, all parties are required to have regard to the Code.

Parental and child participation

Parents have specified rights with respect to the process from identification and assessment through to provision. The 2001 Code emphasizes *child* participation to a much greater extent, although the nature will vary with developmental stage and experience.

Identification and assessment

Identification and assessment form part of a continuum and require multi-professional (and parental) input. The Code specifies four (previously five) stages from the practice of teachers alone through to assessment leading to *a statement* of SEN.

Statements of SEN

Whereas 20 per cent of children may be identified as having SEN, only a small proportion of these will have a statement. Rates vary greatly between local education authorities dependent both on the nature of the population and local policy. Parents and schools have welcomed Statements of SEN as a means of access to improved resources and this has resulted in an increase in the proportion of children with a Statement from about 2 per cent to about 3 to 4 per cent, including more children with less severe difficulties. Government seeks to reverse this increase by enhancement of provision below the level of a statement (School Action Plus). This policy depends on effective and appropriate provision at the earlier stages of the procedure to reassure parents and professionals that this is appropriate and not cost cutting.

Responsibility of health services

There must be clear methods for collaboration between NHS trusts, the local education authority, and social services departments. Primary care and other NHS trusts must consult with the local education authority on how to deliver the health responsibility for assessing and making provision for children with SEN. The responsibility of health professionals is to indicate whether there are health needs or treatment implications which are relevant to the child.

Responsibility of health professionals

Staff may be involved in offering *general* advice and action at Stage 1 (School Action), but are mainly concerned from Stage 2 (School Action Plus) where *individuals* may be assessed in more detail. There are specific time-scales, normally 6 weeks, for providing advice for statutory assessment for the draft statement. Such advice may draw upon or comprise existing written information and advice to the school. When, exceptionally, a longer time is required, perhaps to gather information from several specialists, parents and the local education authority should be informed.

Individual doctors and other health staff may provide oral and written advice on children with SEN at any time, but formal medical advice must be submitted as part of a statutory assessment (*see* HFAC4 website). This should be coordinated by the designated medical officer for SEN and comprise advice from relevant health professionals including the GP, school doctor, therapists, and other specialists (e.g. paediatric neurologists).

Consent and confidentiality

Medical advice for a statutory assessment must be available to the local education authority, other relevant professionals, and parents. Parents must be able to give informed consent to this passing on of information.

Early identification

Children with more severe difficulties will be identified from birth or during the early years, but moderate and milder SEN will become apparent when the child enters pre-school or school provision.

Review

Special educational needs change over time and *reviews* are required of all children on a school's register of SEN. Those with Statements must have at least an annual review, with a medical contribution generally required at key points (e.g. primary–secondary transfer, transition plans). Input to reviews will vary with the importance of medical aspects of the child's SEN.

Inclusion

Inclusion goes beyond *integration*, the placement of children with SEN within mainstream schools. Inclusion requires the school as a whole to change to meet the child's needs and for the child to be placed, as a right, within a main-stream environment. It will require increased resources and changes in atti-tudes and teachers' skills to meet children's special needs.

Individual educational plans

These must be produced for children with SEN. They should be useful for identifying targets and means of achieving these. Individual education plans must be reviewed and amended regularly.

Therapy services

Therapy services, notably speech and language therapy, are increasingly being provided in schools rather than by withdrawing children to clinics. This is more efficient in time allocation and allows therapists to develop collaborative work-ing with teachers to address both specific difficulties (e.g. a language impair-ment) and curricular access (e.g. reading *per se* and literacy skills for other subjects). Therapists are also developing *consultancy* models in addition to *direct treatment* within schools, but both approaches are necessary to meet the range of needs.

Performance targets

Health services must normally respond within 6 weeks of the date of receiving a request for advice from the local education authority for a Statement of SEN. The local education authority will have notified the designated medical officer of the possibility of an assessment. The health services are not obliged to respond within 6 weeks if they had no relevant knowledge of the child concerned prior to the local education authority's informing them that assessment was being considered. Other exceptions to the 6-week rule are as follows:

- where there are exceptional personal circumstances affecting the child or his/her parents (e.g. family bereavement)
- where the parents of the child are absent from the area of the authority for a continuous period of 4 weeks or more
- where the child fails to keep an appointment for an examination or test.

Role of the designated doctor to the local education authority

The designated doctor will require a minimum of two sessions per week per 300 000 total population. The post-holder should be a senior paediatrician who has adequate time allocated in the job plan for committees and supervision. The designated medical officer for SEN must have a strategic and operational role in coordinating strategic and operational activity across PCOs and NHS trusts. The designated medical officer's tasks are summarized in the box. At a strategic level, the Primary Care Organisation should have arrangements for ensuring that trusts and GPs provide appropriate services for children (see box).

Duties of the medical officer

1 Ensure that the responsible body (usually the PCO) is informed about policy development and changes regarding children with SEN and, where appropriate, facilitate policy development arising from such changes; for example, using opportunities to develop pooled budgets and integrated commissioning.

2 Coordinate and ensure the provision of advice to local education authorities, as part of the statutory assessment of children within the statutory time limits.

3 Ensure that all schools have a health contact for seeking advice on the health implications for children who may have SEN.

4 Provide advice and support in conjunction with other relevant health service staff to, for example, GPs, HVs and other primary care workers in preparation of reports on the medical history and health needs of children for schools and local education authorities.

5 Where appropriate, and in collaboration with other relevant health service staff and in consultation with the local education authority, agree standard formats for reports.

6 Ensure coordinated health service provision for a child with special educational needs when, as may be the case with therapy and nursing services, a combination of health authorities, trusts, and other agencies may be responsible for commissioning and providing these services.

7 Make sure through appropriate mechanisms that health advice is provided for annual review meetings and transition plans when appropriate, and for policy development meetings.

Duties of the provider trust

1 Inform the local education authority of particular local arrangements for the early identification of children whom they think may have SEN.

2 Make sure that child health services inform the local education authority about any child who may have SEN.

3 Make sure that all trusts, other providers of health care, and health professionals are aware of the time-scales for statutory assessment and provision of advice as set out in the SEN Code of Practice.

4 Consider, with local education authorities and with a regard to available resources, the health services' contribution to the provision to be specified in a Statement.

5 Consider how the new powers of the Health Act 1999, allowing pooling of budgets and integration of commissioning or providing functions between the NHS and local authorities (including education), can best support services for children with SEN.

6 Meet with senior representatives of local education authorities and health services to plan and coordinate strategic and operational activity.

7 Consider how inter-agency evidence-based planning for children with special educational needs can be an integral part of the Children's and Young People's Strategic Plan and NHS plans.

Summary

- SEN is a *relativistic* concept.
- There is no direct relation between diagnostic categories and provision.

- Multi-agency working is essential.
- Partnership with parents is required by law, as well as being good practice.
- Children must also be meaningfully involved.
- Inclusion is increasing and is the predominant policy.
- Professionals will spend more time in schools and pre-school provision working collaboratively with teachers.
- Consultancy, as well as direct assessment/intervention approaches, is required.

Recommendations

1 There are certain duties which *must* be fulfilled:

 (a) to work with local authorities to **identify children in need** (including those with disability)

 (b) to have regard to the Education Act Code of Practice

 (c) to contribute to the assessment of children with SEN when requested and to **provide advice to local education authorities**

 (d) to provide evidence for assessments within a specified time frame

 (e) there must be a designated doctor to the local education authority.

2 There is ample evidence as to what parents want and need for the diagnosis and care of a child with a disability, and services should be provided in line with that evidence.

3 The identification, care, and support of children with SEN requires multi-agency collaboration; job descriptions must provide sufficient time for this to be undertaken both for individual children and for service planning.

Chapter 15

Child protection programme

This chapter reviews:

- ◆ The Children Act 1989
- ◆ Role of health professionals in child protection
- ◆ Duties of Area Child Protection Committee
- ◆ Designated and named doctor and nurse
- ◆ Categories of child abuse and child protection registers
- ◆ Domestic violence
- ◆ Looked after children
- ◆ Designated doctor and nurse for looked after children
- ◆ Resource implications
- ◆ Private fostering
- ◆ Adoption

In Chapters 2 and 3 we considered the factors that protect against and help to prevent child abuse. Here we examine the management of suspected or actual abuse, and the systems that underpin identification of, and intervention for, children who require protection. We then review the specific needs of children looked after, and the medical contribution to adoption and fostering.

4r **National Service Framework**

The relevant NSF standard is Standard 5 (Core Standards): 'Safeguarding and Promoting the Welfare of Children and Young People'. www.dh.gov.uk/policyandguidance/healthandsocialcaretopics/childrenservices

Child abuse and neglect

'Child abuse consists of anything which individuals, institutions or processes do or fail to do which directly or indirectly harms children or damages their prospects of safe and healthy development into adulthood' (National Commission of Enquiry into the Prevention of Child Abuse, *Childhood matters*, 1996). Child abuse occurs across the spectrum of social class and during any developmental stage of a child, but children under 5 years are at greater risk of serious acute or long-term harm and even death. Cultural differences must be respected and handled sensitively, but are never a reason for accepting inappropriate care, neglect, or abuse.

Every health professional, including those who work largely in adult services, needs to be aware of their duty to recognize and act on concerns about child abuse and of their responsibilities towards the wider group of children in need. The Children Act 1989 provides the legal framework underpinning services for both of these groups.

Children Act 1989

The Children Act 1989 provides a framework of law, determines the jurisdiction of and the approach to decision-making about children's welfare by the courts, and establishes the responsibilities of public agencies to deliver services in order to safeguard and protect children from abuse and neglect and promote their welfare. The Children Act 1989 includes anyone under the age of 18 years old unless they are married. The main points are summarized in the box.

Children Act 1989

When social services are informed that a child who lives, or is found, in their area has been subject to emergency action by social services or the police because of concerns with regard to his welfare or they otherwise

'have reasonable cause to suspect that a child . . . is suffering, or is likely to suffer, significant harm',

they have a duty to:

'make or cause to be made such enquiries as they consider necessary to enable them to decide whether they should take any action to safeguard or promote the child's welfare.' (Section 47(1))

Under Section 17 of the Act, social services have a duty to:

'(a) safeguard and promote the welfare of children within their area who are in need; and

(b) so far as is consistent with that duty, to promote the upbringing of such children by their families, by providing a range and level of services appropriate to those children's needs.'

A child is to be taken to be in need if:

'(a) he is unlikely to achieve or maintain, or have the opportunity of achieving or maintaining, a reasonable standard of health or development ...'

or

'(b) his health or development is likely to be significantly impaired, or further impaired'

without the provision of services by a local authority or

'(c) he is disabled.' (Section 17(10))

Social services are unable to carry out these important statutory responsibilities without access to information and expertise held and services delivered by staff working in other agencies. The Act empowers social services to call upon other agencies to assist them with the delivery of these functions. The agencies that may be required to assist social services include:

◆ any health authority

◆ any special health authority

◆ any national health service trust

◆ any primary care trust.

Guidance on inter-agency working

The Secretary of State has powers under Section 7 of the Local Authority Social Services Act 1970 to require local authorities in their social services functions to act under his general guidance. Such guidance, although it does not have the full force of statute, must be complied with unless local circumstances indicate exceptional reasons justifying a variation. Social services are required to establish and lead inter-agency working, to ensure that statutory welfare and protection functions are effectively carried out. Recent guidance issued under this section has included:

◆ *Working together to safeguard children* (TSO, London, 2006)

◆ Safeguarding children in whom illness is fabricated or induced. TSO, London, 2002

◆ *Framework for assessment of children in need and their families* (TSO, London, 2000)

◆ *Safeguarding children involved in prostitution* (TSO, London, 2000).

The role of health professionals is summarized in the box.

Role of health professionals

'The involvement of health professionals is important at all stages of work with children and families:

- recognizing children in need of support and/or safeguarding, and parents who may need extra help in bringing up their children;
- contributing to enquiries about a child and family;
- assessing the needs of children and the capacity of parents to meet their children's needs;
- planning and providing support to vulnerable children and families;
- participating in child protection conferences;
- planning support for children at risk of significant harm;
- providing therapeutic help to abused children and parents under stress (e.g. mental illness);
- playing a part, through the child protection plan, in safeguarding children from significant harm; and contributing to case reviews.'

(*Working together to safeguard children, 1999*, Paragraph 3.19)

The common assessment framework has been developed to provide a standardised framework for the early assessment of children who have additional needs. (http://www.everychildmatters.gov.uk) It is to be used by all statutory agencies and will cover the three domains of child care: the child's developmental needs, parenting capacity, and wider family and environmental factors (see fig. 1.2, p. 21). This should provide more detailed information to assist decision-making.

Health authorities and primary care trusts are required to:

- ensure that they participate in inter-agency planning and cooperation through Children's Services Plans and Quality Protects Management Action Plans and that there are clear cross references in the Health Improvement Programmes.
- provide services for vulnerable children and contribute fully and effectively to local inter-agency working to safeguard children and promote their welfare.
- contribute to assessments of children in need, including implementing clear service standards.

◆ ensure that all NHS trust staff are alert to concerns about a child's health and development and know how to act upon these concerns in line with local protocols.

Social services are required by the guidance to exercise their powers, in particular those under Sections 47 and 27, to require other agencies to cooperate with the application locally of this national guidance. The interaction of these statutory provisions underpins inter-agency cooperation and the establishment and working of Area Child Protection Committees (ACPCs).

Area child protection committees (ACPCs)

Prior to 2006 there was an ACPC in each local authority area. This was an inter-agency group whose job was to coordinate services to protect children from abuse and neglect. Health services, covering both managerial and professional expertise, were included in the membership. Its responsibilities are summarized in the box. The designated doctor and nurse were members of the ACPC (see page 291).

Duties of the ACPC

◆ To develop and agree local policies and procedures for inter-agency work to protect children, within the national framework provided by this guidance.

◆ To audit and evaluate how well local services work together to protect children, for example through wider case audits.

◆ To put in place objectives and performance indicators for child protection, within the framework and objectives set out in Children's Services Plans.

◆ To encourage and help develop effective working relationships between different services and professional groups, based on trust and mutual understanding.

◆ To ensure that there is a level of agreement and understanding across agencies about operational definitions and thresholds for intervention.

◆ To improve local ways of working in the light of knowledge gained through national and local experience and research, and to make sure that any lessons learned are shared, understood, and acted upon.

- To undertake case reviews where a child has died or, in certain circumstances, has been seriously harmed, and abuse or neglect are confirmed or suspected. To make sure that any lessons from the case are understood and acted upon, to communicate clearly to individual services and professional groups their shared responsibility for protecting children, and to explain how each can contribute.
- To help improve the quality of child protection work and of inter-agency working through specifying needs for inter-agency training and development, and ensuring that training is delivered.
- To raise awareness within the wider community of the need to safeguard children and promote their welfare and to explain how the wider community can contribute to these objectives.

Membership includes:

- The local authority, including social services, education services, and leisure and amenity services
- The National Society for Prevention of Cruelty to Children (NSPCC)
- Health services (managerial and professional) should include the designated doctor and nurse, a representative of the primary care organization and ideally one from adult and child mental health services
- Police
- Probation service
- Other members may include:
  - (i) Other voluntary/independent agencies such as the Soldiers' Sailors' and Airmen's Families Association (SSAFA), National Children's Homes (NCH), Barnardos, Children's Society, etc.
  - (ii) Lawyers
  - (iii) Crown Prosecution Service

Local Safeguarding Children Boards (LSCBs)   4r

From April 2006, these non-statutory bodies were replaced by statutory local safeguarding children boards (LSCBs). These will be heavily based on the pattern of good ACPCs. http://www.everychildmatters.gov.uk/socialcare/safeguarding/lscb/

Duties of the LSCB

- Developing **policies and procedures** for safeguarding and promoting the welfare of children, including on:
  - action where there are concerns, including thresholds
  - training of persons who work with children
  - recruitment and supervision
  - investigation of allegations
  - privately fostered children
  - co-operation with neighbouring authorities
- Participating in the **planning of services** for children in the area of the local authority
- **Communicating** the need to safeguard and promote the welfare of children
- Procedures to ensure a co-ordinated response to **unexpected child deaths**
- **Monitoring effectiveness** of what is done to safeguard and promote the welfare of children
- Undertaking **Serious Case Reviews**
- Collecting and analysing **information about child deaths.**

Membership includes:

Representatives of the Local Authority and its Board Partners:

- District Councils in local government areas which have them.
- The Chief Office of Police for a police area any part of which falls within the area of the local authority.
- The Local Probation Board for an area and part of which falls within the area of the local authority.
- The Youth Offending Team for an area any part of which falls within the area of the local authority.
- Strategic Health Authorities and Primary Care Trusts for an area any part of which falls within the area of the local authority.
- NHS Trusts and NHS Foundation Trusts all or most of whose hospitals or establishments are situated in the local authority area.
- The Connexions Service providing services in any part of the area of the local authority.

- CAFCASS (Children and Family Courts Advisory and Support Service).
- The governor or director of any Secure Training Centre in the area of the local authority.
- The governor or director of any prison in the local authority area which ordinarily detains children.
- Other relevant statutory and non-statutory organizations, including the NSPCC, as appropriate.
- (Adult services from the local health authority and health services should be represented).

Designated and named staff

Each PCO must appoint a designated doctor and a designated nurse for child protection (*see* HFAC4 website). Their role is essentially strategic, ensuring that policies and procedures are in place, ensuring that training is available, and monitoring quality and outcome of services. Each trust must appoint a named nurse and doctor for child protection (*see* HFAC4 website). Their role is essentially operational, ensuring delivery of services, supporting and training staff, and ensuring professional standards of work.

Child protection services and procedures within a PCO should be provided by a team whose membership will be determined by the services delivered and the professional groups employed.

*Child protection categories and registers

Working together (Paragraph 5.99–1999) requires that the social services department keeps a central register of all children resident in the area who are considered to be at continuing risk of significant harm and for whom a child protection plan is required. Agencies and professionals who have concern about a child must have access to the register and be able to make enquiries both in and outside office hours. The categories of registration are physical, emotional, or sexual abuse or neglect as decided by the chair of the child protection conference. These divisions are, to some extent, artificial as there is

---

*See also: Responsibilities of Doctors in Child Protection Cases with regard to Confidentiality. February 2004 www.rcpch.ac.uk

4r

often more than one form of abuse. The category used for registration is the main, but not the only, form of abuse. Tables 15.1 and 15.2 show the numbers of children involved.

From April 2008, Child Protection Registers will cease to exit. Where a child is subject to a child protection plan this should be recorded on the LA Integrated Children's System.

Table 15.1 Numbers of children on child protection registers in England (31 March 2001)

	<1 year	1–4 years	5–9 years	10–15 years	16+ years	All ages
*Numbers**						
Total[†]	2800	8000	8000	7400	600	26800
Boys	1400	4200	4200	3700	200	13700
Girls	1300	3800	3800	3600	40	12900
Rates per 10000 population						
Total[†]	48	33	25	19	5	24
Boys	49	34	25	19	3	24
Girls	48	32	24	19	6	24

* Figures may not add due to rounding

[†] The 'All ages, total' figures include 207 unborn children.

Source: Department of Health (2001), *Children and young people on child protection registers.*

Table 15.2 Registrations to child protection registers in England during the year ending 31 March 2000 by category of abuse: showing the mixed categories incorporated with the main categories

Category of abuse	Number	Percentage
Neglect*	12400	46
Physical abuse*	8000	30
Sexual abuse*	4300	16
Emotional abuse	4600	17
Other	600	3

* Three main categories also feature in the mixed categories. The above table includes these categories with the main categories in order to show the total numbers of children for whom each category of abuse was quoted on the register. The total of percentages will exceed 100 because children in the 'mixed' categories are counted more than once.

Source: Department of Health (2001), *Children and young people on child protection registers.*

The Information Sharing Index (ISI) is a newly introduced approach 4r designed to ensure that professionals concerned about child safety can easily determine which other agencies are involved.

See: http://www.everychildmatters.gov.uk/deliveringservices/index/; also 'Information Sharing: practical guidance', 'Common core of skills and knowledge' also at www.ecm.gov.uk

Physical abuse (Working together, 2006, paragraph 1.30)

Physical abuse may involve hitting, shaking, throwing, poisoning, burning or scalding, drowning, suffocating or otherwise causing physical harm to a child. Physical harm may also be caused when a parent or carer fabricates the symptoms of, or deliberately induces illness in a child. This situation was commonly described using terms such as fictitious illness or Munchausen syndrome by proxy, but now fabricated or induced illness. (see HFAC4 website for more details).

Sudden unexpected death in infancy. Working party report, Chair: Baroness Helena Kennedy, QC. 2004. www.rcpch.ac.uk

Emotional abuse (Working together, 2006, paragraph 1.31)

Emotional abuse is the persistent emotional maltreatment of a child such as to cause severe and persistent adverse effects on the child's emotional development. It may involve conveying to children that they are worthless or unloved, inadequate, or valued only insofar as they meet the needs of another person. It may feature age or developmentally inappropriate expectations being imposed on children. These may include interactions that are beyond the child's developmental capability, as well as overprotection and limitation of exploration and learning, or preventing the child participating in normal social interaction. It may involve seeing or hearing the ill-treatment of another. It may involve serious bullying causing children frequently to feel frightened or in danger, or the exploitation or corruption of children. Some level of emotional abuse is involved in all types of maltreatment of a child, though it may occur alone.

Sexual abuse (Working together, 2006, paragraph 1.32)

Sexual abuse involves forcing or enticing a child or young person to take part in sexual activities, including prostitution, whether or not the child is aware of what is happening. The activities may involve physical contact, including penetrative (e.g. rape, buggery or oral sex) or non-penetrative acts. They may include non-contact activities, such as involving children in looking at, or in the production of, pornographic material or watching sexual activities, or encouraging children to behave in sexually inappropriate ways. See also: Sexual Offences Act 2003, which introduces important new legislation: http://www.opsi.gov.uk/ACTS/acts2003/20030042.htm and guidance following the Bichard Inquiry Report, www.ecm.gov.uk/strategy/guidance.

Neglect (Woring together, 2006, paragraph 1.33)

Neglect is the persistent failure to meet a child's basic physical and/or psycho-logical needs, likely to result in the serious impairment of the child's health or development. Neglect may occur during pregnancy as a result of maternal substance abuse. Once a child is born, neglect may involve a parent or carer failing to provide adequate food and clothing, shelter including exclusion from home or abandonment, failing to protect a child from physical and emotional harm or danger, failure to ensure adequate supervision including the use of inadequate care-takers, or the failure to ensure access to appropriate medical care or treatment. It may also include neglect of, or unresponsiveness to, a child's basic emotional needs.

Domestic violence

This is a common and under-recognized problem (see box). The definition of domestic violence used by the Home Office and adopted in the Department of Health's *Domestic violence: a resource manual for health care professionals* (Department of Health, 2000) is the following:

> domestic violence shall be understood to mean any violence between current or former partners in an intimate relationship, wherever and whenever the violence occurs. The violence may include physical, sexual, emotional or financial abuse.

Domestic violence

- Domestic violence accounts for one-quarter of all violent crime in the UK.

- One in four women and one in six men have experienced domestic violence as defined.

- The likelihood is highest in young people and declines with age.

- Half of those reporting violence in the previous year were living with children under 16; 29% said the children had been aware of what was happening. This proportion increased to 45% in the families of women who were repeatedly assaulted.

- Domestic violence often starts or intensifies during pregnancy and is associated with death, severe morbidity, fetal death, miscarriage, depression, suicide, and alcohol and drug abuse. The characteristics of women suffering violence in pregnancy are well described. See *Why mothers die*, www.cemd.org.uk, pp. 241–51.

- On average a woman is assaulted by her partner 35 times before reporting it to police.

- Risk factors include non-professional background, marital separation, young children, financial pressures, drug and alcohol abuse, disability, and ill health.
- Nearly 35 000 children per year pass through refuges for women victims of domestic violence annually in England and Wales.

Health professionals find it very difficult to ask about domestic violence but there are no acceptable ways of doing this.

The response must be based on respect and confidentiality, but the safety of children is paramount.

Multi-agency planning, local domestic violence fora, and the ACPC are important in addressing the issue of domestic violence.

A useful review of the subject with practical guidance has recently been published:

http://www.dh.gov.uk/PublicationsAndStatistics/Publications

Based on *Domestice violence: a resource manual for health workers* (Department of Health, 2000).

Violence between adult partners occurs in all social classes, in all ethnic groups and cultures, in all age groups, and in disabled as well as able-bodied people. It may involve abuse, accusation, and innuendo, deprivation of freedom, physical or sexual assault, or attacks with deadly weapons. Hearing an assault take place can be as distressing for a child as witnessing one.

Procedures

Each LSCB is responsible for developing local child protection policies procedures, following the guidelines in Chapter 3 of *Working together*. These may vary from authority to authority. (*See* HFAC4 website for further details.)

Quality standards

Child protection is a complex area where legal requirements, local guidance, and the professional practice of many agencies come together within a common framework. The consequences of failure are often tragic in both the short and long term. (*See* HFAC4 website for further details.)

Training

All staff should receive relevant child protection induction and regular updates. This means *every* health worker, including those from adult services who have professional contact with children and young people, parents, or potential perpetrators. Non-clinical managers also require training. (*See* HFAC4 website for further details.)

Looked after children

Looked after children are amongst the most socially excluded of our child population. A series of Government reports have highlighted the extent to which health neglect, unhealthy lifestyle, and mental health needs characterize children and young people living in public care. Looked after children are the epitome of the inverse care law. Their health may not only be jeopardized by abusive and neglectful parenting, but public care itself may fail to repair and protect health and may even exacerbate damage and abuse.

Outcomes of public care have direct and indirect impact on health. In 1997 a Social Services Inspectorate report documented that 75 per cent of care leavers had no academic qualifications, 50 per cent were unemployed, and 17 per cent of young women were pregnant or already mothers. Care leavers are over-represented amongst the prison population (23 per cent of adult prisoners) and 20 per cent experience homelessness within 2 years of leaving care. Of all children they deserve robust health policy and practice and immaculate inter-agency working if the cycle of deprivation is to be broken. This summary outlines the key issues relevant to promoting health in this population.

Definition of looked after children (Fig. 15.1)

The term 'looked after child' was introduced by the Children Act 1989 and describes children in England and Wales in the care of a local authority:*

- as a voluntary agreement between the local authority and those with parental responsibility (*accommodated*, Children Act 1989, Section 20).

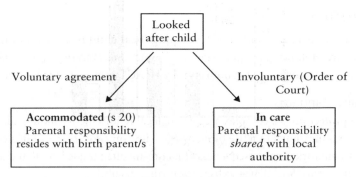

Fig. 15.1 Definition of a looked after child (England and Wales).

* Note the Children Act Scotland 1995 uses the term 'accommodated' to imply a child resident in foster care or a residential children's home who may either be voluntarily accommodated (Section 25) or compulsorily accommodated (Section 70 supervision requirement or order issued by the Sheriff or Children's Hearing). All such children are also referred to as 'looked after'.

♦ as a consequence of a court order where the threshold of 'significant harm' has been established so that parental responsibility is granted to the local authority in partnership with birth parent/s (*in care*).

Epidemiology

During the 12 months to 31 March 2000, a total of 81 500 of England's children had been looked after.[†] This figure[‡] excluded children in agreed short-term respite placements. Of these 81 500 children, a little over half, (41 200) were looked after continuously over the year and a third were new entrants (27 600). This longitudinal perspective gives a clearer insight into actual population need than the commonly quoted snapshot view (58 100 children in England, 11 300 in Scotland, 5371 in Wales looked after on 31 March 2000). Hence, while approximately 1/200 of England's children will be in public care on any particular day, during a year approximately a third as many again will experience the care system. This dynamic picture is more relevant when planning local service provision. In a PCO serving a total population of 100 000, approximately 130 children would be expected to experience public care in a year, of whom approximately 40 would be new entrants.

The following figures and statistics relate to England for children looked after on 31 March 2000. They mask considerable variation between local authorities due to local policy and socio-economic differences. Department of Health statistics provide informative local data. Boys are in a slight majority (55 per cent) and children aged 10 and over are more likely to be looked after

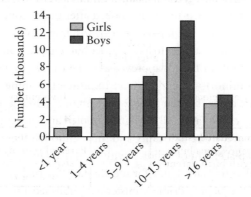

Fig. 15.2 Age/sex distribution of looked after children in England and Wales (March 2001).

[†] Department of Health children's statistical returns, May 2001 (http://www. doh.gov.uk/public/stats1/htm).

[‡] Children receiving local authority respite care: Arrangements of Placements of Children Regulation 13 (HMSO, 1991).

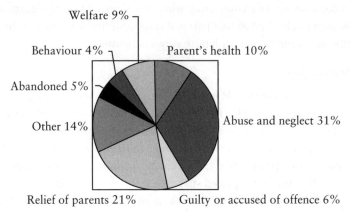

Fig. 15.3 Reasons for being looked after.

(69 per 10 000 child population) than children less than 10 years of age (39 per 10 000 child population) (Fig. 15.2). Data are not currently collected on the ethnicity of children in public care*. However, there is evidence that ethnic minority children are more likely to have adverse health experiences and particular needs in care (*see* HFAC4 website). Data on disabled children are not accurately reported, but at least 9 per cent of allchildren were reported as requiring care (mostly respite) due to their impairment.

Children enter public care for a variety of reasons (Fig. 15.3). Most have experienced parental neglect (by omission or commission) or abuse. Not surprisingly therefore, two-thirds are looked after under court orders. While the majority of children are looked after by foster carers, there is a growing trend for children to be subject to a care order but living at home (11 per cent) or placed with family or friends approved as foster carers (16 per cent of foster placements). A minority of children live in residential homes (11 per cent). Usually these are older children (only 2 per cent of children in residential care are less than 10 years of age). All the figures quoted are subject to considerable variation, both according to locality and time, although there are consistent trends towards placement of children with extended family or near to home, with residential settings used only for specific-task-focused placement.

4r The office of the Deputy Prime Minister has published a report of an investigation into problems encountered in providing looked after children with a good education: A better education for children in care. ODPM, 2003 www.socialexclusion.gov.uk

* It has been collected from the year ending 31 March 2001.

The nature of health problems in looked after children

Until recently there has been no systematic monitoring of health process and outcomes in looked after children. Evidence from local studies (*see* HFAC4 website) suggests neglect of routine immunizations and screening, lack of appropriate care for known acute/ chronic health conditions, and failure to diagnose health and mental health problems (*see* HFAC4 website). However, these studies describe small unrepresentative uncontrolled samples and are unable to distinguish problems preceding or consequent on the child's care experience. Jackson *et al.* (*see* HFAC4 website) compared a group of 119 looked after children with non-looked after population controls. The looked after group fared worse for routine dental care, immunization status, and health-threatening behaviour. Emotional and behavioural problems were more prevalent, and despite a high level of mental health referral few children received treatment. Hill and Watkins studied the records of 49 children over 1–2 years in public care and found that less than 50 per cent of health care plan recommendations had been implemented (*see* HFAC4 website).

More rigorous methodology has been possible in the USA where states have superior health monitoring of 'foster care children' and an enhanced ability to study health care utilization through Medicaid claims. These have shown high utilization of health care, particularly mental health care, compared with socio-economically deprived controls (*see* HFAC4 website).

Policy context

Regulations of the Children Act 1989 recommended a statutory annual medical examination for all children (biannually for children under 5 years old). Local authority performance monitoring has improved uptake rates from earlier estimates of 25–65 per cent. The little evidence available suggests the process may have been ineffective and unpopular with children. New Regulations are now in place (see box).

Amendment of the Arrangement of Placements of Children Regulations 1991 in force from April 2002

Health assessments. Regulation 7

... a responsible authority shall ...

(a) before making a placement, or if that is not reasonably practicable, as soon as reasonably practicable after a placement is made, make arrangements for a registered medical practitioner to conduct an assessment, which may include a physical examination, of the child's state of health;

(b) require the registered medical practitioner who conducts the assessment to prepare a written report of the assessment ...

(c) ... prepare a plan for the future health care of the child if one is not already in existence.

Health reviews. Regulation 6

The responsible authority shall, in respect of each child who continues to be looked after or provided with accommodation by them—

(a) arrange for an assessment, which may include a physical examination, of the child's state of health, to be conducted by a registered medical practitioner, or a registered nurse or registered midwife acting under the supervision of a registered medical practitioner ...

The Quality Protects initiative (England) and the Children First initiative (Wales) aim to improve the welfare of looked after children by a 5-year programme of funding to local authorities. In parallel, the introduction of a national performance-monitoring framework requires local authorities to report annually on 'life health chances' of children in their care. Current health indicators (Table 15.3) remain a crude representation of health.

New arrangements for young people aged 16 or over (care leavers) extend the duties of local authorities to assess and meet the needs of young people up to the age of 18. While statutory regulations currently only require health assessment up to age 16, the need to integrate health care planning into care-leaving pathway plans provides an opportunity for positive health input at this vulnerable age.

Policy in practice

The *Looking After Children* materials, adopted by 98 per cent of local authorities in England and all local authorities in Wales raise the profile of health needs in the overall monitoring and planning for looked after children. They form the basis of the development of the Integrated Children's Services Framework. Carer, social worker, and competent children complete action and assessment records at 6-monthly intervals. In some local authorities these documents are the authoritative record of health status used for performance indicator reporting. The lack of cross-reference to health data sources may undermine the quality and validity of these data. Better integration of the *Looking after children* materials and the statutory medical examination are imperative.

Table 15.3

Examples of potentially useful performance indicators (C19)	Percentage of children in England looked after for at least 1 year on 30/9/01 achieving performance indicator
Immunizations up to date	71
Teeth checked by a dentist in past 12 months	67
Have had annual health assessment	68

In many trusts health professionals work closely with the local authority to promote the health of looked after children. However, at the present time NHS trusts are not accountable for the provision of care other than through local agreements. This situation differs from child protection where in the past health authorities have been charged with the duty to set standards for safeguarding children assisted by the ACPC and designated health professionals. Lack of NHS accountability has resulted in a multiplicity of models of service delivery. At one end of the spectrum there is unregulated use by local authorities of primary care practitioners to perform annual medical assessments; at the opposite end of the spectrum there are multidisciplinary health teams for looked after children. Provision remains a post-code lottery, often funded through short-term initiatives (e.g. Quality Protects) and determined by local political priorities rather than need.

The evolution of primary care organizations may bridge this divide between local authority accountability and NHS provision and allow a truly joined-up approach in the future. At present, although social services have performance targets for the health of looked after children, these performance indicators are not given a high priority in the NHS Plan. It is likely that the NHS will not give them the priority afforded to hospital waiting times.

National consultation was undertaken by the Department of Health during 2000 on how best to achieve health and well-being for looked after children through improved health care planning, assessment, and monitoring. Future guidance is in preparation. However, key themes emerge which are relevant for future practice.

1 Health assessment and health care planning

The principles of health care assessment and planning are:

- to be inclusive of all those caring for the child
- to be child centred, age appropriate, and allow participation of the child

- to ensure advocacy for the child's health, particularly related to waiting-list transfer and access to mental health services
- to integrate with prior assessments, (e.g. if the child has had health needs assessed under the Framework for the Assessment of Children (section 17) or child protection enquiries (Section 47) these findings should not be duplicated)
- to integrate with local authority looking after children reviews (timing 28 days, 4 months post care entry, and then 6 monthly).
- to ensure that the GP record is the child's lead health record, contains a copy of the health care plan and can be fast tracked when children move area
- to ensure consent is achieved for assessment (both from an adult with parental responsibility and wherever possible the child) and confidentiality respected, where appropriate
- to generate social care health records (including genetic background and details of illness and treatments) which can inform care leavers to manage current and future health needs.

Process

It is recommended that a single comprehensive health assessment takes place shortly after the child has become looked after.

- A written report (to include a detailed collation of health information from hospital, community and GP records) and health care plan should be available for discussion at the 28-day local authority review.
- Where there are unresolved abuse or acute physical or mental health concerns this assessment may need to be offered immediately.
- Age-appropriate content recommendations will determine the skills of professionals undertaking assessment (Table 15.4).

2 The role of the designated doctor and nurse

4r

In 2002, the Department of Health issued guidance on the care of looked after children (Promoting the Health of Looked after Children www.dh.gov.uk). Each PCT or group of PCTs should appoint a designated doctor and nurse. It is envisaged that the designated doctor be a senior paediatrician with clinical experience in the field (likely to have experience as a medical advisor to an adoption/fostering agency) and that the designated nurse has senior nurse or health visitor training with experience of the health care needs of children and young people. The roles are designed to be collaborative and complementary

Table 15.4 Principles of good health care assessment and planning

For all children (regardless of age) first assessment should:

♦ Compile an accurate personal health history from available medical records including Personal Child Health Record and child health database. This should identify if the child has received all recommended routine child health surveillance and immunizations and has any outstanding health appointments.

♦ Assess genetic and congenital risk (alcohol, hepatitis/HIV) from available maternal/family (with parental consent). This may be the last opportunity to salvage this information for the child's future.

♦ Examine physical health, dental health, and growth.

♦ Assess emotional/behavioural and mental health status, preferably with validated tool (e.g. Strengths and Difficulties Questionnaire for 3–16 year olds).

♦ Ensure child is registered with a GP and dentist.

The following are age-specific additional recommendations

Assessment of very young (under 5 years)

♦ Health promotion including diet, immunizations, teeth

♦ Behaviour including attachment, sleep, feeding, toileting

♦ Assessment of developmental milestones:
   speech and language
   gross and fine motor function
   vision and hearing
   play and pre-literacy skills
   social and self-help skills.

The middle years (primary-age children)

♦ Communication-skills

♦ Ability to make relationships and to relate to peers

♦ Progress at school

♦ Health promotion about exercise, diet, personal hygiene, basic safety issues including road safety; if appropriate, advice to cope with the physical and emotional changes associated with puberty, access to information about sexual health.

Adolescence and leaving care (secondary-age children and young people)

♦ Ability to take responsibility for health (e.g. independent management of asthma)

♦ Communication and interpersonal skills

♦ Educational and social progress

♦ Health promotion including counselling about available sources of information (and advice) about diet, physical activity, sexual health, substance misuse, and emotional and behavioural problems.

Table 15.5 Roles of designated doctor and nurse

Advisory role

♦ to PCT on questions of planning, strategy, and the audit of quality standards in relation to health services for looked after children

♦ to social services departments, residential children's homes, foster carers, professionals undertaking health assessments, and other health staff on health matters relevant to looked after children including issues of confidentiality, consent, and information sharing

Policy and procedures

♦ to take a strategic overview of the service and ensure robust clinical governance of local NHS services for looked after children

♦ to ensure those providing health care to looked after children are aware of local policy and procedures and their role

♦ to contribute to local children service plans and HImPs*.

♦ To maintain regular contact with local health team undertaking health assessments

♦ To liaise with social service departments and other PCOs over health assessments and health care plans for out-of-area placements.

Training

♦ responsibility for planning local training for health professionals undertaking health assessments for looked after children

♦ contributing where appropriate to local undergraduate and postgraduate paediatric and multidisciplinary training to ensure the health needs of looked after children are addressed

♦ maintaining professional development in the field

Monitoring and information management

♦ ensure an effective system of audit is in place

♦ monitor quality of health care assessments and implementation of health care plans for individual children

♦ review patterns of health care referrals and their outcome

♦ ensure full registration of each looked after child and care leaver with a GP and dentist

♦ contribute to production of health data on looked after children including case-mix analysis

♦ evaluate the extent to which children and young people's views inform the design and delivery of the local health services for them.

The performance of health services and professionals performing health assessments for children and young people looked after should be evaluated annually by the designated doctor.

* Health Improvement Plans

and PCOs and NHS trusts to discharge their duties to comply with local author-ity requests regarding the health improvement of looked after children.

3 Holistic approaches to promoting health

In practice the promotion of health in the spirit of the Children Act as 'a pos-itive state of physical, mental and spiritual well-being' requires far more than health assessment. Young people are known to prioritize different aspects of health to professionals (e.g. housing and personal relationships) and may not respond to health education. Factors such as stable placement, educational inclusion, and school attendance are key to health in the broadest sense. There are many examples of local interventions to promote particular aspects of health in looked after children, although there is a dearth of evidence for effectiveness. The Quality Protects website (http://www.doh.gov.uk/ qualityprotects/index.htm) maintains a good-practice database with a dis-claimer that projects may not be transferable. However, principles can be identified from evidence-based approaches in other areas.

- **Interventions** should be focused with clear aims and outcome measures.
- **Education** should be timely, practical, positive, needs led, and joined up with service provision.
- **Services** should be accessible, joined up, committed, accepting, and respect confidentiality.

Practitioners and commissioners may need to cross traditional boundaries within health to link resources from health promotion, substance abuse, sexual health, genito-urinary medicine, and mental health and school health services to target this group of children and young people. The need to approach health promotion in the spirit of the Ottawa Charter* (box) means

---

Ottawa Charter

- Building healthy public policies
- Creating supportive environments
- Strengthening community action
- Developing personal skills
- Reorienting health services

---

* World Health Organization International Conference on Health Promotion 1986.

that networks need to be established across both statutory and voluntary sectors.

4 Monitoring of outcomes

Early national performance monitoring has encouraged a welcome focus on health. Statistics (see Quality Protects website) suggest improvements in the indicators measured (Table 15.3). However, prospective long-term health status monitoring and measures of both process and process outcomes are required to identify and target areas for improvement in health outcomes (see HFAC4 website).

Resource implications

Delivery of effective services will have resource implications. The following are rough estimates based on Department of Health statistics.

Minimal requirement

PCOs will need to review local arrangements for health assessments and ensure that they are undertaken by suitably trained practitioners. The need for assessment to be completed within 28 days, and possibly urgently, excludes a lone practitioner. The service is probably best delivered by a team of medical practitioners with requisite skills and commitment to training, supported by a designated nurse. These individuals could be paediatricians or GPs with suitable paediatric skills, but might not be the child's own registered GP.

A PCT covering a population of 100 000 would provide about 50 comprehensive assessments and 100 health reviews per year (taking into account the need for biannual reviews in under-fives and the proportion of children who return home within 3 months). Previous estimates have suggested that a comprehensive assessment report takes on average 6 hours. To deliver the statutory role alone such a PCO would need to resource approximately:

- two notional half-days per week of medical time for comprehensive assessments
- one FTE designated nurse (H grade) to undertake and coordinate health reviews
- one session per week for the designated doctor
- administrative and data management support

Economies of scale suggest that the designated doctor role might need to be linked with several PCOs, ideally coterminous with local authority boundaries. This role could also encompass the traditional role of medical advisor to social services which is fully described elsewhere (NB: This time commitment is not included in the above estimates). PCOs will need to determine the best configuration for local services to meet the recommendations for service delivery and designated roles. Truly health promoting services require the coordination of many services and agencies with strong and effective involvement of child and adolescent mental health services. A managed clinical network of health care providers may be required (see HFAC4 website).

Further work required

Providing appropriate and responsive health promoting services to looked after children is no simple task. They are heterogeneous group. Many answers to their health problems lie with early prevention and improving the quality of substitute care itself. Nonetheless, individual health professionals have a duty of care at the point of contact and those with strategic responsibility have a duty to monitor and respond to the call for health-promoting policies. What is clear is that much of current practice guidance is based on fragmented evidence. There is a pressing need to address the following:

(1) to systematically harness population data on health need and outcomes of health assessment;

(2) to develop evidence based health promoting interventions;

(3) to ensure that PCOs and NHS trusts, as well as local authorities, are accountable for the health of looked after children;

(4) to improve integration of health information gathering between the agencies.

Children in private fostering arrangements

Sir William Utting, in his report on the safeguards for children living away from home (see HFAC4 website), recognized private fostering as the care environment that is least controlled and most open to abuse. Private fostering remains a poorly regulated, largely hidden, and poorly understood activity—highlighted recently by the tragic death of Victoria

Climbie. It is defined as the care of a child under 16 years old (or under 18 years if disabled) for more than 28 days by an adult who is not a relative as a private arrangement between the parent and carer. In the context of private fostering the Act recognizes as relatives grandparents, siblings, step-parents, aunts and uncles, or those with parental responsibility.

Children in private fostering include:

- children whose immigrant parents are working and studying in the UK (typically West African, but also Chinese, families)
- adolescents estranged from their families and living with the families of friends
- children from overseas attending language schools, independent schools, and exchange visits
- refugee children accompanied by agents (immigration officials only have to satisfy themselves of the child's status as an asylum seeker and not their relationship to the accompanying adult)
- children brought into the UK from abroad with an intent to adopt— although non-adherence to the regulations of the Adoption (Intercountry Aspects) Act 1999 is now an offence.

The Children Act 1989 offers children in private foster care some protection. Local authorities have duties under the Act to satisfy themselves that the welfare of the child is not at risk by checking the suitability of the placement, making regular visits to the child, and offering advice where required. However, the duty to notify the local authority of the arrangement lies with the birth parent and carer. In practice very few arrangements are notified and few local authorities allocate resources to support and assess private foster care placements. Furthermore, at the present time, the Department of Health does not collect statistics on children in private foster care. Estimates suggest that 8000–10 000 children may be privately fostered in the UK, of whom a majority are believed to be from West African families. Few of these families would choose private fostering in favour of alternative arrangements, but are motivated by lack of choice, income, and cultural beliefs. While some private arrangements may meet the needs of a child and family, there are many examples where children have become estranged from birth parents and their cultural roots, suffer unhappy and neglectful care and in extreme cases are 'lost' or murdered.

Health professionals may be the first to recognize the situation of these children and should notify local councils. As well as protecting the child, notification may offer positive benefits to carers and parents through Section 17 financial assistance, local carers support networks, and social security benefits such as child benefit. It remains to be seen whether the Climbie inquiry will recommend a review of the regulations governing private fostering as originally suggested by Utting (*see* HFAC4 website).

Adoption*

Although children may be adopted from soon after birth, having never been cared for by their biological parents, or adopted from abroad (usually as infants), the great majority of children requiring adoption have been in the care system, sometimes for prolonged periods. In most cases, the child has experienced neglect or abuse, and rehabilitation attempts with his/her family have failed.

Intercountry adoptions

Up to 1999, approximately 300 children were adopted from abroad by UK residents. There were approximately 100 other cases each year where people avoided the adoption procedures and brought children to the UK without approval. The Adoption (Intercountry Aspects) Act 1999 was passed to regulate all adoption of children from abroad. This was followed by guidance, the latest being issued in 2001. The latter included the following provision:

> The prospective adopter is required to undergo assessment by an adoption agency [may be local authority or private], be approved as suitable to be an adoptive parent and have received notification from the Secretary of State that he is willing to issue a certificate confirming that the prospective adopter has been assessed and approved and that the child will be authorised to reside permanently in the British Islands if entry clearance is granted and an adoption order is made. The prospective adopter is required to notify his local authority of his intention to apply for an adoption order, or alternatively that he does not intend to give the child a home, within fourteen days after bringing the child into the United Kingdom.
>
> The Regulations also specify the procedure to be followed by an adoption agency and adoption panel in relation to assessment and approval of a person wishing to adopt a child from overseas, and require the provision of certain information to the Secretary of State. These provisions apply to England only; similar provision is to be made in relation to Wales by the National Assembly for Wales.

Children adopted from abroad will need a detailed medical assessment as they may have been exposed to illnesses not commonly seen in UK and they may not have had the routine care and immunizations that are available in the UK.

* The Adoption and Child Act 2002 replaces/consolidates previous legislation.

Adoption of looked after children

At any one time 58 000 children are being looked after by their local authority, and over a period of a year this rises to around 90 000. Of these, about 40 per cent return home within 8 weeks, over 50 per cent within 6 months, and 70 per cent within a year of entering care. Approximately 28 000 have been in care for over 2 years and 12 000 for 5 years or more. By the time a child has been in care for 18 months or more it is likely that they will still be in care after 4 years. When it appears that return to their family is no longer a viable option, adoption is the best way of ensuring a stable environment for children and young people. However, the use of adoption is very variable, with between 0.5 and 10.5 per cent of children in care being adopted, depending on the council. In the year to 31 March 2001, 3067 looked after children were adopted in England, of whom 67 per cent were 5 years or older at the time of adoption and 5 per cent were 10 years or older.

As adoption is a final process which severs all legal links between biological parents and their child, it is not a decision taken lightly by child protection agencies, adoption agencies, or the courts. However, if the long-term plan for the child does not include rehabilitation into the birth family, it is in the child's best interests to avoid the unsettling effects of multiple foster placements. Therefore once the decision for adoption has been made, a placement should be found as soon as possible. Table 15.6 shows the delay between a child entering local authority care and being adopted. The average is about 20 months to placement and 33 months to legal adoption.

Owing to a shortage of suitable potential adopters, there are often long delays between the decision to place for adoption and a final placement being made. The average delay is 7 months and is longer for children entering care at an older age.

As outlined in the section on looked after children, by the time a child in care reaches the point of adoption, s/he is likely to have numerous problems.

Table 15.6 Length of time looked after before adoption

Length of time	Percentage of children 1999	Percentage of children 2000
Under 1 year	13	20
1–2 years	28	38
2–3 years	28	26
3–5 years	23	13
5+ years	8	3

Therefore placement can be difficult and this is reflected in the fact that approximately 25 per cent of adoptive placements break down before the child has been legally adopted. Once adopted, the children and their new families will continue to need support. The Adoption Act 1976 made allowance for this, but support is often short lived. Adoption allowances were introduced to ensure that monetary considerations would not stop a child being adopted because of limited income of the prospective adopters, disability, or other exceptional needs of the child, such as an existing attachment or a group of siblings requiring placement together being split up (*see* HFAC4 website).

Because of these concerns, a White Paper proposing some changes was published in 2000, and the Adoption and Children Act was passed by Parliament in 2002. Amongst the initiatives are means to reduce delays at all stages and provision for extra support post-adoption. Standards have also been published.

What is the role of the health service?

All adoptions from care should go through an Adoption Panel which is constituted by a registered Adoption Agency, a quasi-autonomous body of a local authority. Every Adoption Agency must have a medical adviser. This person will be called upon to provide a report on the present health (physical and mental) and development of the child. S/he should also comment on any genetic or environmental influences which may be relevant to the child and which may have an effect on the child's future health and well-being. To do this s/he may need to collate reports from a number of sources and sometimes see the child him/herself. As the number of babies being adopted has decreased, proportionately more children have complex medical and emotional problems. Therefore it is essential that the medical adviser is appropriately trained in this field and should be a paediatrician. The role and functions of the medical adviser are described in the service specification and practice standards agreed by the British Agencies for Adoption and Fostering Medical Group (*see* HFAC4 website).

The health of the adopters also needs to be assessed to ensure that they will be able to provide an appropriate stable environment for the child or young person. The medical adviser should counsel potential adopters about any health or developmental issues or risks relevant to the child and be able to advise them on the appropriate management. S/he should advise the panel on the suitability for an adoption allowance on medical and health grounds and the necessity for continuing support post-adoption. The medical adviser is a full member of the panel and, as such, can comment on any matters relating to the welfare of the child.

4r   For further details of legal arrangements such as special guardianship, introduced in 2006 see 'legal arrangements for family and friends care on the 'Every Child Matters' website (www.everychildmatters.gov.uk)

Summary and Recommendations

1   There are important duties in respect of child protection and looked after children, set out in guidance and statute.

2   Inter-agency work is an essential part of planning and providing care for children at risk of being abused or neglected, or who are looked after.

3   Each PCO must appoint a designated doctor and a designated nurse for child protection. Each trust must appoint a named nurse and doctor for child protection. These staff must have adequate time to carry out their duties to a high standard and to maintain their own continuing education in these fields.

4r   4   Each PCO must appoint a designated doctor and a designed nurse for looked after children. These include strategic roles.

5   A substantial professional time commitment will be needed to carry out the assessment and care programmes to the standard envisaged. Priority in resource allocation is justified for looked after children who are among the highest risk groups in our society.

6   Each local authority Adoption Agency will require the services of a medical adviser for adoption.

Chapter 16

Children in special circumstances

This chapter considers the needs of children in special circumstances:

- ◆ Asylum seekers, refugees, and international adoptions
- ◆ Entitlements
- ◆ Emotional health and health care
- ◆ Screening and management of health problems
- ◆ Immunizations for children with no records
- ◆ Health care needs of traveller families
- ◆ Homeless families
- ◆ Children and young people in prison

In this chapter we review the health care needs of children living in special circumstances. Primary care trusts will be responsible for the health care of all children resident within their boundaries, and among these there will often be a significant number of children with exceptional problems and needs who will need additional and often specialized resources.*

Asylum seekers, refugees, and internationally adopted children

To become officially recognized as a refugee, an individual must be judged to have left his or her country 'owing to a well-founded fear of being persecuted for reasons of race, religion, nationality, membership of a particular social group or political opinion'. In the UK an asylum seeker describes someone who has applied for refugee status. Once accepted as refugees all family members will have the same rights to welfare benefits and health care as UK citizens.

Providing health care for asylum-seeking and refugee children must extend beyond ensuring access. A wide range of problems are faced by asylum-seeking and refugee families. Health professionals need some knowledge of

---

* A group of children and adults who have recently gained prominence are those who have been trafficked. PCOs and Trusts should ensure staff are trained to recognise and take appropriate action for such children and adults. (www.ecpat.org.uk)

entitlements and should be prepared when necessary to advocate on their patient's behalf.

Dispersal under the Immigration and Asylum Act 1999 means that some families are now finding themselves in areas unfamiliar with the provision of services to refugees and where health service staff may have had little or no advance warning of their arrival. The proposed Consortia of Service Providers in receiving areas should avoid this and make planning possible. The primary care organization in which the refugees are living will be responsible for their initial health care provision, and so links with the local consortium are vital.

It is unreasonable to expect refugees to slot neatly into existing styles of health care. They need support in accessing and using services, and health professionals require guidance on how to respond effectively. Newly arrived children and their parents usually speak little or no English and will often have witnessed and suffered events outside the experience of most health professionals in this country. Staff training and support are needed. Where numbers are large, consideration should be given to setting up a dedicated service. A good interpreting service is essential. It is not acceptable to rely on the use of children as interpreters for the parents at medical appointments.

Entitlements

Subsistence and housing

The entitlements of asylum seekers and the arrangements for housing and dispersal are kept under review. For up to date information, consult the website of the Refugee Council (http://www.refugeecouncil. org.uk).

Unaccompanied minors

Unaccompanied minors (children under 18 years old) have the right to be 'looked after', to have somewhere to live, and to education and health care. Current initiatives in the UK, within the Government's Quality Protects programme, are seeking to improve the health and educational outcomes for children in public care. Unaccompanied young asylum seekers must be included in such local provision. Currently many 15- to 18-year-olds are placed in adult accommodation and many authorities do not offer this age group full needs assessments leading on to individual care plans.

Health entitlements

All child asylum seekers or refugees have the same rights of access to all health services as any other children in the UK, including referral to specialist services. However, under the new provisions, asylum seekers are not eligible for welfare foods and vitamins for themselves or their babies. This has implications for the child's nutrition and is causing a particular problem for HIV-positive mothers who currently are advised not to breastfeed (though this advice is controversial and may change).

All children are entitled to routine child health surveillance, health promotion, and immunizations, including a primary course if this has not previously been completed. Early permanent registration with a GP should be encouraged to ensure that routine health promotion appointments are sent. Health visitors and school nurses should seek out new arrivals and ensure that they are provided with relevant health information in a format that can readily be understood.

Both children of asylum seekers and unaccompanied children can be considered 'children in need' and both groups are mentioned in the new Department of Health guidance.

Asylum seekers are not eligible to claim Disability Living Allowance either for themselves or for their children. Therefore once refugee status is approved it is important to ensure that the appropriate applications are rapidly made.

Emotional health and well being

While refugee parents and children may be psychologically distressed, it is important that resilience and resourcefulness are recognized and respected. Some families come from cultures with perceptions of mental illness that are very different from those in the UK, and for them the suggestion of 'referral for counselling' is meaningless and unhelpful. Distress should be acknowledged and support may be offered. Some children may exhibit signs of post-traumatic stress. Response to stress might manifest itself with physical signs. For those who are suffering the consequences of torture, help should be sought from specialist services such as the Medical Foundation for Victims of Torture in London (*see* HFAC4 website). Local child and adolescent mental health services need to gain expertise in providing the therapy needed by some of the more severely damaged young people.

Children can also be affected by their parents' psychological state. Parents suffering from the effects of their own traumatic experiences and preoccupied with making sense of life as an asylum seeker will find it difficult to provide their children with a self-confident and strong role model. Nor are they likely to be as emotionally available to support and encourage their children as they might wish.

Young people themselves have identified a number of issues that affect their well being. When groups of young asylum seekers (aged 12 to 16) were consulted in South London they included loss of family members, loneliness, feeling cold, being depressed, lack of money, and language barriers. Bullying emerged as a major concern, as did difficulty in accessing services (not just health). More than half felt that their health had deteriorated since coming to the UK.

Health care

Detailed information is available for PCOs and paediatricians (*see* HFAC4 website).

Specialist advice may be needed for unfamiliar diseases, depending on the country of origin and the length of time spent in camps or in transit. Children may have had no previous child health surveillance or neonatal screening for congenital abnormalities or inherited metabolic disorders. For unaccompanied children, relevant medical details, notably immunization records (p. 318), may be restricted or missing.

Culturally sensitive advice on diet and support for breastfeeding must be available. Children may arrive malnourished, but are also at risk of suffering from an inadequate diet in this country.

Paediatricians should be cautious if asked to make a medical assessment of a young person's age. The Home Office Asylum Casework Instructions acknowledge that anthropometric measurements can be misleading, and consider it is inappropriate to use radiography merely to assist in age determination. Some children and young people may come from cultures where birthdays are not celebrated and may be genuinely uncertain of their exact age.

Refugees and children being adopted from abroad may have similar medical problems. Many of these relate to lack of routine child health surveillance in the countries of origin (e.g. undetected defects of vision, hearing, and speech, and omission of routine immunizations), whereas others will be infections acquired from the child's country of origin. The risk and type of infection depends upon the country from which the child has come.

- Children from the USA, Western Europe, and Australasia will be subject to the same level of care as in the UK and will suffer, broadly speaking, the same infectious diseases (some arthropod-borne diseases may be more common in these countries).
- Children from some countries of Eastern Europe may be at increased risk of diphtheria and tuberculosis. Enteric infections are also more common. Children who have lived in orphanages or received blood transfusions may have acquired HIV and/or hepatitis B infection, especially in Romania.
- Children from Africa, the Indian subcontinent, and some parts of South America may have been exposed to numerous diseases not usually

encountered in the West. Treatment for diagnosed diseases may have been suboptimal, suppressing the illness rather than eliminating the infection. Many infections may be asymptomatic at the time of entry to the country and some (e.g. schistosomiasis and liver flukes) may take years to become apparent. Recurrent fever due to chronic malaria is accepted as the norm in many countries.

Management and screening

In this section the management of asymptomatic children only is considered. (For the management of a child from abroad who has a fever or other symptoms, *see* HFAC4 website.) An intercountry adoption form should be completed for children being adopted from abroad. This includes a thorough history and examination. All other children coming from abroad should, at least, answer a health questionnaire. Any omissions in routine child health surveillance or immunizations should be rectified.

Whether or not to screen asymptomatic children from abroad for infections is unclear (see box).

In 1991, a study at the Hospital for Tropical Diseases, London, screened 1029 asymptomatic individuals (135 less than 14 years old) returning from a prolonged stay abroad. It was difficult to estimate in how many people the abnormalities that were found related to their stay abroad.

- Urine analysis of 830 cases showed abnormalities in 116. In none of these was the abnormality related to the stay abroad.
- Stool microscopy for cysts, ova, and parasites showed abnormalities in 207 of 995 (20.8%). The most common finding was the presence of cysts of *Entamoeba histolytica* or *Giardia lamblia*. Almost all were treated, despite being asymptomatic.
- Out of 852 blood samples, 67 (7.9%) showed an eosinophilia. In 26 people this was associated with parasitosis (schistosomiasis in 18).

The authors concluded that screening for tropical disease can be efficiently carried out by an informed health professional using structured history taking and relevant laboratory tests. A survey of health authorities and boards in the UK, published in 1990, showed a wide variation in policy for screening children from abroad. The authors suggested the following procedure for children entering the educational systems in the UK after spending more than 8 weeks in Asia, the Far East, Africa, or South America.

1 The school nurse should interview the family before the child starts school and review the child's health. A Nautoux test should be performed, and if negative, BCG should be given. Children already in school should be interviewed as soon as possible.

2 If asymptomatic, the child can start school as soon as the interview has been completed.

3 Immunizations should be completed (Table 16.1).

4 If the child does not already have a GP, advice should be given on registering.

5 Consideration should also be given to voluntary confidential testing for children and adults from high-risk areas for HIV and hepatitis B infection.

In the absence of evidence to the contrary, the above procedure is recommended. Screening for other infectious diseases cannot currently be justified.

Vaccination of children with unknown immunization status

Often a child presents with an inadequate immunization history and it is not clear what vaccinations s/he may have had in the past. Apart from the possibility of increased local reactions with excessive doses of tetanus, there is evidence that extra doses of most vaccines will do no harm. Therefore, if it is not clear whether or not a child has had particular vaccines in the past, the best course of action is to give the child all those vaccines about which there is doubt. Table 16.1 is a guide to what would be appropriate at particular ages. There is little research on this topic, so policies may differ.

Travellers

Travellers are defined from a legal perspective as 'persons of nomadic habit, whatever their race or origin' (Caravan Sites Act, 1968). They have become a very heterogeneous group made up of traditional Travellers (English and Welsh Romanichal or Romany Gypsies, Irish Travellers, Scottish Travellers, and a recently increasing number of European Romanichals (Roma) and new Travellers) who have abandoned their settled lifestyle to become nomadic.

The cultures and languages of these different groups make generalizations difficult but they do have some common features. Ofsted estimated that there

Table 16.1** Vaccination of children with unknown immunization status 4r

Age	Primary immunizations required	Booster immunizations required subsequently
Under 12 months	DTaP(5)/Hib/IPV × 3 at monthly intervals Meningococcal C*	As per routine schedule
1–10 years	DTaP(5)/Hib/IPV × 3 at monthly intervals MMR × 2* Meningococcal C × 1	Booster DTap/IPV or dTaP/IPV (if <10 years, or Td/OPV if >=10 years) should be given at least one year after last dose of primary course. Td/IPV 5–10 years later.
10 years or more	Td/IPV × 3 at monthly intervals MMR × 2* Meningococcal C × 1	Td/IPV after 1 year Td/IPV after a further 5–10 years

*Notes:

♦ BCG should be given according to local policy.

♦ Hepatitis B vaccine may be indicated in some instances.

♦ Where a child starts their course of meningococcal C vaccine after 4 months old and less then 12 months old, 2 doses of the vaccine should be given.

♦ The two doses of MMR should be at least three months apart, except in an outbreak when this can be reduced to one month.

Key: DTaP, diphtheria/tetanus/acellular pertussis; IPV, inactivated polio vaccine; Hib, *Haemophilus influenzae* type b; MMR, measles/mumps/rubella; Td, tetanus–low dose diphtheria. Unfortunately, immunization schedules vary between countries, even in Western Europe. They also vary from time to time and it is not easy to publish a paper guide to them as it would rapidly be out of date. Some information is available from websites of individual National Health Departments and also WHO (www.who.int/gpv—surv/sched.xls), but is often very out of date.

** A new immunization schedule is to be introduced in the summer of 2006. These recommendations will need to be altered in the light of the changes.

was a total of 89 000 travellers (70 000 Gypsy Travellers, 10 500 fairground/show people, 2000 circus people, 6000 new Travellers, and 500 bargees/boat dwellers). It is difficult to estimate the number of children in these communities, but this same report quoted a figure of 50 000 children aged from birth to 16 years and felt that this could be an underestimate.

All Travellers tend to be ostracised by settled populations; they are frequently moved on, sites that are provided for them are often unsuitable for any other use (old refuse tips and sites near motorways), and there tends to be a higher morbidity and mortality than found in the settled community. It has been suggested that this difference in mortality could paradoxically be due to constraints on their traditional lifestyle. There seem to be as frequent mental and physical health problems in housed Travellers as in those on established sites.

Travellers often have little access to health and education services. The allocation of specialist health visitors and education personnel can help to alleviate these concerns. Experience suggests that, contrary to popular view, Traveller families value these services. In view of the fact that problems often persist when the families become settled, this extra input should continue even after the nomadic lifestyle has been abandoned.

Homelessness

A distinction is drawn between statutorily and non-statutorily homeless people in the UK. Statutorily homeless households, following assessment by a local authority, qualify for permanent re-housing in council or housing association housing. The homeless households that qualify for assistance include people with dependent children, women who are pregnant and single people who are *vulnerable*, in that they cannot be expected to fend for themselves. In London (and the rest of the UK), statutorily homeless households often have to wait for permanent social housing to become available. While statutorily homeless people are waiting in temporary accommodation (such as leased accommodation, hostels and bed and breakfast hotels) for their permanent homes, they are still regarded as homeless.

Homeless people who do not qualify for assistance under the homelessness legislation are generally single people without children who are not deemed to be vulnerable under the terms of the legislation. These homeless people are usually referred to as single homeless people. Most single homeless people live in short term accommodation such as hostels and bed and breakfast hotels, but a substantial minority live on the streets. People who live for some or all of the time on the street are usually referred to as people who are sleeping rough.

At the end of the first quarter of 2001, there were 75 120 households accommodated by local authorities and categorized as homeless, of which 10 830 were in bed and breakfast accommodation. Of the new households accepted in that quarter, 56 per cent contained dependent children and another 10 per cent included pregnant women; 22 per cent of these new households required accommodation because of a relationship breakdown, of which over two-thirds involved violence. Webb *et al.* estimate that about 35 000 children pass through refuges every year in England and Wales. They found a high incidence of problems and poor uptake of services in a survey of children in refuges in Cardiff.

See HFAC4 website

Children and young people may be affected by homelessness in one of two ways. They may be part of a family unit which is homeless or they may be a single homeless person in their own right. The link between homelessness and poor health is well established. Behaviour problems, acute infections, and accidents have been shown to be more common. The accommodation is often cramped and dirty, with shared toilet and cooking facilities. Opportunities for children to play are severely limited.

Because such families are often moved on to alternative accommodation, it may be difficult for health visitors to keep track of them and be in a position to deliver the core child health promotion programme. Good liaison with the housing department in some areas has ensured that as soon as a new family arrives, a designated health visitor is informed so that s/he can make contact as soon as possible. Of course, it is doubly important that the Personal Child Health Record is fully used in such circumstances as other records are often inaccurate.

Mental health problems are common among homeless children and families. This high incidence of mental health problems in both mothers and children persists even after they have been rehoused. Therefore support needs to continue beyond the period of homelessness.

Many families in temporary accommodation are unable to receive mail and hence do not know about appointments made for them. As with looked after children, these children move frequently and their names may never reach the top of waiting lists for specialist services—they go to the bottom again with each move. Consultations and services should be arranged with these constraints in mind.

Children, young people, and prison

Prison impinges on the lives of children and young people in three possible ways:

- they may be born in prison and perhaps remain there for a variable period
- a parent may spend time in prison and thus be separated from them
- they may be in custody in their own right, either on remand or serving a prison sentence.

Children of women in prison

In 1994 a detailed survey was undertaken of women prisoners to ascertain the numbers who were mothers, the composition of their families, how they kept in contact with their children, and what arrangements had been made to care for them.

Prison is not an optimum environment for babies to be brought up in and they often miss out on routine services, though this is changing. While in prison, mothers find it even more difficult to keep close contact with their children outside than do fathers as there are fewer women's units and so travelling can be difficult. Extended visits and opportunities to cuddle and touch their children improve the quality of visits. It is not always easy for mothers or children to make telephone calls and letter writing can be quite difficult for a population whose standard of literacy is poor.

In 2000, the average daily prison population was 64 602 of whom 3350 were women. Of these, 11 088 were under 21 years old (10 592 males and 496 females), of whom about a quarter were on remand. More than one-third of women prisoners are held on drug charges.

Of the women:

+ 31 per cent had no children
+ 1 per cent had no children but were pregnant
+ 2 per cent had children under 18 years old and were pregnant
+ 58 per cent had children under 18 years old and were not pregnant
+ 8 per cent had children, all over 18 years old

The average number of children for each mother was 2.

+ 55 per cent were teenagers at the time of the birth of their first child (cf. approximately 20 per cent in the general population)
+ 27 per cent were single mothers (cf. 8 per cent in the general population)

Of the children:

+ 30 per cent were under 5 years old
+ 34 per cent were 5–9 years old
+ 21 per cent were 9–13 years old
+ 13 per cent were 13–16 years old
+ 3 per cent were 16–18 years old

In 1997–1998, 72 babies were born to women in prison. Although the number of Mother and Baby Unit (MBU) places has risen from 48 in 1994 to 66 in 1999, it is still limited and there were only four MBUs in the country. The upper age limit to which babies could stay with their mothers was 9 months in two of these units and 18 months in the other two.

See HFAC4 website

There is little research on the effect that this has on children, but that which has been done shows that a high proportion of children have behaviour problems following the imprisonment of their mother. These are more common amongst older children and those who were separated from their siblings. This was much less likely when the father, rather than the mother, is imprisoned.

A number of solutions have been suggested.

- As far as possible, custodial sentences should be avoided for pregnant women and mothers of babies.
- If a custodial sentence is considered essential it could be served in community units, along the lines of those seen in the Netherlands and Australia. These resemble open prisons with weekend leave, and accommodate mothers and children up to 4 or 5 years old.
- Any child detained along with his/her mother should receive the routine programme provided by the health services and be considered a 'vulnerable child'.
- Mothers serving custodial sentences should do so in facilities close to the rest of their family.

Young people detained in prison in their own right

Young people in prison are a vulnerable group. As such, they have often missed out on routine health care and education. The opportunity to rectify these omissions can and should be taken while they are in custody. Contrary to their experience outside prison, many young offenders are very positive about their experience of prison education.

In March 2000 there were 2247 young people (anyone aged under 17 years is referred to legally as a 'child') aged 15–17 in prisons in England and Wales. This is a 75 per cent increase on 1993 and is due both to more people being placed in prison and to the imposition of longer sentences. Almost 20 per cent of young people in prison are black as opposed to about 2 per cent of that age group in the general population. Approximately 75 per cent of the offences of the young people were non-violent. There is a very high rate of re-offending amongst young prisoners: 88 per cent of all 14- to 15-year-olds leaving prison in 1995 were reconvicted, and in 64 per cent the offence was so serious that they were imprisoned again. In 2000, 11 young people under 21 years old committed suicide in prison. The majority of young offenders had ceased full-time education before school-leaving age, the average being at about 14 years.

Recommendations

4r
- ◆ PCOs should be clear who is responsible for the health care of children. In England, PCTs are responsible for the care of all children registered with the PCT's GPs, wherever resident, and children without a GP, but resident in the PCT's geographical catchment area.

- ◆ They will need to determine the number and location of children in the various categories described here for whom they are responsible.

- ◆ The health needs of these children and families are likely to be similar in kind of those of other families, but there is likely to be more unmet need and greater difficulty in establishing a relationship with them and providing services in ways that they are able to use.

- ◆ Allocation of additional resources will be needed for service provision, staff training, and support.

Chapter 17

Personal Child Health Records and minimum dataset

This chapter deals with:

- ◆ Personal Child Health Records: their ownership and use
- ◆ the content and format of the record
- ◆ confidentiality
- ◆ information
- ◆ distribution
- ◆ recommendations for use of a National Personal Child Health Record
- ◆ information collection and management

Personal Child Health Records

Fifteen years ago a model Personal Child Health Record (PCHR) was launched. The ethos behind parents holding their child's records was that it would encourage partnership between health professionals and parents, improve communication between health professionals, leading to enhanced continuity of care, and increase parents' understanding of their child's health and development. This ethos is echoed in the NHS National Plan with its emphasis on patient involvement at all levels of care.

In conducting a review of the PCHR and determining the way forward the sources of information used were published and unpublished literature, the findings from a survey of 166 trusts and health authorities (response rate 84 per cent) on the current use and policies with respect to the record, review of records provided by surveyed districts, discussions which took place at a national conference held in 1999, and the discussions of a PCHR working group (p. vii) and other experts in the field (see HFAC4 website).

Ownership of records

Despite the intent to empower parents, there was a lack of consensus as to whom the PCHR belongs and statements about its ownership varied widely.

In the survey, 53 trusts reported that the PCHR belonged to the trust, 51 to the parent alone, 17 to the parent in partnership with the trust or the Secretary of State and another, 10 to the Secretary of State alone, and one jointly to the Secretary of State and the trust. Only three specifically reported that the PCHR belonged to the child. The strict legal position concerning ownership is unclear, and so we would suggest that wording along the following lines appears at the front of the PCHR: 'This is the main record of your child's health, growth and development and therefore we would ask you to keep it in a safe place'. Somewhere else a note should be made as to who supplied the record, but by separating the two statements the impression that the supplier owns it is lessened.

Use and continuity of records

Studies have shown that retention rates are high, that they are readily accepted, well liked, and well used by parents, that their use is approved by health visitors and general practitioners, and that they are generally adequately completed.

4r However, although a large survey found that overall use was good, effective use was significantly less by mothers living in disadvantaged circumstances and by those whose children were admitted to hospital (Dezateux C, Foster L, Tate *et al*. Children's Health in: Children of the 21st century. From birth to nine months. Eds Dex S, Joshi H. Policy Press, Bristol, 2005). There is evidence to indicate that the use of the PCHR by some professional groups, in particular GPs and hospital-based doctors, is suboptimal. This is in part due to a reluctance to duplicate information recorded elsewhere. To ensure continuity there should be a follow-on from the national maternity record (NMR), with a page provided with details of the birth and immediate post-partum period.

4r A recent report describes how personal child health records have been widely supported though their use remains variable. *See* Hampshire AJ, Blair ME, Crown NS, *et al*. (2004). Variation in how mothers, health visitors and general practitioners use the personal child health record. *Child: Care, Health and Development* **30**: 307–316.

Content and format of records

Format of records

Since the launch of the model PCHR, there has been a proliferation in different formats with many areas designing their own. This has limited the usefulness of the PCHR in a number of ways, making it difficult for parents who move from area to area and for health professionals to navigate around it. Although they have basic similarities, it can be difficult to know where to find a particular piece of information. Development of records at district level is also not cost effective. In an attempt to overcome these limitations, districts have been working together in a number of regions to develop a PCHR which is as far as possible common to all (e.g. the West Midlands and Tyne and Wear). There is now a multidisciplinary national committee, set up to advise on the PCHR under the auspices of the Royal College of Paediatrics and Child Health.

Design of records

Although the PCHR is intended primarily for parents, its appearance is not always user-friendly. For example, the written content of many PCHRs is considerable, with densely printed pages in small font sizes. There are good examples of the use of simple yet attractive drawings, and this should be developed further. Language should be accessible to the majority of readers.

Information on confidentiality and use of personal health information

Just over a half of the trusts reported that information was provided in the PCHR on confidentiality and use of personal health information. This information should be included in records and it is proposed that a standardized statement should be included:

> To provide proper care for your child we need to record information in written records and on computer. Each organization involved in your child's care should be able to give you details of the safeguards and guidelines they use with regard to this. Your health visitor or school nurse will be able to give you further information on local policies.

The use made of multiple self-copying sheets held within the PCHR for transfer of information to computerized data systems was explored, with the majority collecting information regarding programmed child health contacts (94 per cent). Fewer trusts reported using this system for transfer of information regarding immunization (34 per cent) and breastfeeding (53 per cent).

Variation also exists in the coding systems used to record details of routine child health contacts. SPOTRN (satisfactory, problem, observation, treatment, referral, not examined) was the most widely used acronym (74 per cent of areas). However, 28 other recording systems were described from 36 areas. This limits the ability to utilize such data for epidemiological purposes on a national or even a regional basis. This is further limited by the lack of standardized definitions of either what is included in routine child health contacts, or in the use of the categories for recording the details of the contact. In one study examining whether existing information systems could be used to follow up high-risk groups of children, this lack of standardization of terms used was found to be a major limiting factor. For example, it was found that a child with expressive language delay at 18 months could be classified as 'satisfactory', 'problem', 'observe', or 'referred' by different professionals. Further work is required to develop a standardized system for recording such information, and this system should be fully evaluated before widespread introduction.

Information on screening and other health checks and reviews

There is little consistency in the information provided in records about routine screening and other health checks, and indeed many areas do not provide such information at all. It is important that parents are provided with information which describes in simple terms the benefits and limitations of screening and of other health checks and reviews. This information should be standardized to ensure equity and accuracy. An example is given in the box.

Child health checks

Your doctor, health visitor, or midwife will do some simple routine checks on your child.

Some of these are called 'screening' tests and include:

- hearing tests at birth
- blood tests for rare conditions where the body's chemistry does not work properly (*metabolic conditions*)
- checks of your baby's hips
- checks of your baby's heart
- checks of your baby's eyes for cataracts.

Other checks or reviews include:

- checks of height and weight
- checks for undescended testicles
- eye checks
- dental checks.

Screening tests and other health checks and reviews are done to pick up problems before they have been noticed. They can **never** be fully accurate in all cases. This means that sometimes there is a false alarm. In this case you may be told that your baby *may* have a condition. However, further tests may show that she or he does not have the condition. It also means that sometimes a problem may not be picked up. So even if your baby has had a check for a condition, if you think there may be a problem you should still point it out to your health visitor or GP. Do not assume that because the check was 'normal', there can't be a problem.

Health promotion material

Many records contain health promotion material. There is evidence that although it is used by some parents, others are not aware of it. The quantity and quality of such information varies greatly, and in some cases the quality is poor and lacks an evidence base. On the other hand, most first-time parents are issued with a copy of *Birth to five* produced by the Department of Health (DoH). Use of such materials has a number of advantages; not only does it ensure that parents are given information at the appropriate time which is consistent, accurate, and evidence based, but it also means that such information does not have to be developed at a local level, saving considerable resources. To maximize the potential of the PCHR as a record, it is recommended that health promotion material be kept to a minimum, with signposting as appropriate to *Birth to five* or other sources of information such as immunization leaflets produced by DoH. A recent paper showed that even 4r when prepared with professional designer help, the PCHR was not well used by parents as a source of health promotion (Wright CM, Reynolds L. How widely are personal child health records used and are they effective health education tools? A Comparison of 2 records. *Child: Care, Health and Development.* 2006; **32**: 55–61). Where health promotion information is contained within the PCHR, it should be stored at the back and should not interfere with the order of recording pages.

Timing of distribution of record to parents

Policies differ with respect to the timing of distribution of the record. In the majority of areas the health visitor issues the record to parents at the first visit. However, a majority would prefer them to be distributed either in the antenatal period or in the first 48 hours after birth by either midwife or health visitor. Ideally the PCHR should be given out with the *Birth to five* book. The ideal 4r would be for the parents to be provided with an explanation of the record and its uses at the time of issue. However, in practice it may not be possible for this to be carried out until the first postnatal visit by the health visitor, and this should be viewed as the latest opportunity for this information.

Development of records for specific groups

There have been initiatives to develop special records or extra pages to be inserted into the existing record for particular groups of children such as those with specific conditions (e.g. Down's syndrome) or living in specific social circumstances (e.g. looked after children). In some areas records for school-aged children have been developed. These initiatives are in varying stages of development and evaluation. It is helpful if people could ensure that copies of any extra pages are sent to the Royal College of Paediatrics and Child Health where a library of such pages is kept (*see* HFAC4 website).

Recommendations for a National Personal Child Health Record

1 **The design needs to be updated**—this is a task that should be undertaken by experts in design.

2 **Content should be reduced to the bare minimum** to ensure that it is a *record*.

3 **The core pages should be standardized** in line with the recommendations of *Health for all children* (4th edition) and the National Screening Committee (NSC), and informed by the minimum core data set recommended by the Child Health Information Consortium (CHIC) (*see* HFAC4 website and p. 342).

4 **Pages of the record should be kept to a minimum in the same order, well indexed, and numbered.**

5 **Detailed health promotion material should not be included**, but rather should be signposted (e.g. *Birth to five* published by HPE). Health promotion pages that are distributed should be given out at the appropriate time as an adjunct to verbal information rather than included in the book as standard.

6 **Local information can and should be included but should not interfere with the order of the pages.**

7 **The record should be given to parents in the antenatal period with an explanation of its use, or as soon as possible after birth with an explanation by the health visitor at the first postnatal visit.**

8 **Proposed contents and order of contents**

 - Index
 - Biographical details, NHS number
 - Local information
 - Information (standard paragraphs) about: screening; consent to transfer of data; confidentiality
 - Summary of birth, receipt of vitamin K, hepatitis B and BCG vaccinations, newborn examination, neonatal hearing screening

- Feeding information to be collected at standard ages (e.g. 4/8/12/16 weeks) using a standardized question
- Immunizations given by whom, date, site of injection, batch number, signposting to more detailed information in DoH leaflet(s)
- Nationally agreed checks/reviews with standardized coding for results
- Feedback of outcome of referrals
- Nine-centile national growth charts
- Health promotion material—should be a minimum and stored at the back.

Further work to be done

Despite many local evaluations of the record, there is little information on what parents actually want from the PCHR. In future developments of the record, it is important to ensure that there is significant input from parents.

Information

Reliable, accurate, complete, up-to-date, and secure information is critical to the delivery of a high-quality effective child health service:

- to support clinical management and care of ill children
- to monitor development of all children up to age 5 and for selected children (i.e. those with persisting health problems) through school age to adulthood
- as with other client groups, to assess health needs within a district population for commissioning health care and for monitoring the performance of providers in meeting these needs
- for service development (e.g. to evaluate the effectiveness of screening programmes and other health care interventions)
- for management purposes
- for epidemiological research.

What information do we need?

In general, less is more where records are concerned. Often too much data of poor quality and limited usefulness is collected. Definitions need to be agreed and information needs to be standardized—the same items, meaning the same thing to all those involved, should be collected across the country.

Only essential core data should be recorded in computerized child health records, especially if the information is to be used to monitor the health of a child population. Additional information on individual children can be recorded in PCHRs or other easily accessible clinical notes, including individual electronic patient records.

Data sharing and confidentiality

To be useful information needs to be shared. Computer systems need to be electronically linked to exchange data, both within the health service and with other agencies. Appropriate data protection and confidentiality safeguards must be maintained. Parents need to be aware of how data is collected and how important it is, as well as the safeguards in place to ensure confidentiality. There should be a carefully worded statement at the beginning of the PCHR which is clear and applicable wherever the child is in the UK. Parents need to know that data may be used in various ways for NHS purposes. Guidance from the Department of Health as to how this is to be managed is needed. Appropriate access to records should be standardized and non-negotiable.

The electronic health record and the electronic patient record

The Department of Health with the NHS Information Authority is promoting electronic patient records (in general practices, hospitals, and other health service organizations) and an individual electronic health record (EHR) which will contain summary information and, with necessary security safeguards, will be accessible for NHS purposes from anywhere within the UK. Information in this EHR will be derived by automatic electronic transfer from the various electronic patient records and other sources such as the PCHR. The EHR will support routine care and 24-hour emergency care, and will be accessible to the patient. Aggregated anonymized subsets of EHR data will be used to develop health improvement programmes, for clinical governance, and for epidemiological research. Electronic links to the EHR from other agencies (e.g. social care records) are being developed.

Essential core data for child health

The Child Health Informatics Consortium, a national coordinating body, has been working with the Royal College of Paediatrics and Child Health and other professional and statutory bodies to develop an essential core dataset for child health. This should form the basis of a child health EHR. This essential core dataset (ECD) is available on the HFAC4 website. The items in plain text are 'one off' (e.g. birth weight). Those in italics (e.g. vaccinations) need regular updating. Those in bold are in general more complex. Some items are still under development or undergoing field testing. The items included in the ECD are collected as part of normal clinical care and make use of the PCHR and existing manual and computerized information systems.

The 2 year sign-off

Innovations in the ECD which should improve health for all children and facilitate monitoring of individual children include the health summary status for each child (an 'MOT') at key ages. The sign-off at 2 years confirms that immunizations are up to date, documents whether the child has any significant medical conditions, has been admitted to hospital, or has attended accident and emergency department appointments or out-patient clinics. Links with social services departments can record care status and possible child protection registration. Where there are parental or professional concerns, for example if the child is recorded as having a significant condition (*see* HFAC4 website) it is recommended that the child's disability status be documented in a standardized manner. Most of the recommended items for the 2-year sign-off assessment are recorded in present computerized records. Computerized disability registers (special needs modules) are particularly useful sources of information, but are not yet available in all areas.

Similar sign-offs are recommended at school entry and, after further development, at secondary school transfer and at school leaving.

Information from the CHIC-ECD/Electronic Health Record will be abstracted to enable *key indicators of child health* to be used to monitor the health of groups of children, for example, within primary care trusts, within strategic health authority areas, and at national level (*see* www.CHIConsortium.uk).

Research and development

Additional research and development **needed in the information area includes the definition and measurement of:**

- ethnicity
- maternal education and other markers of disadvantage
- disability status
- coding of accidents
- outcomes expected from the pre-school health promotion programme.

The NHS number is a unique anonymous identifier of prime importance in health information. It should be included in all health service records and communications, and could be adopted as the basic identifier by all statutory agencies. This would greatly facilitate inter-agency data-sharing on individuals and populations of children.

4r   The development in England of the NHS Core Records Service will provide a single up to date electronic record of a patient's healthcare through England. This will simplify information transfer across all providers.

Chapter 18

The universal programme

This chapter:

- ◆ Summarizes the justification for providing a universal preventive child health service for families, children, and young people
- ◆ Sets out the general principles which underpin such a programme
- ◆ Summarizes the objectives of a universal programme
- ◆ Describes the core programme of pre-school care and the need for a programme for school-age children and young people
- ◆ Emphasizes the importance of adequate community resources to deal with problems detected and to undertake effective prevention and health promotion strategies.

Developing communities, improving housing and the environment, tackling poverty, and raising the standards of education are the key to improving the lives and health of children. Nevertheless, we should not underestimate the contribution made by high-quality preventive health care for individuals. In constructing this programme, we have taken account of the arguments in favour of universal access to such care as set out in earlier chapters. We have tried to reconcile the research evidence, the scepticism of chief executives and commissioners, the passionately held views of many professionals, the clearly expressed concerns of parents, children and young people, and voluntary organizations, and the duties laid upon statutory authorities by legislation.

The views of children, young people, and parents are not known on every aspect of the topics covered in this book, but where there is evidence it has been considered (see Chapter 5).

4r National service frameworks

The relevant NSF standard is Standard 1 (Core Standards): 'Promoting Health and Well-being, Identifying Needs and Intervening Early'.

www.dh.gov.uk/policyandguidance/healthandsocialcaretopics/children
services

Why we recommend a universal or core programme

The following propositions summarize what we believe to be the common
ground between the many individuals and agencies with an interest in
children's health:

♦ Parents value individual contact with health professionals, when they feel
   the need, in order to express and clarify concerns and access the most
   relevant expertise.

♦ Parents value early diagnosis and intervention whether or not there is
   medical evidence of 'benefit'. They feel let down when the health service
   fails to deliver this.

♦ Parents are clear what they expect from the services when a disorder or
   developmental delay is suspected.

♦ There are many ways of achieving these goals, of which screening is only one.

♦ Screening programmes should be confined to those whose benefits have
   been carefully evaluated and shown to outweigh the hazards.

♦ Screening is of no value unless supported by excellent accessible diagnostic
   and management systems.

♦ Delays in diagnosis are not necessarily attributable to lack of screening
   programmes—they may be due to the failure of professionals to act
   decisively in undertaking appropriate investigations or the reluctance of
   parents to accept referral.

♦ The evidence base for some primary prevention and health promotion
   strategies, incorporating concepts such as social support, parent education,
   and health-promoting schools, is at least as good as that for many other
   medical interventions and is more robust than the evidence for some
   screening tests.

♦ Comprehensive multi-agency intervention strategies on a community-
   wide basis, such as Sure Start, offer the opportunity to combine prevention,
   problem recognition, and intervention.

♦ Vulnerable children are the first priority in planning care programmes.
   This includes children with disabilities and children whose physical safety or
   emotional, cognitive, and language development is being affected adversely
   by their environmental circumstances.

♦ Although there are many socially excluded and disadvantaged children,
   overall the total number of children in 'middle-class' families is much

larger, and among these there will always be a significant number of children with undetected problems.

- The ethos of schools and the quality of teaching and relationships within each school have an important influence on educational and health outcomes.

General principles

1 There should be a universal or core programme available to all (see box for justification), plus additional services targeted to those who need them.

2 The content of the universal programme should be justified as far as possible by evidence of effectiveness, but the views of parents as consumers, where known, are also important.

3 The professional qualification of the person(s) delivering the various aspects of this programme is less important than the quality of their initial and continuing training, audit, and self-monitoring.

4 The delivery of care should be based on what people need and the skills and resources required to meet those needs, rather than being based on traditional professional roles. If new skill combinations are needed, developing these must be the aim. (For these reasons, successive editions of *Health for all children* have been cautious in specifying which particular discipline should provide any particular service unless there is specific evidence that one approach or type of training is superior to others.)

5 Several factors make flexibility and teamwork more important than ever— workforce shortages, the growing realization that skill mix is vital, the increasing complexity of health care, the need for a degree of specialization, the increasing wish of staff to work on a part-time basis, and the importance of developing staff for new roles. Continuity of care cannot always depend on a single individual, and therefore good records and efficient information sharing are vital.

6 Opportunistic detection of health problems makes an important contribution to health care. Primary care staff need training and a high level of awareness for disorders of growth, development and behaviour, and for emotional distress in the child and parents.

The objectives of the universal or core programme

- To ensure that all parents and children have access to, and understanding of, all relevant health care messages that are evidence based and shown to be beneficial.

The benefits of and the justification for a universal programme of preventive health care for all children

Benefits

- It specifies a minimum level of care and support which a parent can expect wherever they may live in the UK.

- It provides a framework that encourages formation of a constructive relationship between professional and family, allowing the promotion of health independent of the stress caused by acute medical problems.

- It provides opportunities for health education and guidance which can be linked to developmental stages.

- It provides a flexible framework of reviews and advice which can be delivered in various ways and with varying levels of professional input, according to the needs of the family.

- It reduces the chances of families with unrecognized needs being 'missed' by the network of services.

- It provides a convenient vehicle for securing high uptake of immunizations.

Justification

- Some procedures, tests, and items of information or primary prevention have a sufficiently sound evidence base and magnitude of benefit that they should be available to all children and families.

- It is not desirable, feasible, or cost effective to provide high levels of support or health professional input to every pre-school child. Some families need more input or support than others in order to achieve equity of outcome, but the identification of children and families needing additional services or support is only achievable if a core programme is universally available.

- There is no individual factor or set of risk factors that would allow sufficiently precise targeting of services to families with problems, and therefore it is necessary to have a process that allows professionals to establish the needs of each family.

- Services that are provided only to selected families have a high risk of becoming stigmatizing and therefore of being rejected by the families. Targeting more resources to more needy areas is preferable to profiling and targeting individuals.

- The concept of social support for families with problems has an increasingly solid research base.

> ◆ Public health work involving community-wide initiatives may be the best way to help many families. Programmes are designed to involve a whole community, but recruiting and involving individuals is intrinsic to successful public health work. Individual care and public health work are not options to choose between—they are both vital.

- ◆ To arrange and deliver immunizations.
- ◆ To carry out the agreed screening procedures.
- ◆ To enable parents with worries about their child to locate the help they need promptly and efficiently.
- ◆ To support the local community in creating an environment at home and at school in which the child can be safe, grow, and thrive physically and emotionally.
- ◆ To identify vulnerable children and families (see below) who may benefit from additional support or services beyond the core programme and negotiate whatever is needed.
- ◆ To ensure that as far as possible children who have or may have special educational needs are identified and referred to the education services and to the appropriate voluntary agency.

Vulnerable children

Chapters 14, 15, and 16 set out the statutory duties placed on the NHS and on social services to provide for certain groups of vulnerable children. This is a responsibility that must be clearly allocated in primary care organizations. The aims of the core programme are firstly to prevent children developing these problems where they are preventable—and to identify and refer them to the right service where they are not. Vulnerable children include:

- ◆ disabled children
- ◆ children with special educational needs
- ◆ abused or neglected children
- ◆ children being looked after by the local authority
- ◆ children being fostered or awaiting adoption
- ◆ homeless children, refugees, asylum seekers, and travellers
- ◆ children who live in poverty or on the edge of poverty and by virtue of their poverty have limited access to health care.

Providing appropriate services for these children is a major challenge for both primary and secondary health care providers, especially as many children fall into more than one of these categories.

Primary care for children

Primary care services for all children and young people provide diagnosis and treatment for the common illnesses and disorders of childhood. At the same time they have many opportunities for the early identification of problems and the promotion of physical health and emotional well-being—see box.

On average, children see their GP:

- 9 times in the first year of life
- 4 times per year between the ages of 1 and 4
- twice per year between the ages of 5 and 14
- 3 times per year between the ages of 15 and 17

Each contact between a primary health care professional and a child should be viewed as part of continuing child health surveillance and used to opportunistically detect health issues and concerns, and where relevant to provide health promotion advice. The professional skills required include:

- systems planning (environment and process) to facilitate optimal consultation with children and young people
- a set of quick methods for eliciting parental concerns
- observational skills for identifying possible problems affecting health, growth, development, and emotional well-being in the child
- sensitivity to parental physical or mental health disorders that might affect the child
- the ability to adapt consultation styles for older children and young people.

Summary of the core programme
Antenatal care

Antenatal care comprises the following: the identification and prevention of pregnancy complications; informing the parents about the birth and, where appropriate, the options available, carrying out agreed screening and monitoring procedures; providing information about early baby care issues, in particular the benefits and technique of breast feeding; developing a relationship between the primary health care team and the family that will facilitate future professional and community support for the family; recognizing social circumstances that may affect the parents' ability to provide optimal care for the infant; making a preliminary assessment of the likely needs of the family for advice, support, and other services after the baby is born.

The core programme as recommended in the National Service Framework for Children, Young People and Maternity Services.   4r

Overview of the Child Health Promotion Programme
This table sets out health promotion services that will be offered to all pregnant women and children and for which there is evidence of effectiveness. Services may change as new evidence emerges, particularly in the area of adolescent health, and in response to new health concerns (including priorities that may be identified in the White Paper on public health).
See Standards 6 and 11 for pre-conception care and advice.

Age	Intervention
Ante-natal	Ante-natal screening and preliminary assessment of child and family needs. Provide advice on breast-feeding and general health and well-being, including healthy eating and smoking cessation where appropriate. Arrangements are put in place, including sharing of information, to ensure a smooth transition from the midwifery to health visiting service.
Soon after birth	General physical examination with particular emphasis on eyes, heart and hips. Administration of vitamin K (if parents choose vitamin K drops, these are administered during the first week after birth). BCG is offered to babies who are more likely to come into contact with someone who has TB. The first dose of Hepatitis B vaccine is give to babies whose mothers or close family have been infected with Hepatitis B.
5–6 days old	Blood spot test for hypothyroidism and phenylketonuria. Screening for sickle cell disease and cystic fibrosis is also being implemented. See www.newbornscreening-bloodspot.org.uk
Within 1st month of life	Newborn hearing screen now being rolled out to all areas. If hepatitis B vaccine has been given soon after birth, the second dose is given
New birth visit (usually around 12 days)	Distribution of `Birth to Five' guide and the Parent Held Child Record if not already given out ante-natally. Home visit by the midwife or health visitor to assess the child and family health needs, including identification of mental health needs. Information/support to parents on key health issues to be available (e.g. support for breastfeeding, advice on establishing a routine etc).

Age	Intervention
6–8 weeks	General physical examination with particular emphasis on eyes, heart and hips. First set of immunisations against polio, diphtheria, tetanus, whooping cough, Hib, and Meningitis C. Review of general progress and delivery of key messages about parenting and health promotion. Identification of post-natal depression or other mental health needs.
3 months	Second set of immunisations against polio, diphtheria, tetanus, whooping cough, Hib, and Meningitis C. Review of general progress and delivery of key messages about parenting and health promotion, including weaning. If Hepatitis B vaccine has been given after birth, the third dose is given.
4 months	Third set of immunisations against pokio, diphtheria, tetanus, whooping cough, Hib, and Meningitis C. Opportunity to give health promotion and advice to parents and to ask about parents' concerns.
By the 1st birthday	Systematic assessment of the child's physical, emotional and social development and family needs by the health visiting team. This will include actions to address the needs identified and agree future contact with service.
Around 13 months	Immunisation against mumps, measles and rubella (MMR). Review of general progress and health promotion and other advice to parents. If Hepatitis B vaccine has been given soon after birth a booster dose and bloodtest are given.
2–3 years	The health visiting team is responsible for reviewing a child's progress and ensuring that health and developmental needs are being addressed. The health visitor will exercise professional judgement and agree with the parent how this review is carried out. It could be done through early years providers or the general practice or by offering a contact in the clinic, home, by phone or email etc. Use is made of other contacts with the primary care team (e.g. immunisations, visits to the general practitioner etc.).
3–5 years	Immunisation against mumps, measles, rubella (MMR) and polio and diphtheria, tetanus and whooping cough. Review of general progress and delivery of key messages about parenting and health promotion.
4–5 years	A review at school entry provides an opportunity to check that: immunisations are up-to-date, children have access to primary and dental care, appropriate interventions are available for any physical, developmental or emotional problems that had previously been missed or not addressed, to provide children, parents and school staff with information about specific health issues, to check the child's height and weight, and to administer the sweep test of hearing. National orthoptist-led programme for pre-school vision screening to be introduced.

	Foundation Stage Profile—Assessment by the teacher to include a child's: >Personal, social and emotional development; >Communication, language and literacy; >Physical development, and >Creative development.
Ongoing support at primary and secondary schools	Access to school nurse at open sessions/drop-in and clinics by parents, teachers or through self-referral. Provision for referral to specialists for children causing concern. Children and young people with medical needs and disabilities may receive nursing care within the school environment according to their needs.
Secondary school	The Heaf test is carried out between 10 to 14 years, and BCG vaccine given to those requiring it.

Key to relevant records

▓▓▓ NHS Care Record Service

░░░ Parent Held Child Record

This schedule is underpinned by a health promotion programme, based on best available evidence, that focuses on priority issues such as healthy eating, physical activity, safety, smoking, sexual health and mental health, and is delivered by all practitioners who come into contact with children and young people, and in all settings used by this age group.

© Crown copyright 2005

Immediately after the birth

Carry out initial inspection of the infant for visible and obvious anomalies or signs of illness.

Within 72 hours of birth

The parent(s) should be interviewed and the baby examined. The consensus is that the target should be to complete this (a) within 24 hours of birth *and* (b) before discharge from hospital. The newborn examination should include inspection of the eyes for cataract, examination of the cardiovascular system for congenital heart disease, and a check for congenital dislocation of the hip. We emphasize that this is a health promotion and information sharing opportunity as well as a screen for abnormalities (see Chapter 7).

Hearing screening

Currently universal neonatal hearing screening (UNHS) is being piloted in 20 sites around the UK. If successful, this will become a countrywide programme. The pilot sites include some where screening will be done in the community. For those districts where UNHS is not yet available, many units are instead offering high-risk screening. Local policy should include planning for UNHS. Meanwhile, if the infant distraction test is being continued it must be done to a high standard, by trained staff, in protected time, and under satisfactory conditions.

Further follow-up of mother and baby

Visits to the family at home are usual on several occasions within the first 10 days of the baby's life. We have not defined any fixed frequency of visits— some mothers may need to be seen twice in one day, whereas others may be visited only once every 2 or 3 days. In addition to monitoring the mother's health and well-being, these visits provide an opportunity to observe the baby's health, feeding, and progress. Where appropriate the baby should be weighed. Support for establishing breastfeeding is important and a contribution to this can be made by lay workers. Additional support may be needed for babies who have special needs or who have needed treatment in the neonatal intensive care unit.

A review of the family's circumstances and needs should be undertaken within the first few weeks in order to make an initial plan with them for what care may be needed over the short to medium term. High-risk situations should be identified. This may require one or several more visits.

At 7 days, the blood spot for PKU and hypothyroidism screening is collected. In due course haemoglobinopathy and cystic fibrosis screening will be offered, and further biochemical screening tests may also be added in the future.

An **examination** should be planned for **6–8 weeks** and the aim should be to *complete* this examination in *all* babies *by* 8 weeks of age. Any baby in whom there is suspicion of the problems listed in Chapter 7, resulting from a check at 6–8 weeks, must be referred with the appropriate degree of urgency. The parents' health, particularly mental health, should also be considered in view of the importance of postnatal depression.

At age 2, 3, and 4 months, the parent should be invited to bring the baby for immunization. The baby is weighed. Whoever is responsible for giving vaccines and for weighing must be able to deal with questions about vaccines and the interpretation of the weight chart, either in person or by passing the queries to someone better qualified. Immunization may be done at home if circumstances warrant this.

Further reviews after 4 months

Previous editions of the UK programme have proposed three further contacts after the age of 4 months—at 6–9 months, 18–24 months, and 39–42 months.

A review between 6 and 9 months was originally recommended because 7–8 months is the optimal age for the distraction test of hearing. This may be a suitable time to identify the infant who is not gaining weight well or has serious feeding problems (p. 178); developmental problems may be emerging and home safety advice can be offered. As this review is long established, staff are very familiar with infant development at around this age. On the other hand, there is no firm evidence base to support this age over any other; for example, it has been proposed that the review might be done at around 12 months to coincide with the MMR vaccine visit.

At 24 months, there are no formal screening measures for which the evidence is so robust that they must be provided universally. Children whose parents are worried about their physical health are likely to have contacted their primary health care team before the age of 2 years, but parents often use the 2-year review as a way of clarifying concerns about behaviour, growth, or development. Given the accumulating evidence of benefits from pre-school high-quality learning opportunities, the contact should also be valuable for informing parents about child development and behaviour.

By 3–4 years, most children with developmental problems have already been identified in playgroup or pre-school, although a few parents may have unresolved worries about their child's progress or be reluctant to accept referral for a variety of reasons. A review at this age might identify some children with previously overlooked disorders affecting health, growth, development, or behaviour, and many parents may be reassured by having the child assessed, examined, and pronounced normal. However, as we have illustrated in this book, there can be no guarantee that abnormalities would be found and the numbers of important positive new findings are likely to be very small.

There are **two opposing arguments**. On the one hand, when resources are limited and skilled professionals are in short supply, it is unquestionably important to minimize routine tasks, whose benefits are uncertain, in order to release time and energy for children with higher levels of need. Establishing contact with the most needy families can be difficult and time-consuming (see discussion of targeting later in this chapter). On the other hand, there are fears that in the absence of any universal programme of contacts, children with developmental, behavioural, or growth problems will be 'missed' and that children may enter school with undetected disabilities. Paraprofessional staff who undertake 'routine screening' need thorough training. As we have shown in this book, evaluation and promotion of development in the family context is not a simple protocol-driven process.

There are significant *potential* benefits from retaining fixed points in the programme. First, the parents may appreciate the opportunity to receive up-to-date advice and information about promoting health and development and to discuss any anxieties they may have; conversely, for children who may have special educational needs, early identification allows time for parents and the education services to consider future plans. Second, a rigorous approach to a high coverage of universal reviews at fixed ages would focus attention on marginalized and excluded children. Areas with adequate data usually find that coverage over 60–70 per cent is hard to maintain after the first year of life, and considerable resources would be needed to maintain or improve this, while simultaneously ensuring that more effort can be devoted to marginalized and socially excluded families. Third, universal review is needed to maintain a minimum public health dataset as recommended in Chapter 17. Fourth, in Sure Start areas data are needed to monitor the programme and it would make sense to follow compatible procedures in other areas.

For some families, particularly those who have already had at least one child and are not disadvantaged by residence or circumstances, these goals might be achieved without a face-to-face contact. Some families may already be receiving frequent support for various reasons, whether from the health visitor or other professionals or from a programme like Sure Start. Some will be frequent attenders at the health centre and will be well known to the GP and the health visitor. Some parents may feel that they do not need any further formal reviews.

A 'best-buy' proposal

Accordingly, we recommended in 2003 that after the third dose of vaccine at 4 months, the health visitor should negotiate the *nature* of subsequent reviews. The National Service Framework modified this and advised that this process of negotiation and planning might need to continue up to the first birthday and we are happy to support this proposal. It is up to parents and professionals together to decide on what should be done, in the light of individual needs and, inevitably, of competing priorities. When there is no formal face-to-face contact, the primary health care team would need to assure itself that, at each stage (8 or 12 months, 2 years, and 3.5 years), no new problems had emerged. Where a family is well known to the primary health care team a formal contact may not be necessary. In other cases contact by telephone or letter may be sufficient, whereas in some families a face-to-face contact may be required. For this to work properly, the primary health care team must truly function as a team and also maintain good liaison with others in contact with children such as nursery staff etc.

Further doses of vaccine are given at 12(Hib/Men C booster) and 13 months (MMR and Pneumococcal conjugate vaccine) and at 3–4 years (pre-school booster and second MMR).

Pre-school vision check

The 'best buy' is for screening of the vision of all children to be undertaken by an orthoptist with the aim of achieving this between the ages of 4 and 5 years. Formal screening for vision defects should not be undertaken on a community-wide basis before 4 years of age, because the failure and recall rates are unacceptably high. There is no need for a second vision test at school entry.

Those districts that cannot immediately achieve this 'best-buy' standard should carry out only one vision screen, and should as a minimum ensure that an orthoptist provides both training and monitoring.

Growth

Serial height measures are carried out in many districts, but the evidence does not currently support routine *monitoring* of height; the only recommended age at which height should *routinely* be measured is at or around 5 years old. In a number of places, the referral criterion is the second centile rather than the 0.4th as we have suggested—this results in large numbers of children being referred, most of whom turn out to need no treatment. Some people are still reluctant to use the 1990 nine-centile charts which have been agreed as the standard by the Royal College of Paediatrics and Child Health. A few teams are still using the Oxford wall chart, which we do not recommend as it does not allow accurate measurement.

Weight should be recorded with height and these measurements used to calculate the body mass index (BMI) for public health monitoring purposes only—the BMI is not intended as a screening test for individual children. Childhood obesity is a major public health problem, but investment in prevention programmes seems likely to be more relevant than screening.

Although we recommended that the height and weight should be measured at around the age of 5, at school entry, we are aware that in some districts staff shortages or other local problems may prevent this from being implemented immediately.

The Department of Health recommends that, for public health monitoring purposes and monitoring of attainment of the Public Service Agreement (PSA) target, the heights and weights of all children in reception classes and year 6 should be measured and reported centrally, at which stage the BMI is calculated. (www.dh.gov.uk)

Many growth problems can be identified before school entry by the primary health care team. If *at any time* there is any parental or professional concern about the child's growth, or worries about possible chronic health problems, height and weight should be checked, charted, and interpreted as part of the clinical evaluation, or alternatively the child should be referred for specialist opinion.

School entry

When the child starts formal schooling (around the age of 5) the following should be done: height and weight (see above); hearing test (under review); vision check if not done previously; identification of children whose immunizations are incomplete or who have not received routine pre-school health care for any reason. Chapter 5 reviews the options for additional procedures at school entry. Children not on the list of any primary health care team are a priority, and the aim should be to secure their primary health care needs rather than merely to carry out a single health review.

Further health checks in school

After school entry, there are no further formal universal routine procedures except for immunization programmes where indicated and information transfer procedures for the core dataset. Districts where vision is checked at 11 years old should continue this pending further review by the National Screening Committee. If not being undertaken, it should not be introduced.

Pre-school health promotion

All *pre-school children and their families* should have access to a health promotion programme. This includes antenatal information and care, early support after childbirth with particular reference to breastfeeding, and information and guidance about issues where the evidence supports universal intervention.

Child development and behaviour

Sure Start and related programmes aim to promote parenting, support parents, and encourage parents to work with their children and tackle behavioural problems before they are entrenched. Additional benefits may include improved home safety and enhanced injury prevention programmes, and better nutrition and dental care.

The more children are enrolled in pre-school programmes that also engage parents, the less we will need to treat aberrant development or difficult behaviour as pathological entities for which screening is needed. Parents and pre-school professionals who are well informed about child development in all its aspects will be effective in identifying problems and judging when specialist evaluation might be indicated.

Promoting health in schools

Developing policies such as the Healthy Schools initiative requires multi-agency collaboration and has the potential to make substantial improvements in the mental and physical health and the educational outcomes of all young people. Older children and young people have particular and clearly expressed needs for health care, summarized in Chapter 5. Children may be vulnerable for many reasons at different points in their pathway through school, and support for vulnerable children in school is an important part of the universal service.

Community resources

Preventive programmes are of little value unless there are adequate resources to deal with problems identified and to undertake effective prevention initiatives. Thus we stress again the vital importance of providing multi-agency services of high quality, and in sufficient quantity, for children who are at risk or vulnerable because of social circumstances, disabilities, mental health problems, or educational difficulties. In a twenty-first century health service, children deserve more than the minimalist service needed to fulfil statutory duties, and all communities should guarantee the necessary investment in personnel, training, and facilities.

Targeting child health promotion programmes

The concepts of targeting and resource allocation were introduced in Chapter 1. We believe that an argument for universal access to preventive health care does not imply that all families must receive the same service. On the contrary, in order to achieve greater equity of outcome some families may need substantially more input than others.

Some parents need considerable personal help and support either at specific times or for a continuous period; others need only appropriate information and ready access to professional advice when they have concerns. It follows that, although the aims of child health promotion programmes should be the same for all parents, they may be achieved in various ways.

Targeting—a summary of the evidence

- The distribution of health visitors across the UK shows little correlation with deprivation levels.

- Most health visitors target their time according to the perceived needs of their clients but the extent of this, measured by the ratio of time devoted to the most versus the least needy clients, varies widely.

- Taking into account caseload size and deprivation levels of each caseload, there are substantial differences between the workload of individual health visitors.

- Allocation of health visitors (and other similar resources) should be based on a formula using these parameters.

See HFAC4 website

The allocation of health professional time is driven by two main types of influence. The first are ***managerial*** influences—they affect the allocation of health visitors to practice populations, which is largely determined by the historical distribution of health visitors, contractual decisions by health authorities, and managerial decisions by the trusts which employ health visitors. The second type of decision is best described as ***professional***—the judgements of health visitors, as a professional group and as individual practitioners, about the allocation of their time between types of case (e.g. child protection, postnatal depression, community development) and between individual cases.

Decisions about targeting can be made at three different levels:

- In the geographic sense—some parts of a health district will have much higher levels of need than others. Even within a single post-code district there can be dramatic differences in poverty and in health.

- Within the case-loads or practices of individual practitioners or primary health care teams (see box and Figs 18.1 and 18.2).

- In working with individual families or small groups, it may be necessary to focus on particular themes and problems and to defer others which have a lower priority.

Sheffield health visitors developed a system of reviewing needs and then prioritizing their clients into three groups (Fig. 18.1). High-priority clients received substantially more contacts than those rated low priority (Fig. 18.2). The extent of targeting varied significantly between health visitors after controlling for other possible factors such as case-load size. Mothers rated as low priority were asked if they were satisfied with the service they received.

Mothers of children who at 8 weeks of age were thought to need only the core programme of child health surveillance services were asked about the health visitor service. Most felt that they had seen their health visitor often enough and were 'fairly' or 'very' satisfied with the support they had received for their baby, but only 72 per cent expressed the same level of satisfaction with the support they had received from the health visiting service for themselves. Furthermore, over half expressed dissatisfaction with some aspect of the service, with requests for more support in the first few weeks following the birth, more home visits, improved appointment system, more appropriate advice, and more time to talk.

Conclusions

1 The results suggest that even 'coping' mothers appreciate more support in the early weeks of the baby's life.

2 The core programme is acceptable but only if the responsive service is satisfactory.

See HFAC4 website

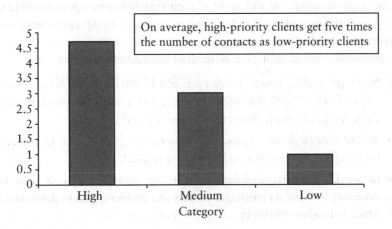

Fig. 18.1 Ratio of contact rates by priority rating.

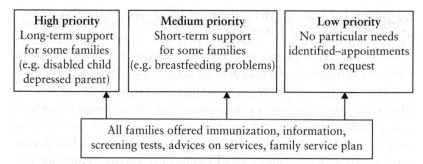

Fig. 18.2 Classification of priority ratings used in the study shown in Fig 18.1.

Geographic targeting—using locality needs and deprivation levels

A good case can be made for allocating more resources to localities that make greater demands on professional staff by reason of areas or pockets of poverty, linguistic barriers, low population density, or perceived threats to personal safety. Information about the relative needs of different areas of a district is required.

Community profiling provides an information base on the health of children for practitioners and purchasers. It involves identification of local factors that affect health, and reviewing access to and availability of statutory and voluntary services. Local and national data should be used along with information on demographic and social characteristics, health status, statutory and voluntary services, transport, and the physical environment. This can be analysed according to electoral ward or enumeration district, health localities, primary care team boundaries, or school. Local authority data can be useful and may be more up to date than national census data. Further work is required to develop systems that can generate and utilize these data more easily. Without both commitment to action and resource allocation, the exercise is of limited value.

A commitment to action

Many districts have a stated policy of discrimination in favour of the poorest areas, in the use of community health care resources—yet inability to initiate staff redistribution, difficulties with recruitment and morale in the most needy areas, and distortions introduced by changing patterns of funding often result in no net changes occurring or even an increase in resource allocation to more prosperous areas.

Targeting by the identification of 'high-risk' families using checklists or formulas

There have been many attempts to streamline recognition of 'vulnerable' or 'high-risk' families in order to save time and reduce investment in supposedly low-risk families. Checklists and formulas do not seem to achieve this. They may have a place in some situations, as *aides mémoire* or prompts, and may also offer a means by which staff can demonstrate the magnitude and extent of the social difficulties their clients face (see box for example). However, they are deservedly unpopular with many clinicians as a routine tool. There are several reasons for this.

Firstly, there is no agreed definition of what is meant by 'vulnerable' or 'high risk'. 'Vulnerability' for a few families might be a permanent state, but for many others it is transient and changes with life circumstances and events.

Secondly, health professionals develop an intuitive sense about the health and the needs of their patients or clients, based on knowledge and experience,

---

Example of checklist

- First pregnancies and first-time parents
- Breastfeeding mothers
- Mothers recovering from difficult delivery (e.g. Caesarean section) or suffering postnatal depression or mood disorders, particularly if partner unhelpful or absent, or mother lacking in other social support networks
- Unsupported young poor parent, particularly in substandard housing; any family in temporary accommodation
- Domestic violence; drug or alcohol misuse
- Concern about possible child neglect or abuse; past or present concerns identified by the child protection system
- Parent(s) with learning disability, poor skills in managing their affairs, lacking in confidence, or with low self-esteem
- Child who is premature, low birth weight, disabled, or chronically sick
- History of previous 'cot death' or other infant death
- Infant with 'difficult' temperament, irregular sleep patterns, difficult feeding, etc.

familiarity with a family's previous history, and an understanding of the local neighbourhood. Stress factors may be internal (depression, poor health, disabled child) or external (housing problems, financial difficulties). Checklists may overemphasize vulnerability factors and ignore protective resources, such as a supportive partner or a close relationship with a friend or relative, yet the latter are at least as important in determining needs (see below). The weight which should be attached to each adverse and protective factor would have to be fixed in a formal checklist approach but can be assessed individually by an experienced professional.

Thirdly, although some needs may be identified by the parent or obvious to the professional, some problems are only identified by leading questions and may be acknowledged by the parent only after a relationship with the professional has been established. Sensitivity is essential in raising personal matters—this cannot easily be done in one visit or by using a formal checklist.

Effective targeting and health needs assessment

This is dependent on a number of factors.

1 It is essential that staff have the time and the skills to listen to what parents are saying and try to develop a genuine sense of partnership, rather than imposing their own agenda or that of their managing authority. Health care staff (who are still predominantly white and middle class) do not have a monopoly of wisdom in matters of child care, child rearing, or family life. The insights of developmental psychology, linguistics, and child psychiatry do not guarantee that we now know the 'right' or 'best' way to bring up children. Unsolicited advice may not always be welcome. In the UK, the historical context of health visiting, coupled with public and professional anxiety about child abuse and neglect, can result in the role of health promoter being confused with that of the social worker, police officer, hygiene inspector, or NSPCC officer. Although health visitors are usually welcomed by parents, their perceived responsibility to identify child abuse can place them in a difficult position.*

2 All professionals need to be aware of, and resist, the tendency to assess and act on the perceived 'social worth' of patients and clients. 'Worthiness' in this sense does not refer to their social status; it is a more complicated concept involving estimates of how deserving clients are of help, whether their needs

---

* This is said to be a less prominent problem in countries like France, where the division of responsibility between health visitor and social worker is much sharper and there is more support for families with young children, so that their care is shared between parents and other adults.

are a legitimate call on the professional's time, and whether clients are responsive to the offers made by the professional.

3 Health professionals are often wary of discussing needs for which no service exists, particularly if, as is often the case, they have no direct means of influencing the planning of services. In this situation, it is important that unmet needs *are* acknowledged, documented, and brought to the attention of managers, public health physicians, and other relevant authorities. This advocacy role may not be perceived as important or effective by the family concerned but its long-term benefits should be stressed (see Chapter 1).

4 Alternatively, there is a risk that clients may be matched to the service which comes closest to meeting their needs, even if it is not the ideal. Health professionals may be tempted to construe problems in terms of health care needs that can be met by the health service, when sometimes other solutions might be more appropriate. This can result in disappointment and time-wasting for the individual, and reduces the efficiency of the service in question.

5 Cultural, religious, ethnic, and language barriers may prevent accurate needs assessment in precisely those families who are likely to benefit the most from a variety of different services.

6 Children's own perceptions of need are often ignored or are not taken seriously. It is important that professionals learn to listen to children's concerns. Current evidence shows that even very young children can be involved in this process. Chapters 1 and 5 summarize current work on involving children and young people in policy making.

Individual work and community-wide approaches

Our assessment of the current literature and the experience of practitioners strongly support an integrated care approach that incorporates both individual client work and a community-wide approach. This implies the need to re-examine the roles of the staff who traditionally work with children and families in the community—health visitors, school nurses, and a range of other professionals. The concept of a public health nursing team, able to handle the individual client contacts and the challenges of community development and inter-agency working, is gaining favour.

The role of non-qualified staff ('paraprofessionals')

Professionals are not essential in every situation. The needs of some families can be met as effectively, or in some cases more effectively, by non-qualified or lay staff. This has obvious advantages; individuals can be selected from their own community and therefore are familiar with its lifestyle and its problems, and they bring an income into their family and into their community.

Not surprisingly, this option has attracted much interest for both financial and philosophical reasons (see box). Nevertheless, it is not necessarily simple or cheap. To be successful, paraprofessional staff need training and support. Their case-loads are usually smaller than those of professionals, and their ability to cope with stressful problems may be reduced, particularly if they themselves are subject to similar life stresses. Some families may be reluctant to disclose problems to lay workers (although others may be equally reluctant with professionals). Lay workers and the members of voluntary organizations such as Homestart, Newpin, and breastfeeding support groups provide a valuable service and should be encouraged and supported. They are neither a threat to nor a substitute for professionals.

Selected points from a systematic review on role of peer/paraprofessional one-to-one interventions

- Peer/paraprofessional one-to-one interventions are frequently embedded in interventions with multiple components and/or intervenors, some of whom are professionals.
- Most studies targeted high-risk populations.
- Peers/paraprofessionals can have a positive impact on child development and parent–child interaction, particularly when the intervention is high in intensity (weekly or biweekly visits for at least a year) and part of a multifaceted intervention which includes professionals.
- Evidence of the long-term effectiveness of these interventions has not yet been established and there are no high-quality cost-effectiveness studies in the literature.
- Peers/paraprofessionals can have an impact on parent-child interaction and child development. Peer/paraprofessional intervention should begin during the prenatal period, be high in intensity (weekly or biweekly visits for at least a year), and embedded in multifaceted interventions comprised of multiple components and/or intervenors, some of whom are professionals.
- Peers/paraprofessionals should receive extensive training in all areas of the intervention as well as the peer/paraprofessional role, have ongoing professional supervision, and utilize a curriculum to guide the intervention.

www.Health.Hamilton-went.on.ca

See HFAC4 website.

Conclusions

Our review suggests that the ideal model is a universal preventive service for children and young people. Resource allocation should aim to reduce inequalities by targeting resources to more needy areas. Professional staff should allocate their time and skills according to assessments of need that are negotiated with individual clients and the local community.

Recommendations

- We recommend a universal programme of preventive health care for all children including screening tests as summarized on p. 342.
- This should be available to every family.
- Resources should be allocated according to the needs of neighbourhoods; thus needy localities may need significantly more staff than more favoured areas in order to deliver the same outputs in terms of coverage and health gain.
- The core programme set out here assumes universal access to pre-school health reviews at specified ages but allows a degree of flexibility among health care teams as to how this is delivered for individual families.
- Investment in prevention, health promotion, and support for school-age children and young people is essential.
- Primary care organizations should ensure that all children have access to a full range of specialized services when they are needed.

Chapter 19

Implementing the programme

This chapter:

- outlines the issues involved in implementing the programme set out in this book
- suggests that the same principles apply whatever the structure and management of the health care system

Organization and management of health care for children varies both within and between the four countries of the UK. Other countries provide health care in many different ways and there is little evidence that any one system is superior. A universal theme is competition between the immediate demands and pressures of acute and emergency curative care on the one hand and the longer-term and less visible challenges of long-term care of people with disability, health protection, prevention, health promotion, and advocacy on the other. This chapter sets out some principles which are relevant to the tasks and objectives described in this book, whatever the structure of the health care system.

4r National service frameworks

The relevant NSF document is 'Key Issues for Primary Care' www.dh.gov.uk/policyanduidance/healthandsocialcaretopics/childrenservices

Principle 1 *The programmes of health care described in this book should be made available to the whole population*
While most parents will make full use of the services on offer, this is not the case for everyone. Additional resources must be committed and alternative means of providing care must be devised to ensure that the many socially excluded groups in our society benefit from and participate in these programmes.

In order to achieve this, information must be acquired and made available about these groups of children and their families. The numbers will vary widely in each area, but the difficulties in mapping their distribution and their needs are common to all such groups. By definition, socially excluded children and

The vulnerable and socially excluded groups include:

- Children in transition (e.g. moving from one location to another, changing schools, changing from paediatric to adult health care)
- Children not registered with any general practitioner
- Children living away from home
- Children excluded by language barriers
- Traveller families
- Families living in temporary or bed and breakfast accomodation
- Children of troubled, violent, or disabled parents
- Children who care for disabled parents
- Children who are involved with, or whose families are involved with, substance abuse, crime, or prostitution.
- Runaways and street children
- Asylum seekers and refugees, particularly if unaccompanied
- Children locked up
- Children of parents in prison

families are not part of the regular health care system and are unlikely to be registered with any part of it. Local networks of health visitors, school nurses, social services staff, housing officers, and religious and community leaders are likely to know many of them, but there is no single reliable source of information.

A fundamental requirement is access to a locality-based primary care service for those who are socially excluded, provided in a way that is acceptable to and used by these families. There are also many children and young people who are not socially excluded but are vulnerable because of their circumstances. The aim is to ensure that, as far as possible, all these groups of children and young people can access health care, education, and local services and facilities. Primary care organizations now have a defined responsibility for the whole population, not just those who are registered.

Principle 2 *Responsibility for the provision and linking of the services described in this book must be clearly identified*
Some of them are statutory (see below) and the duty to provide the services is placed on one particular agency. Many of the care programmes we have recommended are interlinked and depend on individuals and facilities in many different organizations. Each service must ensure that mechanisms are in place to link

the various component parts of the care pathway. There is, for example, no value in establishing an excellent screening programme if the children identified have to wait for months after referral for their definitive assessment, or if after assessment there are no facilities for them to receive appropriate care or education.

Partnerships both within the health service and with other agencies are fundamental to improving the health of children and young people. These include links with education (both at local authority level and with individual educational establishments), social services, housing departments, roads and transport, police and youth offending teams, and voluntary organizations and groups. The nature of these partnerships varies widely according to local and national policies, but all areas will need to develop such collaborative frameworks.

Recent Government statements support the concept of identifying one person in each health care organization to be responsible for children's services. This person might be responsible only for health services, but an alternative model would incorporate social care as well. In view of the magnitude and complexity of these tasks, the individual who is assigned these responsibilities will need an extensive background of experience in child health and, preferably, in social care as well. S/he will need the confidence and energy to undertake extensive networking and liaison with a range of professionals and the ability to act as advocate and champion with management boards.

Lead clinicians need to have sufficient time for developing and improving the service as well as monitoring quality and progress. While structures will vary in detail, input will be needed from a wide range of advisory groups—for example, local expert groups on hearing impairment, child protection, mental health, and many other issues. These groups must be coordinated in order to avoid duplication and to ensure maximum efficiency in delivery and monitoring.

Principle 3 *Prioritization of service provision should be based on statutory duties, evidence of what works and the views of children, young people and their families*
Historical accident, rather than any explicit or coherent plan, often determines the pattern of children's health care and the prioritization of service provision in the local community. We have indicated in this book where there is good evidence that various health care interventions are effective, but do not think that the data exist to attempt any economic analysis in terms of cost–benefit ratios.

Government statute and guidance set out certain duties which must be undertaken (box).

The screening procedures we have described were debated at some length by the National Screening Committee and are as far as possible based on research,

- Designated and named doctor and nurse for child protection
- Named health professional with responsibility for looked after children
- Designated doctor for liaison with the education authority
- Immunization coordinator

NB: *There is no statutory requirement for a named coordinator for screening, but in view of the scope for errors and litigation, a strong case can be made for such a post.*

systematic reviews, and consensus. We think that they are all justified by the available evidence and, while some may wish to expand the programme further, we doubt that any major reduction of our package is justifiable. We propose that the introduction of new screening procedures or an extension of the programme should be justified by a literature review setting out the reasons for the modification and, until accepted as a national programme, should be regarded as a research project requiring appraisal by an ethics committee.

There is growing evidence to underpin the approach we have outlined in earlier chapters to family support in the pre-school years and to a service for children and young people in the school years.

Consultation with children, parents, and young people to ascertain their views on health care is rightly becoming part of mainstream practice. However, much is already known about what they want. There is ample evidence to specify the standards expected of services for children with many types of long-term illness or disability and for young carers, children looked after, and abused children. Consultations with teenagers show a consistent pattern of concerns about how they receive health care. There is also abundant evidence about the major preoccupations of children and families with regard to the wider aspects of health, such as safe play and leisure facilities, protection from bullying, and information on healthy eating. Implementation lags behind knowledge and consultation must not become a substitute for action.

Recognition of an issue or identification of a concern for children, parents, and young people cannot always be addressed by direct health care or related provision. For example, children's and young people's access to a healthy diet will include not only measures such as consideration of school meals and health promotion advice but also addressing the difficulty that many families experience in accessing local supplies of reasonably priced fresh fruit and vegetables. Such provision will be dependent on complex collaborations and advocacy by health professionals with other agencies.

Principle 4 *There should be an explicit focus on and commitment to prevention*
As shown in this book, there are multiple opportunities for prevention in child health. These were summarized in chapters 2, 3, and 4. Failure to prevent conditions that could be prevented is unacceptable and in addition carries increasing legal hazards. Examples involving front-line clinical staff include not explaining or failing to follow up the need for vitamin K to prevent bleeding in the infant (p. 99), and failure to offer correct advice in respect of preventing infectious diseases (p. 77). Prevention is also a public health issue, for example with respect to injury prevention (p. 86), child abuse (p. 66), educational failure and exclusion from school (Chapter 5), and prevention of teenage pregnancy (p. 121).

Principle 5 *Standards of care should be accepted and implemented by providers wherever possible and should use existing agreed standards set by professional and consumer groups unless there is good reason to the contrary*
These standards address a range of issues, including for example the requirements for hearing screening and assessment, the quality indicators for provision of care in a child development centre, and good practice in child protection work.

Standards that specify the allocation of time required to undertake a particular task to an acceptable level are often more difficult to justify with firm objective evidence, but are generally based on the experience of practitioners who are acknowledged by their peers to provide a quality service and whose advice therefore deserves serious consideration.

There are as yet no explicit standards for the provision of primary care for children. Most young children attend their primary health care providers on several occasions in the early years. We commented in Chapter 6 on the importance of opportunistic identification of problems affecting health, growth, development, and emotional well-being. The need for all primary health care team members to receive thorough and relevant initial training and continuing education in the health care of children, for preventive care and for acute, chronic, and non-urgent problems, is, we believe, self-evident.

Risk management should take account of the vulnerable areas in community child health and ensure that appropriate training and monitoring are in place to minimize risks. Complaints and litigation may also arise with respect to dissatisfaction with provision of services for children with disabilities or learning problems, particularly with regard to therapy and access to education. Child protection work is increasingly subject to criticism from parents, legal advisers, and indeed other professional colleagues. Staff training and support are vital to avoid distressing and often high-profile problems.

Principle 6 *Services should be planned to improve equity of provision and the reduction of inequalities in health*

Equity of outcome is the goal: between social groups, between different localities of the same health care district or area, and between different parts of the UK. This may mean that varying levels of resource will be needed for individual groups, service, or areas, and that existing resources should be redistributed.

There are no data to show, in absolute terms, what would be the optimal level of provision of, for example, physiotherapy, mental health services, or community nursing staff. However, as discussed in Chapter 18, there is good evidence that extensive variation in provision of community services for children is widespread and that these variations cannot be justified solely on the basis of varying indicators of need such as deprivation scores. The most extreme examples of variation seem to be in child and adolescent mental health services, but there are also unacceptable variations in both quantity and quality of care in many other aspects of the care programmes set out in this book.

Principle 7 *The provision of quality care depends on recruitment and retention of well-trained staff, continuing provisional development, strong leadership, and adequate supporting resources*

Families expect and deserve care provided by professionals who have a sound basic training and are up to date with the latest developments. In recent years there have been important advances in many areas of child health, including the medical and interdisciplinary assessment and management of child abuse, the care of children with disabilities, and prevention and early intervention with regard to child mental health problems. Continuing education and participation in professional networks are as vital in community child health as in any other branch of health care. No professional should work in isolation.

Shortages of professionals with the requisite training are increasingly a problem in community child health. It is important to plan ahead and, in view of the long lead time to recruit and train staff, to consider what will be needed over a period of several years. There is scope for more extensive skill mix, using nurses and other staff to provide care traditionally delivered by doctors. Similarly, good administrative support can reduce the burden on professionals and enable them to use their time more effectively and efficiently.

Principle 8 *Information for parents and families should be available and accessible*

So that partnership working can be a reality, it is essential that all involved are provided with the information that is appropriate to their level of understanding. This may primarily be verbal, but wherever possible should be reinforced with a more permanent medium (e.g. paper or computer based). All such information should be presented in a comprehensible and unbiased way and based on hard evidence where possible. The Personal Child Health Record (PCHR) is currently one of the best ways of ensuring that carers are fully aware of the care given their child. Increasingly, carers are being provided with copies of reports and letters. In future this should be the norm with professionals prepared to justify any exceptions.

Questions of consent and privacy cause much concern, and staff training in these issues is essential. In particular, the guidance governing the provision of health care to teenagers and the principles surrounding informed consent, including the concept of Fraser (previously known as Gillick) competence, must be understood.

Other important issues include providing interpreter services where needed, ensuring that parents understand the process in child protection proceedings and in assessments for children with special educational needs, and facilitating links with voluntary agencies and parent groups where relevant.

Principle 9 *Information should be collected to monitor the processes and outcomes of these programmes*
When everyone has an electronic patient record, easy and rapid transfer of information will allow for more efficient care. Until that time comes, use has to be made of a combination of paper and computer records. Brief entries in the PCHR will allow all professionals involved in the care of a child to have ready access to an overview of their care.

Where computer-based systems are in place, every effort should be made to collect only useful information that can be used for patient care, audit, and management of services. Some data may need to be collected for a limited period for particular audits or research projects. It is essential that all data that is collected can be accessed and manipulated to produce useful information. Where available, common national or internationally recognized data coding systems should be used to allow comparison of data between trusts. The core dataset for child health was outlined in Chapter 17, though much remains to be done before this can be fully implemented.

All staff will need training in the difficult issue of confidentiality and the transfer of data between agencies. This is a particular cause of anxiety for staff involved in child protection work.

Principle 10 *There should be a plan for using information to undertake audit and monitoring of activity and outcomes*
To ensure the continuing proper provision of services, audit is essential. Useful measures should be examined with an emphasis on outcomes where possible. Adverse outcomes may be uncommon or may only occur many years after the health care was provided (or omitted), and so process measures that are known

to correlate with outcome may need to be monitored. An example would be the measurement of uptake of immunizations (process) rather than the incidence of diseases such as tetanus or diphtheria (outcome).

Critical incident analysis is a useful technique that should be used when an unusual adverse outcome occurs or is narrowly averted. Audit should be conducted in a constructive manner with concentration on learning from sub-optimal outcomes. Where screened conditions are uncommon and/or may come to light some time after the screening process, it is important that appropriate disease registers are in place and audit is conducted on large populations.

Appendix

Policy framework, legislation, and policy*

Special units

Cabinet Committee on Children and Young People's Services

The Cabinet Committee on Children and Young People's Services aims to coordinate policies to prevent poverty and underachievement among children and young people, coordinate and monitor the effectiveness of delivery, and work with the voluntary sector to build a new alliance for children. The Cabinet Committee is supported by the cross-cutting Children and Young People's Unit.

The Children and Young People's Unit (CYPU)

The Unit will administer the Children's Fund and monitor how well Whitehall departments work together to serve vulnerable children. The Children's Fund has allocated £450 million to tackle child poverty and social exclusion (2001–2004), particularly focusing on preventive work with children aged 5 to 13 years and their families, helping them before they hit crisis. The Unit will establish and oversee mechanisms for consulting with and listening to children and young people, with the assistance of voluntary organizations. Information on the CYPU is at www.dfes.gov.uk/cypu

The Social Exclusion Unit (SEU)

The Social Exclusion Unit was set up by the Prime Minister in December 1997 to help reduce social exclusion by promoting better inter-departmental and inter-agency working. Between 1997 and 2001, the SEU published reports in five areas: truancy and social exclusion, rough sleeping, neighbourhood renewal, teenage pregnancy, and opportunities for 16–18-year-olds not in

---

* We thank the Library Services of the National Children's Bureau for their help in preparing this appendix.

education, training, or employment. The SEU is currently working on young runaways, reducing reoffending by ex-prisoners, children in care and education, and transport and social exclusion. Information on the Social Exclusion Unit is at www.cabinet-office.gov.uk/seu

Teenage Pregnancy Unit

The Teenage Pregnancy Unit is a cross-Government unit located within the Department of Health. The Unit was set up to implement the Teenage Pregnancy Strategy, which came out of the Social Exclusion Unit's report on Teenage Pregnancy launched by the Prime Minister in June 1999. It is jointly funded by the Department for Education and Skills, the Department for Transport, Local Government and the Regions, the Department for Work and Pensions, and the Home Office. The objectives of the Teenage Pregnancy Unit are to oversee the implementation of the Government's Teenage Pregnancy Strategy, coordinate activity at national level, and provide support for local activity. The two main goals of the Teenage Pregnancy Strategy are to halve the rate of conceptions among under 18-year-olds in England by 2010, and to achieve a reduction in the risk of long-term social exclusion for teenage parents and their children by getting more teenage parents into education, training, and employment.

At local level, every area in England has a Local Teenage Pregnancy Coordinator in place, jointly nominated by Health and Local Authorities. There are 141 Local Coordinators in total, and funding of £11.5 million is available for local projects in 2001–2002. Local targets have been set and no local authority is to have a rate higher than 41 per 1000 women aged 15–18 by 2010. A national media campaign began in October 2000, including advertisements in teenage magazines and a radio campaign publicizing the national Sexwise young people's telephone advice line and a young people's website called www.ruthinking.co.uk. Information on the Teenage Pregnancy Unit is at www.teenagepregnancyunit.gov.uk

Cross-cutting policies

Children's Commissioner (Wales)

Following the recommendations of Sir Ronald Waterhouse in his report *Lost in care*, Part V of the Care Standards Act 2000 established the role of Children's Commissioner in Wales. The Commissioner's functions extend to all services for children to be regulated by the Act: children's homes, residential family centres, local authority fostering and adoption services, fostering agencies, voluntary adoption agencies, domiciliary care, private and voluntary hospitals/clinics, the welfare aspects of day care and child-minding services for all children under the age of 8, and the welfare of children living away from home in boarding schools. The Commissioner's responsibilities include the reviewing and monitoring of arrangements by service providers for dealing with complaints, provision of advice and information, examination of particular cases of children in receipt of services, provision of assistance, including financial assistance, and representation in respect of proceedings and disputes. The Children's Commissioner for Wales website is at www.childcom.org.uk, the Children's Commissioner for Wales Act is at www.hmso.gov.uk/acts/acts2001/20010018.htm, and the Care Standards Act 2000 is at www.hmso.gov.uk/acts/acts2000/ 20000014.htm

In England, a Children's Commissioner was appointed in 2005.

4r Children's Rights Director (England)

The Children's Rights Director post was created in response to widespread abuse and mistreatment in the care system. It was first announced in November 1998, in the *Modernising Social Services* White Paper and was created by the Care Standards Act 2000 (Schedule 1, Section 10). The principal duty of the Children's Rights Director is to ensure that the National Care Standards Commission (NCSC), to be operational from April 2002, safeguards and promotes the rights and welfare of children who are provided with regulated children's services. About 200 000 children use regulated services (there are 11.3 million children in England).

The draft Children's Rights Director Regulations 2002 were issued on 18 January 2002. These regulations will in due course set out in some detail the core role and functions of the Children's Rights Director.

Connexions

The Connexions service, a cross-Whitehall initiative located in the Department for Education and Skills, was first outlined in the White Paper *Learning to Succeed* in 1999. The service was launched in 2000 and is intended to be fully operational from April 2002. Connexions will provide personal advisers for all 13–19 year olds, targeting those most at risk of underachievement. It seeks to deliver advice and guidance to young people to make a step change in learning achievement, raising aspirations and providing opportunities for young people to achieve their potential. Advisers will be expected to work closely with other agencies (e.g. Youth Offending Teams, housing and health services) to ensure that vulnerable young people receive a coordinated service suited to their individual circumstances. Advisers will also be responsible for planning transition post-16 for young people with special educational needs and offering robust support to care leavers. Information on the Connexions Service is at www.connexions.gov.uk

Excellence in Cities

Excellence in Cities was designed to raise standards in comprehensive schools in inner-city areas. The programme has been rolled out in three phases since September 1999, and involved 58 authorities. There are seven main policy strands: City Learning Centres, Specialist Schools, Beacon Schools, Gifted and Talented, Learning Support Units, Small Education Action Zones, and Learning Mentors. Excellence in Cities has been linked with the Excellence Challenge, an initiative announced by the Secretary of State in September 2000. This aims to improve access to higher education for bright students from disadvantaged backgrounds. Information on Excellence in Cities is at www.standards.dfes.gov.uk/excellence

Local Strategic Partnerships

The Government has made a commitment to the development of Local Strategic Partnerships (LSPs), a new form of governance at a local level. This development creates an umbrella organization for the delivery of the Government's programme for reducing inequalities of health and education and tackling social deprivation. LSPs are expected to bring together the public, private, voluntary, and community sectors to provide a single overarching local coordination framework within which other, more specific, local partnerships can operate.

Guidance on LSPs was issued by the Department for Transport, Local Government and the Regions in March 2001. Councils are required under the Local Government Act 2000 to publish community strategies that set out how the social, economic, and environmental well-being of the community will be promoted. LSPs are not mandatory, but they are seen as necessary to oversee the development of Community Strategies and also the vehicle for delivering Neighbourhood Renewal strategies.

In May 2001 the guidance on Co-ordinated Service Planning for Vulnerable Children and Young People in England was issued. It proposes the creation of local Children and Young People's Strategic Partnerships to oversee planning activity for vulnerable children. *Local strategic partnerships: government guidance* is at: www.local-regions.detr.gov.uk/lsp/guidance; *The Local Government Act 2000* is at www.hmso.gov.uk/acts/acts2000/20000022.htm; *Co-ordinated Service Planning for Vulnerable Children and Young People in England* is at www.doh.gov.uk/scg/childplan.pdf

National Childcare Strategy

The National Childcare Strategy was launched by the Department for Education and Employment in May 1998 as a Green Paper *Meeting the Childcare Challenge*. It aims to ensure good-quality affordable childcare for children aged 0 to 14 in every neighbourhood. This includes formal childcare, such as playgroups, out-of-school clubs, and childminders. It also includes support for informal childcare, for example relatives or friends looking after children. The main delivery agents are Early Years Development and Childcare Partnerships (EYDCPs). Early Excellence Centres have also been funded to develop good practice. Information on the National Childcare Strategy is at www.dfes.gov.uk/childcare

Neighbourhood Renewal

In January 2001 the Government published *The New Commitment to Neighbourhood Renewal: National Strategy Action Plan*. The strategy aims to reduce unemployment and crime in the poorest neighbourhoods and improve health, skills, housing, and the physical environment. It links with the NHS Plan for reducing health inequalities. Information on Neighbourhood Renewal is at www. neighbourhood.dtlr.gov.uk

Linked to the National Strategy is the Neighbourhood Renewal Fund, which was established to support the targets that have been set across departments. It aims to enable the 88 most deprived authorities to improve services, narrowing the gap between deprived areas and the rest of the country. The fund is worth £200 million in 2001–2002, £300 million in 2002–2003 and £400 million in 2003–2004. Information on the Neighbourhood Renewal Fund is at www.neighbourhood.dtlr.gov.uk/fund

New Deal for Communities (NDC)

In September 1998, the government launched a £2 billion, 10-year programme led by the DTLR, to help turn round the poorest neighbourhoods. It aims to bring together local communities, voluntary organizations, public agencies, local authorities, and business in an intensive local focus to turn round problems and make improvements that last. NDC partnerships must address five key issues: worklessness and poor prospects, improving health, tackling crime, raising educational achievement, housing, and the physical environment. Information on New Deal for Communities is at www.regeneration.dtlr.gov.uk/ndc.htm

On Track

'On Track' is a programme aimed at children at risk of becoming involved in crime. The programme was launched at the end of 1999 as part of the government's overall Crime Reduction Programme and is based at the Home Office Family Policy Unit. In May 2000, 24 areas were selected to develop On Track projects. The projects are based in high-crime high-deprivation communities and each receives around £450 000 a year to spend within an area the size of a secondary school catchment area. Funding is expected to be available for a total of 7 years. Each area is expected to develop a range of core evidence-based services for 4–12-year-olds, i.e. structured preschool education, home visiting, home–school partnerships, parent education, and family therapy. On Track's key aims are to create areas of excellence in early prevention, to evaluate the core interventions in terms of their effectiveness and cost-effectiveness, and to identify the best models for inter-agency cooperation. Information about On Track is at www.homeoffice.gov.uk/cpd/ fmpu/ontrack.htm. For information on the Children's Fund, see Working to Prevent the Social Exclusion of Children and Young People: Final Lessons from the National Evaluation of the Children's Fund. Research Report 734 University of Birmingham & Institute of Education DfES 2006. www.dfespublications.gov.uk

Sure Start

Sure Start was a major UK Government programme with the aim of 'ensuring that a child is ready to benefit from education when he starts school'. It built on early intervention research, mainly from the USA, research on nursery education, and ideas about community development and ownership. The aim of the programme is to work with parents and children to promote the physical, intellectual, and social development of pre-school children through better access to family support, advice on nurturing, health services, and early learning, so that children are ready to thrive at school. Early identification and support of children with learning difficulties is emphasized. Information on Sure Start is at www.surestart.gov.uk

Every child matters

The *Every child matters* series discusses and takes forward a wide range of policies including: early intervention and safeguarding; multi-agency approaches such as Children's Centres and Extended Schools; improved data sharing across agencies; a Children's commissioner. See www.everychildmatters.gov.uk and follow link to publications:
Every child matters (Green paper) (2003); *Every child matters: next steps* (2004); *Every child matters: change for children* *(2004).
Choice for parents, the best start for children: making it happen. DfES and DWP 2006. http://www.everychildmatters.gov.uk/resource-and-practice/IG0058/

NB: This document includes a comprehensive list of relevant Government publications (England) up to late 2004—See final section of the document. Many of the proposals were incorporated into the Children Act 2004: See http://www.opsi.gov.uk/acts/acts2004/20040031.htm

Education policy
Education Action Zones (EAZs)

These were proposed in the White Paper *Excellence in Schools* as a way of tackling educational underachievement and raising standards. EAZs are set up in response to applications from groups of around 15–25 secondary, primary, and special schools in a local area. The EAZ is run by a forum of businesses, parents, schools, the local authority, and community organizations and their partners. Applicants set out how they will raise standards, and set themselves demanding targets for improvement. Improvement could include raising pupils' achievement, improving attendance, reducing school exclusions, or creating opportunities for out-of-school activities. In return, the EAZ gets priority access to other initiatives such as specialist schools, early excellence centres, and literacy summer schools. Each EAZ receives up to £1 million each year, £500 000 from the Department for Education and Skills as a baseline and up to £250 000 more in return for funds raised from private partners. In November 2001, Stephen Timms, the Minister for Schools, told the Education Action Zones' annual conference that EAZs would be phased out and not continued beyond their initial 5-year terms, which for some ends in 2003, because of the failure to attract significant business sponsorship. Information on Education Action Zones is at www. standards.dfes.gov.uk/eaz/

Fair Funding

Fair Funding builds on Local Management of Schools by allowing schools to develop further their capacity for self-government by increased delegation of responsibility through funding. The system was introduced in April 1999 and is used by local education authorities (LEAs) to calculate the budgets of all schools maintained by them. It also sets the framework for the financial relationship that operates between schools and their LEAs. Higher delegation targets from April 2001 will put strong pressure on LEAs to delegate substantial SEN resources to schools, although some may still be retained centrally. Information on Fair Funding is at www.dfes.gov.uk/fairfunding/

Education Act 1996

The arrangements for identifying and providing for children with special educational needs are set out in the 1996 Education Act. This is supplemented by a statutory Code of Practice which sets out a staged process for identifying and meeting special educational needs.

Revised Code of Practice on the identification and assessment of pupils with Special Educational Needs

The revised SEN Code of Practice seeks to streamline the identification process of children with special educational needs, reducing it from five to three stages, and emphasizing the role of school-based support and monitoring. It provides practical advice to LEAs, maintained schools, early education settings, and others on carrying out their statutory duties under Part IV of the Education Act 1996 to identify, assess, and make provision for children's special educational needs. The Code also takes account of the SEN provisions of the Special Educational Needs and Disability Act 2001: a stronger right for children with SEN to be educated at mainstream school; new duties on LEAs to arrange for parents of children with SEN to be provided with services offering advice and information and a means of resolving disputes; a new duty on schools and relevant nursery education providers to tell parents when they are making special educational provision for their child; a new right for schools and relevant nursery education providers to request a statutory assessment of a child. This Code of Practice is effective from January 2002 and replaces the 1994 Code in England. The Code of Practice is at www.dfes.gov.uk/sen/

Special Educational Needs and Disability Act 2001

The Act strengthens the right of children with SEN to be educated in mainstream schools, requires LEAs to establish parent-partnership schemes and arrangements for conciliation in case of dispute over statements, and places new duties on LEAs and schools not to treat disabled pupils less favourably than others. The Special Educational Needs and Disability Act 2001 is at www.hmso.gov.uk/acts/ acts2001/20010010.htm

The Standards Fund

The Standards Fund is the main channel for targeting funding towards national priorities to be delivered by LEAs and schools. It provides funding for such initiatives as Excellence in Cities, the National Grid for Learning, the literacy and numeracy strategies and New Deal capital support for schools. Information on the Standards Fund is at www.dfes.gov.uk/standardsfund/

Health policy

Health Act 1999

The Health Act 1999 introduced the duty of partnership, the option for budget pooling by different agencies, lead commissioning, and money transfer powers. The Health Act 1999 is at www. hmso.gov.uk/acts/acts1999/19990008.htm

Health Action Zones (HAZs)

Announced in 1997, HAZs target areas with high levels of ill health, improving the health of the worst off at a faster rate than the general populations. They have three main aims:

+ to identify and address the health needs of local people
+ to increase the effectiveness, efficiency, and responsiveness of local services
+ to develop partnerships to improve health and health services

As well as tackling key priorities such as coronary heart disease, cancer, and mental health, and issues such as teenage pregnancy, drug prevention in vulnerable and young people, and smoking cessation, HAZs are addressing other interdependent and wider determinants of health such as housing, education and employment. Information on Health Action Zones is at www.haznet.org.uk

Health and Social Care Act 2001

This will allow the formation of Care Trusts to integrate the delivery of health and social services in England. Section 60 addresses the issue of how confidential patient information can be used within the NHS. The Health and Social Care Act 2001 is at www.hmso.gov.uk/acts/acts2001/20010015.htm

Health Improvement and Modernization Plans (HImPs)

Health Improvement and Modernization Plans (HImPs) were introduced in the White Paper *The New NHS Modern, Dependable* in December 1997. Their principle was further developed in the *Saving Lives: Our Healthier Nation* White Paper published in July 1999. HImPs are a joint strategy for improving health, reducing inequalities and delivering faster and more responsive services of a consistently high standard. They are developed by health authorities with the support of the local authority, NHS trusts and primary care groups, other primary care professionals, the public, and other partner organizations. Information on HImPs is at www.doh.gov.uk/himp/

Mental health

The legal framework that doctors, nurses, social workers and the police must follow is set by the Mental Health Act 1983. The *Mental Health Act 1983: Code of Practice* (TSO, London, 1999) gives guidance on how the Act should be applied. Section 31 of the Code gives guidance on a number of issues of particular importance affecting children and young people under the age of 18. The White Paper *Reforming the Mental Health Act*, published in December 2000, sets out the Government's plans for new mental health legislation. Part One—*The new legal framework* explains how new mental health legislation will operate for patients generally. Part Two—*High risk patients* sets out specific arrangements for the small minority who pose a significant risk of serious harm to other people as a result of their mental disorder. The Government proposes the introduction of additional measures where existing safeguards for patients are not sufficiently robust and recognizes that there must be special measures to safeguard and promote the welfare of children and young people with mental health problems. Under new legislation, the Mental Health Tribunal will be required to obtain specialist expert advice on both health and social care aspects of the proposed care plan and to consider, in particular, whether the location of care is appropriate. Decisions taken in respect of children will be subject to a clear principle that the interests of the child must be paramount. There will be changes in the provisions regarding the right of a young person between the ages of 16 and 18 to refuse consent to care and treatment for mental disorder. *Reforming the Mental Health Act* is at www.doh.gov.uk/mentalhealth

National Healthy School Standard

The National Healthy School Standard (formerly known as the National Healthy Schools Scheme) was proposed in the Green Paper *Our Healthier Nation* in 1998 and launched in October 1999. It is a national programme funded by the Department of Health and the Department for Education and Skills, and is part of the Government's drive to improve standards of health and education and to tackle health inequalities. Its major aim is to support schools in developing and maintaining a healthy school ethos. This ethos supports pupils and teachers in learning and teaching across the curriculum. It establishes PSHE and Citizenship as central to a school's purpose and children's achievements personally, socially, and academically.

Each LEA has formed a local partnership with health authorities and trusts to take forward the healthy schools programme in their area. Local healthy schools partnerships can gain national accreditation if they meet the national quality standards. These standards are organized in three sections: partnership, management of programme, and working with schools. The national standard gives guidance on the criteria that local partnerships should use in order to make judgements about school success in relation to different themes such as healthy eating and physical activity. Schools that have demonstrated a commitment to becoming a healthy school by participating in a nationally accredited local programme can use the national Healthy Schools' logo. Information on the National Healthy School Standard is at www.wiredforhealth.gov.uk/healthy/healsch.html

National Screening Committee (UK) (NSC)

This was established to address the variability in provision and quality of existing screening programmes and to ensure that new programmes meet stringent standards set out by the Committee. It has two sub-groups dealing with child health and antenatal screening issues. In forming its proposals the NSC draws on the latest research evidence and the skills of specially convened multidisciplinary expert groups which always include patient and service user representatives. The NSC assesses proposed new screening programmes against a set of internationally recognized criteria covering the condition, the test, the treatment options, and the effectiveness and acceptability of the screening programme. Assessing programmes in this way is intended to ensure that they do more good than harm at a reasonable cost. Information on the National Screening Committee is at www. doh.gov.uk/nsc

National Service Framework for children, young people and maternity services (England) (NSF)

This was announced in February 2001 and published in 2004. It set out standards for provision of services for children under six main headings— maternity care, acute and hospital services, disabled children, vulnerable children, mental health services, and universal services. The NSF looks at prevention, care, and treatment and sets out general principles and standards for children's services. In particular it deals with tackling inequalities and access problems, supporting children with disabilities and special needs, involving parents and children in choices about care, integration and partnership, including breaking down professional boundaries, and children growing up, for example the transition to adult services. Information on the National Service Framework for Children is at www.doh.gov.uk/nsf/ children.htm

4r   *The National Service Framework for children, young people and maternity services* published in September 2004. *See* www.dh.gov.uk/policyandguidance/ healthandsocialcaretopics/childrenservice

The standards set out in NSF address a wide range of issues and the individual standards are mentioned in the appropriate chapters.

A consultation paper, *The National Service Framework for children, young people and maternity services in Wales* was published in 2004. This is available from the Children and Families Directorate, Welsh Assembly Government, Cathays Park, Cardiff, CF10 3NQ.

Policy development in Scotland with regard to child health surveillance programmes is discussed in: *Health for all children 4e: Guidance on implementation in Scotland*, published in 2005. http://www.scotland.gov.uk/consultations/health/hfac-00.asp

NHS Plan (England)

The Children's Taskforce is one of 10 Department of Health Taskforces established to work on reforming the NHS and social care services, as proposed in the NHS Plan (July 2000). The Children's Taskforce was created in November 2000 to take forward the NHS Plan with respect to its implications for children. Its objectives are the improvement of services for children with disabilities, the implementation of Quality Protects, improving safeguards for children, improving adoption services, developing child and adolescent mental health services, and maximizing NHS and social care input to cross-government programmes for children. Information on the Children's Taskforce is at www.doh.gov.uk/childrenstaskforce/ and the NHS Plan is at www.nhs.uk/nationalplan

NHS Plan for Wales

The NHS Plan for Wales (January 2001) emphasizes the commitment made to partnership working in the National Assembly's December 2000 consultation document *Children and Young People—A Framework for Partnership*. Information on the NHS Plan for Wales is at www.wales.nhs.uk

Sexual Health and HIV strategy

The National Strategy for Sexual Health and HIV was published in 2002. The strategy has set a programme of action on sexual and reproductive health for England. It has joined up the Social Exclusion Report into Teenage Pregnancy and the developing HIV/AIDS strategy into an overarching strategy and will also coordinate across with the work of the Teenage Pregnancy Unit. Funding of £47.5 million is proposed for initiatives set out in the strategy during the first two years.

The main aims of the strategy are to:

- reduce the transmission of HIV and sexually transmitted infections
- reduce the prevalence of undiagnosed HIV and sexually transmitted infections
- reduce unintended pregnancy rates
- improve health and social care for people living with HIV
- reduce the stigma associated with HIV and sexually transmitted infections

Information on the Sexual Health and HIV Strategy is at www.doh. gov.uk/nshs/index.htm

Social care policy

Carers and Disabled Children Act 2000 and National Carers Strategy

The Carers and Disabled Children Act 2000 introduced the right for those with parental responsibility for a child with disabilities to an assessment of their ability to care, an extension of the direct payments scheme to parent carers, and the power for councils to run voucher schemes for them. The direct payments scheme was also extended to 16- and 17-year-old disabled young people to purchase their own care. The Carers and Disabled Children Act 2000 is at www.hmso.gov.uk/acts/acts2000/20000016.htm and the National Carers Strategy is at www.doh.gov.uk/carers.htm. Information for carers is at www.carers.gov.uk

Children First

A social-services-led programme, Children First (total estimated funding of £66.4 million over 1999–2004), is the Welsh counterpart of Quality Protects. The key elements of the Children First Programme are All-Wales objectives for children's services and associated performance indicators related to clear outcomes for children, targets to be set either across Wales or locally against each of the indicators, partnership between central and local government, an important role for elected members in ensuring the delivery of the programme and ensuring as the corporate parents of children looked after that they receive services of the highest quality, and an annual evaluation of local authority Children First Management Action Plans which set out how they intend to improve their services. Information on Children First is at www.childrenfirst.wales.gov.uk

Children (Leaving Care) Act 2000

This imposes new duties on local authorities to help care leavers until they are at least 21 years old. Its main aims are to improve the life chances of young people who are about to or have left the statutory care system, and to improve the social, educational, and employment outcomes of young people leaving care. The Act's main provisions are: local authorities must assess and meet the needs of eligible 16- 17-year-olds who are in care or are care leavers; local authorities must keep in touch with care leavers until they are at least 21; every 16-year-old should have a clear Pathway Plan, which maps a care leaver's route to independent living; each care leaver should have a young person's advisor who will coordinate, support, and offer help, especially regarding employment and training; local authorities will implement a new financial system for care leavers to ensure they are properly supported; care leavers will be supported and assisted into employment/ training, even past the age of 21. The Children (Leaving Care) Act 2000 is at www.hmso.gov.uk/acts/acts2000/ 20000035.htm

Quality Protects

The Quality Protects social services programme for children in England (total funding £885 million over 1999–2004) has introduced a multidisciplinary assessment framework for children in need and their families (*Framework for the Assessment of Children in Need and their Families 2000*), with earmarked grants of £60 million for services for children with disabilities. It is intended to transform the management and delivery of services for children. All local authorities are expected to strengthen their management and quality assurance systems to provide safe, effective, and high-quality children's services, and every local authority has a statutory duty to produce a Quality Protects Management Action Plan, setting out how they intend to improve their services. Evaluations of local responses to the Quality Protects Programme were published in 1999, 2000, and 2001 by the Department of Health and are available at www. doh.gov.uk/ qualityprotects/info/publications/index.htm. Information on Quality Protects is at www.doh.gov.uk/qualityprotects

Reports
Health service of all the talents

This examines the human resources within the NHS and argues the case for more flexibility and greater use of skill mix. *A health service of all the talents: developing the NHS workforce. Consultation document on the review of workforce planning* is at www.doh.gov.uk/pdfs/workforce.pdf

The Carson Report and 'Reforming Emergency Care'

Both reports review out of hours and emergency care in the light of new developments such as NHS Direct and changes in provision of primary care. *Raising standards for patients. New Partnerships in out-of-hours care. An independent review of GP out-of-hours services in England. Commissioned by the Department of Health* is available at www.doh.gov.uk/pdfs/ooh.pdf *The Department of Health response to the independent review of GP out-of-hours services in England. Raising standards for patients. New partnerships in out-of-hours care* is at www.doh.gov.uk/pdfs.oohgov-resp.pdf; *Implementing the OOH review: Raising standards for patients. New partnerships in out-of-hours care. The 'Exemplar' programme*, is at www.doh.gov.uk/pricare/implementooh.pdf *Reforming emergency care: first steps to a new approach* is at www.doh.gov.uk/capacityplanning/ reformingemergencycare.pdf

The Kennedy Report

The Kennedy Report on the Bristol Enquiry makes a number of recommendations. It stressed the need for care to be provided by staff trained in working with children, and commented on the tension between convenient access and centralization of facilities and services. *Learning from Bristol: the report of the public inquiry into children's heart surgery at the Bristol Royal Infirmary 1984–1995* is at www.bristol-inquiry.org.uk; the government's response to the Kennedy Report *Learning from Bristol: the Department of Health's response to the report of the public inquiry into children's heart surgery at the Bristol Royal Infirmary 1984–1995* is at www.doh.gov.uk/bristolinquiryresponse/. In its response the government agreed in full or in part with 187 of the Kennedy Report's 198 recommendations, and stated its agreement with Professor Kennedy's recommendation that there should be stronger leadership and integration at all levels in dealing with issues relating to children. Accordingly it has appointed Professor Al Aynsley-Green to the post of National Clinical Director for Children. Professor Aynsley-Green is also Chair of the Children's Taskforce.

The Redfern Report

The Redfern report on Organ Retention at the Alder Hey Hospital highlighted issues of consent and parent involvement which go beyond the immediate question of post-mortem examination. The *Royal Liverpool Children's Inquiry* is at www.rlcinquiry.org.uk/download

The Carlile Report

The report *Too serious a thing* was commissioned to review safeguards for children treated by the NHS in Wales, following the Waterhouse Report. It is available at: www.wales.gov.uk

Shifting the balance of power

This report describes the shift in management of resources and commissioning to primary care trusts. *Shifting the balance of power within the NHS: securing delivery* is at www.doh.gov.uk/shiftingthebalance/shifting thebalance.pdf; *Shifting the balance of power: the next steps* is at www.doh.gov.uk/shiftingthebalance/nextsteps/pdf

Index

6–8 week examinations 129, 144–5, 156
abduction, limited 152, 161
absence, management of 43, 112
abuse 172, 174, 175
see also child abuse
Accidental Injury Task Force 94
accidents 12, 61, 122, 321
ACD vitamin drops 205
achievement 42
achondroplasia 187
acquired conductive hearing loss 208–10
acquired hearing loss 218, 221
activity 242
acylCoA dehydrogenase deficiency, medium-
    chain 194
added value from baseline assessment 125
Administration of Medicines in Schools
    Project 114
adolescence 262, 263
adoption 309–12
    health service, role of 311–12
    intercountry 309
    see also asylum seekers, refugees and
        internationally adopted children
    looked after children 310–11
Adoption Act 1976 311
Adoption Agency 311, 312
Adoption and Children Bill 311
Adoption (Intercountry Aspects) Act 1999
    308, 309
Adoption Panel 311
adrenal hyperplasia, congenital 172, 177
adult health issues and impact on children
    10, 41–51
    children as young carers 43–5
    communication difficulties 50–1
    HIV 45–7
    learning difficulties 45
    mental health 41–3
    physical disability 45
    substance misuse 47–50
    successful programmes and projects 51–2
adult services, transition to 272
advocacy 8
Africa 316, 317
African-Caribbean origin 167
AIDS/HIV 45–7, 316, 318, 377–8
air pollution reduction 159
alcohol abuse 42, 48
allergic disease 95, 209

alpha-1 antitrypsin deficiency 196
ALSPAC study 203
amblyopia 226, 228, 229, 231, 232, 237
Amendment of the Arrangement of
    Placements of Children Regulations 1991
    299–300
amenorrhoea 171
American Academy of Paediatrics 197
American Commission on Chronic Illness
    132
ametropia 225
amphetamines 48
anaemia 121, 195, 201
anaphylactic shock 114–15
anisometropia 225
antenatal care 340–3
antenatal health surveillance and health
    promotion 245
Antenatal Subgroups 137
anticipated decision regret 136
anticonvulsants 113
antisocial behaviour disorders 42
anxiety 43
    screening 136
aortic coarctation 156, 158
aphasia 243, 256
area child protection committees 288,
    289–91, 295, 301
Asia 317
Asian origin 100, 101
assessment framework 21–2
asthma 114, 158–9, 162
astigmatism 225
asylum seekers, refugees and internationally
    adopted children 52, 120, 313–18
    emotional health and well being 315–16
    health care 316–17
    health entitlements 314–15
    management and screening 317–18
    minors, unaccompanied 314
    subsistence and housing 314
    vaccination and unknown immunization
        status 318
atrial septal defects 156, 157
attachment behaviour 59
attendance, poor 115
attention deficit hyperactivity disorder 55
audiology services 219–20
audiology working group 219
audit 188–9, 193

auditory agnosia 253
auditory response cradle 213
Australia 88, 117, 246, 252, 316, 323
autism 130, 185, 239, 244, 245, 246–7, 253, 277
    spectrum disorder 146, 245, 246–7, 256
automated auditory brainstem responses
        212–13, 214, 219, 220, 222
automated otoacoustic emissions 212, 213,
        214, 220, 222

baby blues *see* post-natal depression
baby care 143
Baby Friendly initiative 97
baby-walker injuries 90
Back to Sleep campaign 84
bacteriuria, asymptomatic 198
balance, temporary impairment of 210
Bangaldeshi origin 38
Barlow or Ortolani test 161
baseline assessment process 148–9
Bayley test 202
BCG vaccines 143
Beacon community regeneration project
        (Cornwall) 31
behaviour/behavioural 12, 61, 348–9
    difficulties 55
    disturbance 210
    problems *see* developmental and
            behavioural problems
benefits 40
'best-buy' concept 22–5, 149, 346–7
bias 170
bicuspid aortic valve 157
bicycle injuries 88, 92
biliary atresia 144
bilirubin 196
biotinidase deficiency 194
birth, immediately after 343
Birth to five 329
birth weight 12
birth weight, low 95, 121, 159, 201, 204, 206
    developmental and behavioural problems
        247
    early intervention 73
    vision defects 235
birth, within 72 hours of 343
blood transfusion 195
blood-spot-based programmes *see* neonatal
body mass index 180, 181, 183, 187,
        189, 347, 348
bone dysplasia 172
bottle-feeding (infant formula) 102, 173,
        174, 197, 204, 205
breakfast clubs 117
breast cancer 95
breast milk jaundice 95, 197, 199
breastfeeding 95–8, 122, 173, 174, 197, 204, 205
    hearing defects 209

intention 96–7
lactation establishment 97
    maintenance 97
    prolonged 102
    support programmes 356
breech presentation 150, 151, 153
Bristol Child Development Programme 71
Bristol Enquiry 380
British Agencies for Adoption and Fostering
        Medical Group 311
bullying 107, 115, 177
buoyancy 33

Cabinet Committee on Children and Young
        People's Services 366
CAFCASS 289
Caldicott Report 277
Canada 75, 195, 204
cancer 179, 181
car accidents 88, 92, 93
Caravan Sites Act 1968 318
cardiovascular collapse 114–15
cardiovascular disease 174, 181, 182
cardiovascular system 156, 157, 162, 343
care packages 272
Care Standards Act 2000 367, 368
Care Trusts 374
Carers and Disabled Children
        Act 2000 378
carers, support for 55
Caribbean origin 101
Carlile Report 381
Carson Report 380
cataracts 144, 235, 343
    congenital 132
centile crossing 173–4
cerebral palsy 130, 153, 239, 243, 244, 247,
        248, 253
Checklist for Autism in Toddlers (CHAT)
        246, 261
checklists 353–4
chest infection 155
Chief Office of Police 288
child abuse 61, 71, 76, 107
    prevention 66–9
    see also child abuse and neglect
child abuse and neglect 284–95
    area child protection committees 289–91
    child protection categories and
            registers 291–5
    Children Act 1989 285–6
    designated and named staff 291
    domestic violence 294–5
    emotional abuse 293
    inter-agency working 286–9
    local safeguarding children boards,
            duties of 288–9
    neglect 293

physical abuse 292–3
quality standards 295
sexual abuse 293
training 295
child development 60–3
normal 244
services, standards for 274–5
Child Health Informatics Consortium 332
child health promotion 6–7
programme 7, 23, 25, 33, 68
Child Health Promotion Coordinator 140
Child Health Subgroups 137
Child Health Surveillance 3, 7
child prostitution 69
child protection 12
child protection programme 284–312
adoption 309–12
national service framework 284
private fostering arrangements,
children in 307–9
see also child abuse and neglect;
looked after children
child protection registers 292
Childcare Partnerships 370
Children Act 1989 17, 18, 19, 45,
66, 69, 129, 285–6
child protection programme 296,
299, 305, 308
disabilities and special educational needs
270, 276, 277
Children Act 2004 19
Children Act Scotland 1995 296n
Children Can't Fly programme (US) 92
Children First 300, 378
Children (Leaving Care) Act 2000 378–9
children in need 19–22
children as young carers 43–5
*Children and Young People-A Framework for
Partnership* 377
Children and Young People's Plan 19
Children and Young People's Strategic
Partnership 369
Children and Young People's Unit 366
Children's Centres 108–9, 371
Children's Commissioner (Wales) 367–8
Children's Eye Health Working Party 234
Children's Fund 366
children's rights 18
Children's Rights Director (England) 368
Children's Rights Director Regulations 2002
368
children's service plans 18–19, 273
Children's Services Framework 300
Children's Services Plans 287, 289
Children's Special Grants 19
Children's Taskforce 377
Children's and Young People's Strategic Plan
282

choking 93
circumcision 159, 163
Citizenship 375
City University test 233
Clarke-Harcke dynamic method 152
cleft palate 209, 258
Climbié, V. 19, 307–8, 309
clinical audit 276
'clumsiness' 243, 249, 259–60
Co-ordinated Service Planning for Vulnerable
Children and Young People 369
Cochrane review 40
codes of practice 278, 372
coeliac disease 171, 198, 200
cognition 61
cognitive deficits 247, 256
cognitive development 95, 174
'cold chain' 78
colour vision defects 233–4, 237
Common Assessment Framework for
Children and Young People 21, 272
communication difficulties,
parents with 50–1
community development 8–9
Community Fire Service 94
Community Mothers Programme 71
community profiling 352
community resources 349
Community Strategies 369
Community-wide approaches 41, 355
comorbidity 254–5
comprehension 255
Comprehensive Behaviour Support Plans 60
concepts 6–9, 10–16
conditional reference 190
conductive hearing loss 207, 208
confidential advice and support 118
confidentiality 110, 279, 327–8, 332
CONI (Care of Next Infant) 104
conjugated hyperbilirubinaemia 199
Connexions Service 289, 368–9
consent 110, 279, 364
Consortia of Service Providers 314
constitutional delay in growth and
puberty 178
Consultant in Communicable
Disease Control 78, 82
continuing care criteria 272
contraception, under-age 122
conversations, structured 131
coordination 65–6
coronary heart disease 179, 197
cortical visual impairment 235
counselling 33, 50, 128
cow's milk (doorstep milk) 201, 204, 205
crack cocaine 48
craniostenosis 185
Crime Reduction Programme 371

criminality 42, 43
critical path 67
crowding phenomenon 228
CSNHL 216
cultural differences 285
culture 120
cyanosis 155
cystic fibrosis 128, 139, 195–6, 198, 344
cytomegalovirus 212

data sharing 332
day care 72
deafness *see* hearing impairment
death *see* mortality
definitions 6–9
Denmark 14
dental care 348
dental caries 101–3
Dental Health of Five-Year-Old Children 103
Dental Health Survey (2003) 102
dental and oral disease 100–4
Denver Developmental Screening Test 251, 252
Department for Education and
    Employment 370
Department for Education and Skills 60, 110,
    120, 273, 367, 368, 372, 375
Department of Health 100, 124, 183, 329,
    332, 367, 375, 379
  child protection programme 294, 297, 301,
    302, 306, 308
  special circumstances 315
  universal programme 347
Department of Trade and Industry 90
Department for Transport, Local Government
    and the Regions 367, 369, 370
Department for Work and Pensions 367
depression 42, 43, 75–6, 115, 123, 143, 179
  parental 60–3
  paternal 61
  see also postnatal depression
deprivation 35–6, 174
  levels 352
  see also poverty and deprivation
designated doctor 281–2, 302, 304, 305
designated nurse 302, 304, 305
detection *see* early detection
DETR index 11
development 12, 333–4, 348–9
developmental and behavioural problems 70,
    146, 238–68, 321
  definitions 240, 242
  epidemiology 240–1
  identification 241–4
  national service frameworks 240
  normal child development 244
  prevention 58–60
  psychological problems, minor 263–6
  services provision 266–8

services and systems required for early
    identification 239
  see also high-prevalence low-severity
    conditions; low-prevalence high-
    severity conditions
developmental coordination disorder 259–60
developmental dysplasia of the hip (DDH)
    129, 130, 132, 136, 144, 150–3, 160–1, 343
  causes 150
  definition 150
  early detection 150
  hip instability, management of 151
  incidence 150
  practical aspects 153
  screening 151–3, 161
developmental language disorders *see* speech
    and language acquisition, delay in
developmental problems 146, 345
diabetes 179, 181
dialogic reading 66
diet 64, 158, 182
  see also nutrition
diphtheria 316
Director of Public Health 140
disabilities 43, 52, 187, 269–77, 298, 349
  joint agency working 271–3
  legislation and statutory duties 270–1
  national service framework 269–70
  registers 276–7
  service planning 273–5
  service provision 271
Disability Living Allowance 315
disease prevention 7
disorders:
  detection 29, 170–2
  and head circumference 185
  specific 197–8
distraction test 214–16, 220
District Councils 288
divorce 42
DMF index 102
dog attacks 91
domestic violence 68, 70–1, 76, 143, 294–5
Down's syndrome 129, 139, 154,
    162, 187, 197–8
  disabilities and special educational needs
    277
  hearing defects 209
Down's Syndrome Medical Interest Group 154
Drinking-water supplies 117
Drop-in clinics 116, 117, 126
drowning 88, 92
drug abuse 69, 107, 123
dual pathology 216
Duchenne muscular dystrophy 128, 196, 199,
    244, 259
duplication reduction by
    information sharing 125

dyslexia 45, 146, 234, 236, 249, 260
dysmorphic syndromes 129, 177, 184, 187, 208, 235, 247
dyspraxia 66, 146, 259
  see also developmental coordination disorder

early detection:
  developmental dysplasia of the hip (DDH) 150
  heart disease 154
  vision defects screening 223–4
  see also secondary prevention: early detection and screening
Early Development Instrument 75
early diagnosis 128, 211
Early Excellence Centres 370
Early Years Curriculum 64
Early Years Development 370
Eastern Europe 316
eating disorders 176
eclampsia 121
Edinburgh Postnatal Depression Scale 62
Education Act:
  1981 129
  1993 129
  1996 17, 129, 271, 277, 372, 373
  Code of Practice 283
  (Scotland) 1980 276n
Education Action Zones 372
education/educational 12, 305
  attainment and poverty 64
  difficulties 207, 349
  for parenthood 56–8
  plans, individual 280
  policy 372–3
  provision 29
  services, access to 129
elasticity 32
electronic health record 332
electronic patient record 332
emmetropic eye 225
emotional abuse 291, 292
emotional development 61
emotional distress 179
emotional health and well being 115, 315–16
emotional literacy 59
emotional problems 55, 146, 239, 261–3
empathy 34
encephalitis 130
encephalopathy 130, 158, 247
endocrine deficiency disorders 158, 176
energy intake and expenditure 179, 180
Entamoeba histolytica 317
enteric infections 316
environment, role of 65–6
environmental change and childhood injury prevention 92–3

environmental deprivation 210, 258
Environmental Health Officer 82
epidemiology and disability registers 276
epilepsy 244
equity 11
ethnic minority groups 38–9, 100, 101, 167, 185, 205, 298
Europe 88, 99, 204, 316
Every child matters 371
evidence:
  correlational 65–6
  necessity for 22–5
  observational 65–6
evolutionary diagnoses in low-prevalence high-severity conditions 248
Excellence in Cities 369, 373
Excellence in Schools White Paper 372
excluded pupils 120
experimenting, necessity for 25
Expert Working Party 1986 152
Extended Schools 108, 371
extrahepatic biliary atresia 196–7
eye anomalies 129

facial malformation syndromes 209
failure to thrive– 68, 155, 174–5, 177, 189, 195
  see also non-organic failure to thrive
Fair Funding 372
falls 90, 92
familial hypercholesterolaemia 197
family:
  disturbances 174
  health 10
  history 130, 150, 151, 153
  structure 43
  support 111
Far East 317
farm injuries 88–9
fathers 63
feedback in phenylketonuria and congenital hypothyroidism screening 193
feeding 143
  problems 345
  see also bottle-feeding; breastfeeding; nutrition
female genital mutilation 69
fire and flame injuries 89, 91, 92
fire guard injuries 90
First Parent Visiting Programme 71
First Words, First Sentences test 256
fluoride 102–3
follow-on milks 204
foot deformities 150, 151
forced-choice preferential looking methods 227
Ford Foundation 71
formula feeding *see* bottle-feeding
formulas 353–4
foster care placement 175

fostering arrangements, private 307–9
Framework for assessment 16, 52, 55, 68, 302
Framework for the Assessment of Children in Need and their Families 17, 21, 379
Fraser (previously Gillick) competence 364
friendships 43
fulminating pneumococcal infection 194
fundoscopy 235

galactosaemia 194, 196
gall bladder disease 179
gastroenteritis 122
gender issues 43
genetic counselling 128, 172
genetic factors 64, 173, 179
  developmental and behavioural problems 253, 261
  hearing defects 210
genital mutilation 69
genitalia, abnormalities of 159–0, 163
genuineness 34
geographic targeting 352
Giardia lamblia 317
glass injuries 91, 93
Graf static approach 152
Griffiths Scales of Mental Development 203
growth 195, 347–8
growth disorders 146
growth hormone deficiency 171, 173, 177
  idiopathic 178
growth hormone replacement therapy 177
growth impairment 171, 174
growth monitoring and nutrition 164–91
  accuracy and reproducibility 169–70
  audit 188–9
  disorders, detection of 170–2
  growth charts 166–8
  health promotion 172
  height 170, 177–8
  length 176–7
  obesity 178–84
  occipito-frontal head circumference 184–5, 187–8
  parents, focus of interest for 172
  prematurity, correcting for 178
  public health aspects 172
  regression to the mean 189–91
  research 189
  screening or monitoring 164
  single measurement as screen versus multiple measurements over time 178
  usefulness 164–5
  weight 168–9, 173–6
growth velocity estimations 170

haematoma 184
haemoglobinopathies 194–5, 198, 344
  see also sickle cell disease; thalassaemias
hard to reach children and families 36–7

harm minimization of children 49
head circumference 144, 164
  see also occipito-frontal
head injury 130
Head Start 36–7, 73
Heaf test 318
health 13–14
Health Act 1999 282, 373–4
Health Action Zones 374
health assessment for looked after children 301–2
Health Authorities 270, 367
health care of individuals, determining needs of 16
health care plans 113, 301–2
health care programme at school entry 109
health checks 328
health consequences in teenage pregnancy 121–2
health education 8
health entitlements 314–15
Health Improvement and Modernization Plans 374
Health Improvement Plan 119
Health Improvement Programmes 287
health interview 148
health issues *see* adult health issues
health needs assessment 354–5
Health needs of school age children 4
health policy 373–8
health problems, detection of 29
health professionals 279, 287
health profiles 118
health promotion 6
health protection 8
health questionnaire 147–8
Health and Safety at Work Act 1974 110
Health and Safety Executive 88
health and safety policy and school-age children and young people 113
Health service of all the talents 379
health services 279, 311–12
Health and Social Care Act 2001 374
health visiting 29, 34–41, 365
  deprived and socially excluded populations 35–6
  hard to reach children and families 36–7
  help and support in the home 40–1
  housing problems 37–8
  literacy, low 39–40
  'middle class' parents 38
  minority ethnic groups 38–9
  'new to area' 38
  poverty and benefits 40
  progammes, intensive 70–1
  social support and community-wide approaches 41
  training 79
healthy alliances 8
Healthy Schools initiative 181, 349

Healthy Schools programme 111
Healthy Schools Standard 119
hearing 141
hearing behaviour 255
hearing defects screening 146, 207–22, 343–4
  acquired hearing loss 218, 221
  arguments in favour of screening 211–12
  audiology services 219–20
  behavioural testing during first year of life
    214–16
  coordinator 221
  deaf community, views of 211
  distraction test 220
  evaluation of programmes 222
  impedance measurement 218
  'intermediate' screening 217, 220–1
  monitoring and outcomes 222
  neonatal screening 212–14, 220
  organization and equipment 221
  parental observations 214
  research 221–2
  school entry 'sweep' test of hearing 217-18
  testing between 18 and 42 months 216–17
  updates 218–19
hearing impairment 64, 130, 132, 135,146,
    197, 244, 247, 253, 256
  congenital 136
  parents 50, 52
  permanent 207–11, 214
  and visual defects 236
hearing test 344–5, 348
heart defects, congenital 132
heart disease 153–7, 162, 197
  6–8 week examination 156
  congenital 129, 153–4, 156, 157, 162, 343
  early detection 154
  further examinations 156
  identification 154–5
  innocent murmurs 157
  primary prevention 157
  referral 157
  routine examination 155–6
heart murmurs 144, 157
heat stroke 91
height 164, 177–8, 186, 187, 189, 348
  gain 178
  parental 170
  velocity 178
help and support in the home 40–1
hepatitis 196
  B 143, 316, 318
  B vaccine 80–2
hernia 159, 163
heroin 48, 49
hierarchy 13–14
high-prevalence low-severity conditions 243,
    249–63
  borderline or mild learning disabilities
    258–9

'delay' in speech and language acquisition
    253–8
developmental screening 250–3
motor delay and 'clumsiness' 259–60
opportunistic intervention 250–1
Platforms (Australia) 252
primary prevention 250–1
psychological, emotional and behavioural
    problems 261–3
specific learning disabilities 260–1
tests for use by non-specialists 251
high-risk families 353–4
high-risk follow-up and low-prevalence high-
    severity conditions 247
holistic approaches to promoting health
    305–6
Home Office 107, 294, 367
  Asylum Casework Instructions 316
  Family Policy Unit 371
home safety advice 345, 348
home visiting programmes, structured 71
homelessness 52, 320–1
Homestart 72, 356
homicides 43
homosystinuria 194
hormonal deficiencies 177
horse riding accidents 89
hospital admission 175
Hospital for Tropical Diseases (London) 317
House of Commons Select Committee 183
housing 314
  problems 37–8
  see also homelessness
Human Rights Act 4–5, 271
humility 34
hydrocele 159, 163
hydrocephalus 184, 185
25-hydroxy-vitamin D 100
hyperlipidaemia 179
hypermetropia 225, 227, 229
hypernatraemic dehydration 96
hypertension 121, 157–8, 162
hypertrophic cardiomyopathy 155
hypo-and hyper-nasality 258
hypoglycaemia 130, 171, 196
hypoplasia, mid-facial 171
hypospadias 159
hypothyroidism 128, 136, 171, 173, 177, 195,
    197
  congenital 192–4, 198
  screening 344

idiopathic short stature (short normal
    children) 172
illness 43, 52, 174
Immigration and Asylum Act 1999 314
immunity, impaired 194
immunization 82, 144, 344, 348
  advice clinic 79

immunization (*contd.*)
  BCG 143
  coordinator 78–9
  MMR 345, 347
  new vaccines 82
  and unknown immunization status 318, 319
  uptake, increasing 77–80
impairment 242
  see also hearing; visual
impedance measurement 218
impedance tests 221
incidence 7
income 43, 249
incremental yield 134, 135, 216
independence, reduced prospects for 208
India 316
inequalities 11
Infant Health and Development Program 73
infant mortality 12, 122
infection 95
  acute 321
  congenital 208
infectious diseases, reducing incidence of
    77–82, 316
  hepatitis B vaccine 80–2
  immunization uptake, increasing 77–80
  tuberculosis, prevention of 80
  vaccines, new 82
inflammatory bowel disease 171
information 331–4
  necessity for 136–7
  sharing 272–3
  sharing index 292
informed consent 364
injury, unintentional, prevention of 86–95,
    348
  baby-walker injuries 90
  bicycle injuries 88, 92
  community level strategies 93–4
  current status 94
  dog attacks 91
  drowning 88, 92
  environmental change 92–3
  falls 90, 92, 93
  farm injuries 88–9
  fire and flame 89, 92
  glass injuries 91, 93
  horse riding accidents 89
  local accident data 87
  misconceptions 92
  motor vehicle accidents 88, 92
  nationwide strategies 92–3
  playground injuries 91
  poisoning 90, 93
  practitioner, possible roles of in prevention
    93–4
  scalds 89, 92
  stair gates and fire guards 90
  suffocation and strangulation 90
  sunburn and heat stroke 91
  surveillance systems 87
innovation, necessity for 25
institutional racism in NHS 39
Integrated Urban and Rural Models 71
intellectual deficits 64
inter-agency working 286–9
inter-professional collaboration 19
International Classification of Functioning,
    Disability and Health 240, 241
International Classification of Impairment,
    Disability and Handicap 240
International Task Force on Obesity 180
internationally adopted children *see* asylum
    seekers, refugees and internationally
    adopted children
interprofessional working 17
intervention 9, 305
  'delay' in speech and language acquisition
    256–8
  early, delivered in educational sector 72–3
  early for low birth weight infants 73
  obesity 180
  permanent childhood hearing impairment
    211
  programmes 70–1
  psychological problems 265–6
intra-uterine growth retardation 177
inverse care law 251, 266
iron chelation therapy 195
iron deficiency 100, 201–6
  anaemia 201
  definition 201
  effects 201–2
  prevalence 202
  primary prevention 204–5
  research 206
  screening 203
iron supplementation 204, 206
irradiation, cranial or total body 171
Ishihara test 233
Israel 65

Jamaican origin 194
jaundice 171, 196
  due to biliary atresia 144
  see also breast milk jaundice
joint agency reviews 271
joint agency working 271–3
joint assessments 271–2
joint commissioning 272
joint plans 271

Kawasaki disease 154, 157, 162
Kennedy Report 380

laboratory and radiological screening tests
    192–200
  specific syndromes and disorders 197–8

urine infections 198, 199
see also neonatal blood-spot-based
  programmes
labour, difficult 121
Laming report 19
language 120
  acquisition 64–5
  see also speech and language acquisition,
    delay in
lead poisoning, subclinical 197, 200
learning difficulties 143, 239, 244, 249, 277–8
  borderline or mild 258–9
  parents with severe *see* mental handicap
  specific 260–1
  and vision defects 233, 235
Learning from Bristol 380
Learning to Succeed White Paper 368
Leicester Height Measure 169, 186
length 176–7
lifestyle 158
limp 161
linear charts 228
linear logMAR tests 228–9, 237
lines of letters tests 228
literacy 66
  emotional 59
  low 39–40
Literacy Trust 14
litigation and screening 136
liver disease in infancy 196–7
liver flukes 317
local authorities 273, 288, 367
Local Authority Social Services Act 1970 286
Local Coordinators 367
local education authorities 270, 279, 281–2,
  372, 373, 375
Local Government Act 2000 369
Local Management of Schools 372
Local Probation Board 288
local safeguarding children boards 288–9, 291
Local Strategic Partnerships 369
Local Teenage Pregnancy Coordinator 367
localities, prosperous 125
locality needs 352
locality-based primary care service 359
loneliness 62–3
looked after children 295–307
  adoption 310–11
  definition 296
  designated doctor and nurse 302, 304, 305
  epidemiology 297–8
  further work required 307
  health assessment and health care planning
    301–2
  health problems 298–9
  holistic approaches to promoting health
    305–6
  minimal requirement 306–7
  monitoring of outcomes 306

policy context 299–300
Losing the thread 112
low-prevalence high-severity conditions 243,
  244–9
  detection 245–9
  evolutionary diagnoses 248
  management 248–9
  periconceptional and antenatal health
    surveillance and health promotion 245
  prematurity, correction for 248
  primary prevention 244
lower limb abnormalities 153

Macarthur Communicative Development
  Inventory 65, 251, 256
McCormick Toy Test 216
mainstream schools 242
malaria 317
malnutrition 165
managerial influences 350
*Managing Medicines in Schools and Early Years
  Settings* 114
maple syrup urine disease 194
Marfan's syndrome 155, 172
marital discord 42
matching toys tests 227
maternal deaths 60
maturity onset diabetes of the young 179
mean length of utterance 254
media print 66
Medical Foundation for Victims of Torture in
  London 315
medical model approaches 30
medical needs, special 110–11
medical officer, duties of 281–2
medication 112–14
medicines and dental and oral
  disease 102–3
Meeting the Childcare Challenge Green Paper
  370
meningitis 85, 130, 208, 218
meningococcal C vaccine 82
mental handicap 130, 243, 247, 248, 253
mental health 374–5
  parents 41–3
  problems 143, 207–8, 319, 349
  services, tiered structure of 267
Mental Health Act 1983 374
Mental Health Tribunal 375
mental illness and mortality 61
methadone maintenance programmes 49
microcephaly 184–5
microphallus 171
midazolam, buccal or intranasal 113
middle childhood (6–12) and
  psychopathology 263
'middle class' parents 38
middle-ear disease 85, 216
Minimeter 169

Minister for Public Health 124
minors, unaccompanied 314
mitral valve, prolapsing 157
MMR vaccine 345, 347
Modernising Social Services White Paper 368
monitoring:
    hearing defects screening 222
    looked after children 306
    occipito-frontal head circumference 185
    phenylketonuria and congenital
        hypothyroidism screening 193
    see also growth monitoring and nutrition
mood disorders 60
morbidity 86, 194, 195, 319
mortality 60, 61, 86, 194, 195, 319
    infant 12, 122
    mental illness 61
    see also sudden infant death syndrome;
        suicide
motor delay 259–60
motor development 65–6
motor impairments, severe 247
multiple pituitary hormone deficiency 171
multivitamin supplements 101
mumps 208
Munchausen syndrome by proxy 293
muscle disease 244
muscular dystrophy 130, 196, 247
    see also Duchenne muscular dystrophy
myocarditis 154
myopia 225, 231, 235

National Audit Office 183
National Care Standards Commission 368
National Carers Strategy 378
National Childcare Strategy 72, 370
National Curriculum for English 64
National Deaf Children's Society 219
National Fruit Scheme 117
National Grid for Learning 373
National Healthy Schools Programme 117, 119
National Healthy Schools Standards 126,
    375–6
National Institute for Clinical Excellence 96,
    177, 199
national maternity record 326
National Plan for Safeguarding
    Children from Commercial Sexual
    Exploitation 69
national register 222
National Screening Committee 62, 220, 348,
    360–1, 376
    Fetal, Maternal and Child Health 142, 192
    laboratory and radiological screening tests
        193, 195, 196
    physical examination 153
    secondary prevention 133, 137
national service frameworks 6, 335–6, 341,
    346, 358–65, 376–7

child protection programme 284
developmental and behavioural problems
    240
disabilities and special educational needs
    269–70
explicit focus on and commitment to
    prevention 362
information collected to monitor processes
    and outcomes of programmes 364
information for parents and families
    available and accessible 363–4
information used to audit and monitor
    activity and outcomes 364–5
prioritization of service provision based on
    statutory duties, evidence of what
    works and views of children and
    families 360–1
programme of health care should be made
    available to whole population 358–9
quality care provision depends on
    recruitment and retention of well-
    trained staff, continuing provisional
    development, strong leadership and
    adequate supporting resources 363
responsibility for provision and linking of
    services to be clearly identified 359–60
services to be planned to improve equity of
    provision and reduction of inequalities
    in health 363
standard 2 55
standard 3 18
standards of care to be accepted and
    implemented by providers wherever
    possible 362
National Society for the Prevention of
    Cruelty to Children 47
National Strategy 370
near vision 229
needs assessment 16, 28–9
neglect 66–9, 71, 174, 175, 291, 292
    see also child abuse and neglect
Neighbourhood Renewal Fund 370
neonatal blood-spot-based programmes 141,
    192–7, 344
    cystic fibrosis 195–6, 198
    familial hypercholesterolaemia 197, 199
    haemoglobinopathies 194–5, 198
    lead poisoning, subclinical 197, 200
    liver disease in infancy: extrahepatic biliary
        atresia 196–7, 199
    muscular dystrophy 196, 199
    neuroblastoma and coeliac disease 200
    phenylketonuria and congenital
        hypothyroidism screening 192–4,
        198
neonatal examinations 129, 142–3
neonatal screening and hearing defects 220
Netherlands 88, 323
neuroblastoma 200

neurodevelopmental problems 230, 235
neurological disorders 64, 129–30, 153
New Commitment to Neighbourhood Renewal 370
New Deal for Communities 370, 373
New NHS Modern, Dependable, The White Paper 374
'new to area' 38
Newcastle Project 93
Newpin (New Parent Infant Network) 72, 356
Newpin Teenage Mums' Project (Peckham) 125
NHS 11, 18, 103, 106, 129, 267, 374, 379, 380
    child protection programme 301
    disabilities and special educational needs 273, 282
    Information Authority 332
    institutional racism 39
    number 334
    universal programme 339
NHS Act 1999 19
NHS Direct 84, 379
NHS Foundation Trusts 289
NHS Plan (England) 282, 301, 325, 370, 377
NHS Plan for Wales 377
NHS registers 276
NHS Trusts 270, 277, 279, 281, 288, 289, 305
nine-centile growth charts 167, 186
non-organic failure to thrive 175, 189
non-qualified staff (paraprofessionals) 71, 355–6
Noonan's syndrome 187
North America 99
    see also Canada; United States
nursery nurses, role of in detection of illnesses 131
nutrition 12, 95–100, 117, 123, 348
    breastfeeding 95–8
    and dental and oral disease 101, 102
    vitamin K 99–100
    see also growth monitoring and nutrition

obesity 95, 117, 172, 173, 175, 178–84, 187, 189, 347
    body mass index 180
    diet and nutrition 182
    government action 183
    identification 180
    intervention 180
    physical activity 182
    prevention 181–3
    screening 181
    skills and self-esteem 182
    updates 183–4
occipito-frontal head circumference 169, 184–5, 187–8
Ofsted 318
oligohydramnios 150
On Track 370–1

ophthalmoscope 235
opiates 48
opportunistic detection 131
opportunistic intervention and high-prevalence low-severity conditions 250–1
organ retention at Alder Hey Hospital 380
orthopaedic problems 179
Ortolani and Barlow screening tests/manoeuvres 150, 151, 153
osteogenesis imperfecta 244
otitis media with effusion 208, 209, 210, 216, 217–18, 220, 222
Ottawa Charter 305
Our Healthier Nation Green Paper 117, 375
outcome measures 25
Oxford wall chart 347

Pakistani communities 38
palatal dysfunction 258
paracetamol 114
paraprofessional staff 71, 355–6
parasitosis 317
Parent Adviser Model 56, 58
parental and child participation and special educational needs 278
parental depression 60–3
parental heights 170
parental observations and hearing defects 214
parenthood, education for 56–8
parenting 49–50
parenting, helpful 55–6
parenting programmes 70
parents 27–52
    holistic approach 29–31
    listening to and low-prevalence high-severity conditions 247–8
    role of in detection of illnesses 130
    social capital 31–2
    social networks 32–4
    support for 55
    see also adult health issues; health visiting
Parents' Evaluation of Developmental Status 65, 251, 252, 256
Partnership in Action 19
passive smoking 85, 159
patching (eyes) 229, 232
patent ductus arteriosus 154
paternal depression 61
Pathway Plan 379
patients, individual care of 276
Pears Early Education Partnership 66
peer networks 43
penicillin prophylaxis 194
performance 42, 43
    targets 280–1
periconceptional health surveillance and health promotion 245
periodic medical inspections 145

periodontal (gum) disease 103
permanent childhood hearing impairment
    207–11, 214
    acquired conductive hearing loss 208–10
    early diagnosis and intervention 211
    impact 207–8
    unilateral hearing loss 210–11
Personal Child Health Records 81, 321,
    325–31, 364
    design 327
    development for specific groups 329–30
    disabilities and special educational needs
        274
    format 326–7
    growth monitoring and nutrition 186
    health promotion material 329
    hearing defects 213, 214, 220
    information on confidentiality and use of
        information 327–8
    information on screening and other health
        checks and reviews 328
    ownership 325–6
    physical examination 152, 153, 161, 162
    recommendations 330–1
    timing of distribution to parents 329
    use and continuity 326
    vision defects 235
Personal Development Programme 72
personal, social, health and citizenship
    education (PSHCE) programme 123, 375
personality disorder 43
pervasive developmental disorder 246–7
phenylalanine control 193
phenylketonuria 128, 192–4, 195, 198, 344
physical abuse 291, 292
physical activity 182
physical disability, parents with 45
physical disorders 125, 146
physical examination 142–63
    8 week examination 144–5
    after 8 weeks 145
    asthma 158–9, 162
    developmental dysplasia of the hip (DDH)
        150–3, 160–1
    genitalia, abnormalities of 159–60, 163
    heart disease 153–7, 162
    hypertension 157–8, 162
    neonatal 142–3
    neurological disease 153
    routine reviews 160
    school entrant medical examination 145–9
physical health problems 319
physical symptoms 115
picture card tests 228, 229
Platforms (Australia) 252
playground injuries 91
playgroup leaders, role of in detection of
    illnesses 131

pneumococcal vaccine 82, 194
poisoning 86, 90, 93
    lead 197, 200
policy framework, legislation and policy
    366–81
    cross-cutting policies 367–71
    education policy 372–3
    health policy 373–8
    reports 379–81
    social care policy 378–9
    special units 366–7
Polnay Report 4
polygenic hypercholesterolaemia 197
population, determining needs of 16
Portage programme 259
post-natal depression 42, 60, 61, 62, 75–6,
    122, 344
potential harm and screening 134–6
poverty 14, 40, 172, 174
    and deprivation 12–14, 210, 258
    and educational attainment 64
practical help 29
pre-conception counselling 50
pre-school children and psychopathology
    262–3
pre-school health promotion 348
pre-school programmes, desired outcomes of
    74–5
pre-school vision check 347
pregnancy 48
    and smoking 159
    violence during 61
    see also teenage pregnancy
prematurity 201, 204, 206, 230, 247
    correction for in low-prevalence high-
        severity conditions 248
    and growth monitoring and nutrition 178
    retinopathy 235
prevention:
    and obesity 181–3
    see also primary; secondary; tertiary
primary care for children 9, 340
Primary Care Organizations 5–6, 19, 21, 25,
    26, 268
    child protection programme 291, 297, 305,
        306–7, 312
    disabilities and special educational needs
        273, 281
    primary prevention 78
    school-age children and young
        people 123
    special circumstances 316, 324
Primary Care Trusts 289, 302, 324
primary health care team 9
primary prevention 7, 67
    asthma 159
    on community-wide scale 73–4
    heart disease 157

high-prevalence low-severity conditions 250–1
iron deficiency 204–5
low-prevalence high-severity conditions 244
programmes 70–5
see also primary prevention opportunities
primary prevention opportunities 77–105
dental and oral disease 100–4
nutrition 95–100
smoking by parents, reduction of 85–6
special situations 104–5
sudden infant death syndrome and sudden unexpected death in infancy, revention of 82–4
see also infectious diseases, reducing incidence of; injury, unintentional, prevention of
prison, children detained in 323
prison, children of women in 321–3
privacy 364
see also confidentiality
process measures 25
professional advice, role of 131–2
professional sensitivity, necessity for 132
professional support services 43
professionl influences 350
promoting child development 53–76
behavioural and psychological problems, prevention of 58–60
child abuse and neglect, prevention of 66–9
education for parenthood 56–8
language acquisition 64–5
motor development and coordination 65–6
parenting, helpful 55–6
parents or carers, support for 55
pre-school programmes, desired outcomes of 74–5
primary prevention programmes 70–5
social isolation, parental depression and child development 60–3
proteinuria 198
provider trust, duties of 282
pseudobulbar palsy, congenital 253
pseudosquint 230
psychiatric disorder 60
psycho-social development 43
psychological development 95
psychological distress 179
psychological pathology, minor 243
psychological problems 249, 261–6
identification 265
intervention 265–6
inverse care law 266
persistence 265
predisposing factors 264–5
prevention 58–60

psychopathology in childhood and adolescence 262–3
psychosis, acute 42, 43, 60
psychosocial factors 175
puberty, precocious 177
public health nurse 29
Public Service Agreement target 347–8
pulmonary function 195
pulmonary stenosis 157
pyelonephritis, chronic 198
pyrexia 198

qualitative indication 227
quality of life, improved 128–9
Quality Protects 19, 119, 276, 287, 300, 305, 314, 379

racism 39, 107, 115
radiological screening tests see laboratory and radiological screening tests
Raising standards for patients 379–80
REAL-Raising Early Achievement in Literacy 66
recession, persistent 155
red reflex 235
Redfern Report 380
referral criteria 229
referral pathways and vision defects screening 234
'Reforming Emergency Care' 379–80
Reforming the Mental Health Act White Paper 375
refractive error 226, 230, 231–2, 234
refractive state 225
refugees see asylum seekers, refugees and internationally adopted children
refuges for female victims of domestic violence 68
registers and disabilities 276–7
regression to the mean 173, 189–91
Relative Needs Index 11
relatives, role of in detection of illnesses 130
religion 43
renal disease, silent 158
renal failure, chronic 171, 198
reports 379–81
research 189, 333–4
base in health promotion 23–4
and disability registers 276
hearing defects screening 221–2
iron deficiency 206
vision defects screening 237
residential care 242
residential schools 242
resource allocation 11, 28
Resource Allocation Working Party 11
respect 34
respiratory illnesses 85

respite 272
retinopathy 235
Review of Services for Young Children (1998) 54
rheumatic heart disease 154
rickets 100
Romania 316
Royal College of Paediatrics and Child Health 167, 332, 347
rubella, congenital 212
Russell-Silver syndrome 171, 176

Saving Lives: Our Healthier Nation White Paper 374
scalds 89, 92
Schedule of Growing Skills 251, 252
schistosomiasis 317
schizophrenia, chronic 42
school:
    entrant medical examination 145–9
    entry 348
    entry sweep test of hearing 217–18, 221
    health promotion 349
    meals 117
    nurse 29, 116
    preparation for 108
    readiness 74–5
    starting 108
    see also school-age children and young people
School Action 279
School Action Plus 279
school-age children and young people 60, 106–26
    absence, management of 112
    added value from baseline assessment 125
    anaphylactic shock and cardiovascular collapse 114–15
    bullying and racism 115
    children's views 107–8
    confidential advice and support 118
    duplication reduction by information sharing 125
    emotional health and well being 115
    good practice 114, 116
    health care plans 113
    health profiles 118
    health promotion 116–18
    health and safety policy 113
    localities, prosperous 125
    medication 112–14
    physical disorders, detection of 125
    pre-school services 108–9
    public health focus 118
    screening, formal 125
    social exclusion 125
    special medical needs 110–11
    starting school 108, 125

targets 112
vulnerable children and young people 118–20
young mothers and teenage pregnancy 120–5
scotopic sensitivity syndrome 234
screening 7, 132–41
    anxiety 136
    asylum seekers, refugees and internationally adopted children 317–18
    criteria for appraising viability, effectiveness and appropriateness 138–9
    criteria for programmes and tests 133–4
    cystic fibrosis 139
    definition 132–3
    developmental dysplasia of the hip (DDH) 151–3, 161
    formal 125, 132, 134
    genetic 137
    growth disorders 146
    growth monitoring and nutrition 164
    high-prevalence low-severity conditions 250–3
    information, need for 136–7
    iron deficiency 203
    litigation 136
    low-prevalence high-severity conditions 245–7
    monitoring and supervision 140–1
    neonatal sickle cell anaemia 193
    obesity 181
    occipito-frontal head circumference 185
    opportunistic 134
    Personal Child Health Records 328
    planning and purchasing 140
    postnatal depression 62
    potential harm 134–6
    referral 141
    secondary 231
    ultrasound scanning 152
    see also hearing defects screening; laboratory and radiological screening tests; secondary prevention: early detection and screening; vision defects screening
secondary prevention: early detection 7, 67, 69, 127–32
    dental and oral disease 103
    early diagnosis, value of 128
    educational and social services, access to 129
    family history of disorder, close observation of 130
    formal screening, role of 132
    neonatal and 6–8 week examinations 129
    neurological illnesses 129–30
    opportunistic detection 131
    outcome, improved 128
    parents and relatives, role of 130

playgroup leaders and nursery nurses 131
professional advice, role of 131–2
professional sensitivity, necessity for 132
quality of life, improved 128–9
Secretary of State 17, 286, 309, 326
secular trend 167, 172
Secure Training Centre 289
selective methods and physical examination 148
self-empowerment model 7
self-esteem 182
sensorineural hearing loss (SNHL) 130, 207, 208, 209, 212, 213, 217, 221, 222
and vision defects 235
serum ferritin 201
serum iron 201
service planning 276
disabilities 273–5
service provision and disabilities 271, 273–5
services 305
sexual abuse 68, 291, 292
Sexual Health and HIV strategy 377–8
sexual maturation, premature 172
Sheridan's graded balls 227
Shifting the balance of power within the NHS 381
short stature 172
sickle cell anaemia 141, 194
neonatal screening 193
sight *see* vision; visual
SIGN guidelines 103
single assessments 272
single-gene disorders 64
single-letter charts/tests 228, 229
skeletal dysplasias 176
skills 182
mix 29
skin creases, asymmetric 152, 161
smiling 144
smoking 123
by parents, reduction of 85–6
during pregnancy 159
parental 209
see also passive smoking
Snellen chart 228, 229
social adversity 43
social anxiety 13–14
social capital 15, 31–2
social care policy 378–9
social circumstances 173, 349
social class 38, 249
gradient 11, 86, 89
social communication 255
social exclusion 14–15, 120, 121, 125
Social Exclusion Report into Teenage Pregnancy 377
Social Exclusion Unit 366–7
social inclusion initiatives 120

social inequalities 172
social isolation 60–3, 207
social networks 32–4
social services 69, 129, 276, 279, 288, 339
Social Services Inspectorate 296
social support 27, 29, 41
socially excluded populations 35–6
socio-economic deprivation 205
sociopathic personality disorder 43
somatizers 60
South America 316, 317
Southampton Behaviour Resource Service 268
special circumstances, children in 313–24
homelessness 320–1
prison, children detained in 323
prison, children of women in 321–3
travellers 318–20
see also asylum seekers, refugees and internationally adopted children
special educational needs 19, 20, 66, 277–83
code of practice 278, 282
consent and confidentiality 279
coordinators 111
definition 277–8
designated doctor, role of 281–2
health professionals, responsibility of 279
health services, responsibility of 279
identification and assessment 278, 280
inclusion 280
individual educational plans 280
legal basis 277
medical officer, duties of 281–2
parental and child participation 278
performance targets 280–1
provider trust, duties of 282
review 280
revised Code of Practice 373
special educational provision 278
statements 111, 278–9, 280, 282
therapy services 280
Special Educational Needs and Disability Act 2001 373
special schools 242
special units 366–7
spectacles 232
speech discrimination tasks 216
speech and language acquisition, delay in 146, 210, 239, 243, 249, 253–8
causes of delayed development 253
comorbidity 254–5
current best policy 255–6
identification 255
intervention 256–8
normal variation 253–4
outcomes assessment 255
referrals 257–8
specific language impairment 254, 258

spina bifida occulta 136
splenic sequestration crises 194
SPOTRN coding system 327
squint 224, 225, 227, 229, 235
    see also strabismus
SSD 270
staff, designated and named 291
stair gate injuries 90
Standards Fund 373
Standards in Scotland Schools etc. Act 2000
    276n
Statewide Child Injury Prevention
    Campaign (USA) 93
statutory duties 16–17
stools, pale 196, 197, 199
strabismus (manifest squint) 225, 226, 230
straight-eyed anisometropia 229
strangulation 90
Strategic Health Authorities 289
strategic level management and teenage
    pregnancy 124
stress 64
stroke 179
subcultural deprivation 258–9
subdural effusion 184
subsistence 314
substance abuse 43, 47–50, 52, 61, 64, 143
sudden infant death syndrome 24, 61, 82–4,
    85, 95, 143, 174
suffocation 90
sugar-based medicines 102
sugars 102
suicide 61
    attempts 115
sunburn 91
Supporting pupils with medical needs 110
suppurative otitis media, chronic 208–9
Sure Start 5, 28, 36, 53, 54, 58, 65, 70, 73, 75, 371
    developmental and behavioural problems
        244, 251, 256
    Local Programme 54, 74
    primary prevention 85
    school-age children and young people 108,
        121
    secondary prevention 131
    Unit 15
    universal programme 346, 348
surveillance systems 87
swaddling, too tight 150
sweating 155
Sweden 93
syndromes, specific 197–8

tachypnoea 155
tall stature 172
Tanner-Whitehouse growth charts 167
targeting 15–16
    by identification of high-risk families 353–4

effective 354–5
    teenage pregnancy 124–5
teachers, knowledge of to identify problems
    148–9
teenage pregnancy 120–5
Teenage Pregnancy Strategy 367
Teenage Pregnancy Support Group (St
    George's Hospital) 124–5
Teenage Pregnancy Unit 367, 377
teeth *see* dental
temperament 210
terms used 10–16
tertiary prevention 7, 69, 103
testes 144
    undescended 159, 160, 163
tetanus 318
thalassaemia 141, 194, 205
    homozygous 195
therapy services 280
thrive lines 174, 189
thyroid-stimulating hormone 193
thyrotoxicosis 172, 177
Too serious a thing 380
torticollis 150, 151, 153
total iron-binding capacity 201
toxaemia 121
transferrin receptor concentration 201
transferrin saturation 201
Transport Research Laboratory 94
travellers 52, 318–20
truancy *see* absence
tuberculosis 80, 316
tumours, intracranial 171
Turner's syndrome 171, 177, 178, 187, 209
two year sign-off 333
type 1 diabetes 179
type 2 diabetes 179

ultrasound scanning 152
UN Convention on the Rights of the Child
    4–5, 18, 69, 107, 270
undernutrition 174–5
UNICEF 97
United States 7, 9, 31, 36, 156, 246, 299, 316, 371
    New York state demonstration project 213
    promoting child development 56, 65, 66,
        70, 71
    Rhode Island study 213
    Task Force on screening 158
    see also Head Start
universal neonatal hearing screening 343
universal programme 335–57
    action, commitment to 352
    antenatal care 340–3
    benefits and justification for 338–9
    birth, immediately after 343
    birth, within 72 hours of 343
    child development and behaviour 348–9

community resources 349
further health checks in school 348
further reviews after 4 months 344–7
general principles 337
geographic targeting-locality needs and
    deprivation levels 352
growth 347–8
hearing screening 343–4
individual work and community-wide
    approaches 355
mother and baby, further follow-up of 344
national service frameworks 335–6
non-qualified staff (paraprofessionals) 355–6
objectives 337–9
pre-school health promotion 348
pre-school vision check 347
primary care for children 340
recommendations 336–7
school entry 348
schools, health promotion in 349
summary of evidence 350
targeting by identification of high-risk
    families 353–4
targeting, effective and health needs
    assessment 354–5
vulnerable children 339–40
universal screening 230–1
universal vision screening of all pre-school
    children 231
urban anxieties 30
urinary tract infection 198, 199
user involvement 17–18
Usher's syndrome 236

vaccination see immunization
valvular stenosis 154
variability, short-term 170
vegetarianism/veganism 100
ventricular septal defect 154
vesico-ureteric reflux 198
views of children 107–8
violence 107
    during pregnancy 61
    prevention 59
    see also domestic violence
vision defects screening 146, 223–37, 347, 348
    amblyopia 224, 226–7
    colour vision defects 233–4, 237
    community screening-evidence and options
        230–3

definitions 224, 225
    and dyslexia 234
    early detection 223–4
    non-disabling defects 236
    pre-school child: 3–5 years 228
    pre-school screening 229
    referral pathways 234
    research 237
    school-age children 228–9
    severe visual impairment 235
    stabismus (squint) 230
    updates 232–3
    visual acuity in children under 3 years 227
vision disorders 130, 146, 158
visual acuity 225, 228–9, 231–2
visual following 144
visual impairment 51, 130, 244, 247
vitamin C 204
vitamin D supplements 101
vitamin K 95, 99–100, 143
    -dependent bleeding 99, 196
vitamin supplements 101, 204, 205, 206
vulnerable children and young people 21,
    118–20, 339–40

Waterhouse Report 380
weaning 174, 204, 205
weight 144, 158, 164, 186, 187, 189, 344, 345,
    347, 348
    distance centiles 190
    faltering 174–5
    see also obesity; weight monitoring
weight monitoring 168–9, 173–6
    centile crossing 173–4
    'overweight' baby 175
    undernutrition, faltering weight gain and
        'failure to thrive' 174–5
    weight in older children 176
Welfare Food scheme 101, 204, 205
West African origin 194
work, individual 355
Working Party 77, 146, 147, 156, 231,
    245
Working together to safeguard children 17
World Health Organization 95, 174

young mothers 120–5
Youth Offending Team 289

zinc protoporphyrin 201

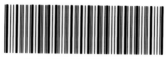